EYE MOVEMENTS: COGNITION AND VISUAL PERCEPTION

EYE MOVEMENTS: COGNITION AND VISUAL PERCEPTION

edited by

DENNIS F. FISHER
RICHARD A. MONTY
U.S. Army Human Engineering Laboratory

JOHN W. SENDERS
University of Toronto

SPONSORED BY THE U.S. ARMY
HUMAN ENGINEERING LABORATORY

LEA LAWRENCE ERLBAUM ASSOCIATES, PUBLISHERS
1981   Hillsdale, New Jersey

Lawrence Erlbaum Associates, Inc., Publishers
365 Broadway
Hillsdale, New Jersey 07642

Library of Congress Cataloging in Publication Data
Main entry under title:

Eye movements.

    "This volume represents the edited proceedings of the
third symposium on eye movements and behavior sponsored
by the US Army Human Engineering Laboratory . . . held at
the Bayfront Concourse Hotel, St. Petersburg, Florida,
on February 11–13, 1980."
    Bibliography: p.
    Includes index.
    1. Eye—Movements—Congresses.   2. Visual perception
—Congresses.   3. Cognition—Congresses.   I. Fisher,
Dennis F.   II. Monty, Richard A.   III. Senders, John W.,
1920–   IV. United States. Army Human Engineering
Laboratories. [DNLM: 1. Cognition—Congresses.   2. Eye
movements—Congresses.   3. Visual perception—Congresses.
WW 400 L349e 1980]
QP477.5.E95   152.1′4   80-27876
ISBN 0-89859-083-3

Printed in the United States of America

Participants and Contributors

Jack A. Adams, University of Illinois, Chicago, Illinois
James R. Antes, University of North Dakota, Grand Forks, North Dakota
Richard N. Aslin, Indiana University, Bloomington, Indiana
Janette Atkinson, University of Cambridge, England
Joshuah Borah, Gulf + Western, Waltham, Massachusetts
Oliver Braddick, University of Cambridge, England
Dennis Carmody, Temple University, Philadelphia, Pennsylvania
Roger H. S. Carpenter, Caius College, Cambridge, United Kingdom
Karen M. Cohen, Bell Laboratories, Holmdel, New Jersey
Stanley Coren, University of British Columbia, Canada
Robert Ditchburn, 9 Summerfield Rise, Goring, Reading, United Kingdom
Peter Dunn-Rankin, University of Hawaii, Honolulu, Hawaii
Jean M. Ebenholtz, University of Wisconsin, Madison, Wisconsin
Sheldon M. Ebenholtz, University of Wisconsin, Madison, Wisconsin
David C. Edwards, Iowa State University, Ames, Iowa
John Findlay, University of Durham, England
Dana G. Fisher, Bell Laboratories, Holmdel, New Jersey
Dennis F. Fisher, US Army Human Engineering Lab., APG, Maryland
Lois E. Flamm, Bell Laboratories, Whippany, New Jersey
Maurice Fleury, Laval University, Quebec, Canada
Alinda Friedman, University of Alberta, Canada
Samuel Y. Gibbon, Jr., Childrens' Television Workshop, 1 Lincoln Plaza, New York, New York
Louise Hainline, Brooklyn College, Brooklyn, New York
Howard Hock, Florida Atlantic University, Boca Raton, Florida
Helene Intraub, Bucknell University, Lewisburg, Pennsylvania
Robert L. Kershner, National Bureau of Standards, Washington, D.C.
Robert H. Lambert, US Army Human Engineering Lab., APG, Maryland
George W. Lapinsky, National Bureau of Standards, Washington, D.C.
Lester A. Lefton, University of South Carolina, Columbia, South Carolina
George S. Leonard, Gulf + Western, Waltham, Massachusetts
Smadar Levin, McLean Hospital, Belmont, Massachusetts
James L. Levine, IBM Research Center, Yorktown Hts., New York
Ariane Levy-Schoen, Laboratoire de Psychologie Experimentale, Paris, France

Terri L. Lewis, McMaster University, Hamilton, Ontario, Canada
E. Llewellyn-Thomas, University of Toronto, Ontario, Canada
S. M. Luria, SMRL Subase, Groton, Connecticut
Daphne Maurer, McMaster University, Hamilton, Ontario, Canada
Joseph Mazurczak, US Army Human Engineering Lab., APG, Maryland
Richard A. Monty, US Army Human Engineering Lab., APG, Maryland
Michael J. Morgan, University of Durham, England
Kevin O'Regan, Laboratoire de Psychologie, Paris, France
Richard K. Olson, University of Colorado, Boulder, Colorado
Lawrence C. Perlmuter, VA Outpatient Clinic, Boston, Massachusetts
Ernst Z. Rothkopf, Bell Laboratories, Murray Hill, New Jersey
J. Edward Russo, University of Chicago, Chicago, Illinois
Allan M. Schrier, Brown University, Providence, Rhode Island
John W. Senders, University of California, Santa Barbara, California
Wayne Shebilske, University of Virginia, Charlottesville, Virginia
David Sheena, Gulf + Western, Waltham, Massachusetts
Joseph B. Sidowski, University of South Florida, Tampa, Florida
Lawrence Stark, University of California, Berkeley, California
Van K. Tharp, Southern California Research Institute, Los Angeles, California
John Tole, Massachusetts Institute of Technology, Cambridge, Massachusetts
Jonathan Vaughan, Hamilton College, Clinton, New York
Frances C. Volkmann, Smith College, Northampton, Massachusetts
Bruce Whitehead, University of Louisville, Louisville, Kentucky
Laurence R. Young, Massachusetts Institute of Technology, Cambridge, Massachusetts
Helmut T. Zwahlen, Ohio University, Athens, Ohio

Contents

Preface

This volume represents the edited proceedings of the third symposium on eye movements and behavior sponsored by the US Army Human Engineering Laboratory. The conference, titled "The Last Whole Earth Eye Movement Conference" was held at the Bayfront Concourse Hotel, St. Petersburg, Florida on February 11–13, 1980. As the conference approached, seizure of the American hostages by the Iranian militants, the Russian invasion of Afghanistan, and the uncertain economic outlook around the world made it appear as though the title was a self-fulfilling prophecy. But the meeting proved highly successful and people throughout the world seem to be adapting to the stresses of international tension, making the possibility of subsequent meetings more likely.

The present volume is intended to serve as a complementary text to R. A. Monty and J. W. Senders (Eds.), *Eye Movements and Psychological Processes*, 1976, and J. W. Senders, D. F. Fisher, and R. A. Monty (Eds.), *Eye Movements and the Higher Psychological Functions*, 1978, both published by Lawrence Erlbaum Associates, rather than a revision and update of them.

We wish to thank the US Army Human Engineering Laboratory for sponsoring the symposium. In particular, we once again wish to express our deep appreciation to Dr. John D. Weisz, the untiring Director of the Human Engineering Laboratory for his continued encouragement and support, and for his recognition of the need for and support of basic research efforts in eye movements as they relate to cognitive and perceptual processes.

Again, special words of thanks to Mrs. B. Diane Barnette who has worked with us on all of these conferences and on the resulting volumes. We continue to be amazed at her ability to handle the myriad of details surrounding each of these efforts. Finally, we are also indebted to Mrs. Colleen Pustola for a magnificent job of organizing the references and retyping hundreds of manuscript pages.

DENNIS F. FISHER
RICHARD A. MONTY
JOHN W. SENDERS

EYE MOVEMENTS:
COGNITION AND
VISUAL PERCEPTION

INFANT AND DEVELOPING MECHANISMS

Saccades, smooth pursuit, and optokinetic nystagmus—when do they begin? Is the ability to perform the various eye movements innate, or must their development correspond to changes in sensitivity of the visual system and the maturation of the visual cortex? What are the implications of the developing eye movement system for perceiving form, adapting to moving stimuli, and perceiving eccentric stimuli? Are there methodological problems in matching the measurement device to the infants' capability of being a cooperative participant? These are some of the questions of concern that are addressed in Part I.

Hainline, in Chapter I. 1 examines the form perception of infants and finds that there is significant variability between infants' scanning patterns. Some infants show very narrow or restrictive patterns, while others show broad scanning patterns with little regularity, irrespective of the size of the form viewed. Procedural implications weigh heavily in her research, both in the handling of infant methodologically and as related to past research findings.

In Chapter I. 2, Maurer and Lewis take issue with the traditional perceptual learning theorists notion that the shape of a stimulus can be resolved only after a thorough scanning, by presenting infants with various "interesting" patterns 20° or 30° in the periphery. Although there may be some question about the infants' selectivity as far out as 30°,

1

lesser eccentricities prove compelling stimuli to the infants except when shown in the presence of competing centrally viewed stimuli. Further, it is their contention that decisions about peripheral stimuli can be made as early as 3 months and these are purely perceptual without cognitive interference. Maurer and Lewis also express their concern over the high degree of poor "voluntary" participation of these infants, generally concluding that they make bad subjects.

In Chapter I.3, Aslin reports on a highly successful monitoring technique in which infants from 3 weeks to 4 months old are tested for the presence and efficiency of smooth pursuit movements, one of the so-called more primitive eye movements. He examines various aspects of the smooth pursuit system by age of emergence, tracking accuracy of various velocities, possible evidence for predictive tracking, and any evidence for a velocity gain mechanism in this smooth pursuit system independent of saccades. While providing many answers to these concerns, the overriding issue of an independent smooth pursuit movement system receives confirmation.

In the final chapter of this section, Atkinson and Braddick describe the development of optokinetic nystagmus in infants as highly correlated with cortical binocularity. In the four experiments described, OKN is related to development, abnormal visual development i.e. strabismus and amblyopia, and to its relationship with other systems like smooth pursuit. For infants under 3 months of age, an asymmetry occurs for nasal-temporal and temporal-nasal direction of the stimulus motion for elicitation of OKN. This asymmetry generally seems to dissipate as the infants grow older. Qualifications were made also on short and long OKN, but a general independence of the OKN system and smooth pursuit system seems confirmed. Somewhat cautiously, these data are interpreted as suggesting that binocular cortex is a necessary condition for symmetrical OKN, but there is as yet little direct evidence that the development of cortical binocularity is the critical factor for the onset of symmetrical OKN in infancy.

I.1 Eye Movements and Form Perception in Human Infants

Louise Hainline
Brooklyn College of C.U.N.Y.

Infancy stands at the beginning of a long course of psychological development. Human infants are faced with the task of appreciating a complex environment with what appears to be a limited set of resources. Vision is obviously one of these resources and infants can be observed actively scanning their environment with organized sequences of eye movements and fixations within minutes after birth. Visual information is an important factor in cognitive and social development, as evidenced in studies of the concept of the permanence of objects and attachment to a caretaker (Fraiberg, 1977). However, an understanding of perceptual development at the beginning of life may also contribute to an understanding of perceptual processes at other stages in the life span. For example, one might study visual development as a means of addressing hoary theoretical questions about the nature of perception as expressed in the polarization between a Gestalt position on innate organization versus a ''constructionist'' approach supporting the role of learning and experience in perception.

For many years the infant was regarded as a largely reflexive creature at the mercy of environmental exigencies. Infants probably haven't changed significantly in the past decade, but developmental psychology's conception of them has. New research on infant psychological processes has generated a revised view of the competent infant, almost hungrily grappling with and trying to master the environment. To some extent, this change in perspective has resulted from methodological innovation and technological advances. Even brief exposures to infants allow the observation of characteristics that make them poor candidates for subjects in psychological research. Evanescent states of wakefulness, unbridled emotions, and periodic dampness pose real challenges to the researcher, who has needed a battery of behavioral and psychophysical techniques to make headway.

3

Since the pioneering work of Fantz (1956, 1958), it has been reasoned that one way of learning what the infant sees is to study what he looks at. This line of reasoning has led from studies of visual choice behavior (the so-called visual preference technique) to increasing sophistication in the measurement of actual eye movement patterns. Early techniques developed by Salapatek and Kessen (1966), Salapatek (1968), and Haith (1978) were based on corneal reflection photography, were painfully slow, and involved various techniques for hand scoring characteristics of the scanning eye "frozen" for analysis one to four times a second. Calibration data on the accuracy of the technique were difficult if not impossible to obtain, but allowed relatively precise specifications of eye position during scanning.

SYSTEM DETAIL

The research technique used in my laboratory is based on the principles of this earlier work on infant eye movement measurement, but allows greater speed and potentially greater accuracy. The system is based on a low light level television system originally designed for measuring adult eye movements, a Gulf + Western, Applied Sciences Laboratory (ASL) Model 1994 Eye View Monitor. Extensive modifications to the apparatus have been made for work with infants, and, in view of its unique nature, it will be described in more detail, although the basic technique is a familiar one. The system's principle of operation is show schematically in Fig. 1. It has a low light level invisible infrared source whose light is collimated so that rays are parallel when they reach the subject's eye, after reflection by an IR reflecting, visible transmitting dichroic mirror. A small amount of the light that enters the pupil is reflected by the retina, and is photographed by a very sensitive television camera. The camera provides an image of the eye with a bright pupil enlarged on a monitor. Actually, only part of the incident light enters the eye; a fraction is reflected by the cornea and appears on the television image as a small bright virtual image, the corneal reflection or first Purkinje image, superimposed on the bright pupil. As the eye rotates to look at a portion of the visual field, the corneal reflection moves differentially with respect to the pupil, but if the entire head moves, within limits, the pupil and corneal reflection move together. Thus if the position of the head is stabilized, analysis of shifts of the corneal reflection relative to the pupil can specify direction of regard. The ASL Eye View Monitor automates this estimation so current eye position is available 60 times a second.

During testing, the infant is held against the shoulder of an experimenter who gently stabilizes the infant's head; the infant looks through the dichroic beam splitter at a rear projection screen on which the stimuli appear. Figure 2 illustrates more clearly the other elements of the system. The "eye camera" as described forms an image of the corneal reflection and the pupil. The "face camera" provides the experimenter with a picture of the infant's face, and so permits the

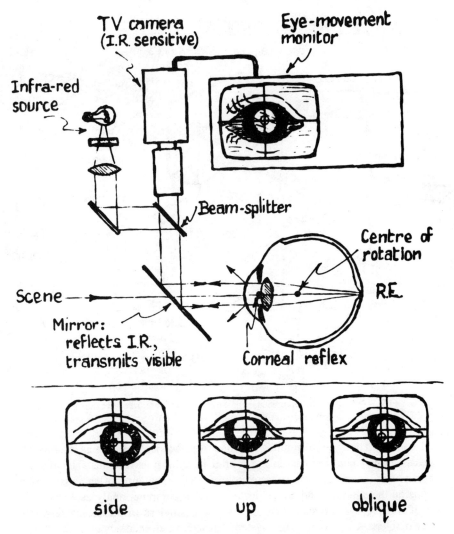

FIG. 1. A schematic representation of the essential elements and principle of operation of a television based infrared eye movement recording system. The lower portion of the figure illustrates the differential movement of the corneal reflex with respect to the center of the pupil during eye movements that is the basis for the calculation of eye position.

proper positioning of the eye. The experimenter cannot see the stimuli and so bias any of the responses. The "scene camera" photographs the stimulus viewed by the infant. Outputs of both the scene and eye cameras are fed into the eye movement monitor, which calculates direction of the infant's regard every 60th of a second and relates it to the stimulus. Data on eye position are fed into a minicomputer that provides some on-line analysis, data storage, and experimen-

Infant eye-movement monitor

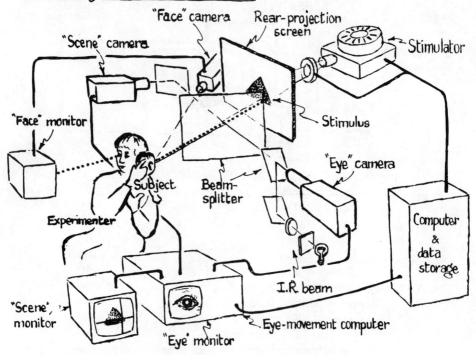

FIG. 2.   A schematic representation of the elements of an infrared eye movement recording system for use with infants.

tal control. The system minimizes subjective decisions by human scorers and gives a large amount of data even for brief stimulus presentations. The digitized eye movement records are subsequently plotted as patterns of successive fixations on the stimulus and are subjected to other computer analyses.

If relative eye movement information is desired as in measuring responses like optokinetic nystagmus, this system can achieve an accuracy of under .5° with infants, but for many research questions, like those involving pattern perception, data on absolute position in space are required. When using older subjects, they can be told to fixate a few specifiable points in the field, and calibration is accomplished by adjusting gains on the apparatus or performing mathematical corrections on the data. True fixation could differ from obtained estimates of fixation for several functionally distinct reasons—for example, instrument error, corneal irregularities, or because the fovea is not actually on the eye's optic axis, which intersects the center of the pupil which is used as the reference point for eye position calculations. The technique further assumes that the fovea is the most relevant portion of the retina for information about the point of regard; for young infants, data on retinal development suggest this may be an improper assumption (Mann, 1964). To estimate the extent of the sum of these errors in infants, we have developed techniques for calibrating the eye movements of subjects who cannot be instructed to fixate points A, B, and C in sequence.

THE CALIBRATION ALGORITHM

Since the attention span of infants is notoriously brief, our strategy has been to collect scanning information to the stimuli of interest first, and then, if the infant is still cooperative, to move into the calibration procedure. The calibration results are later used to adjust the fixation estimates. A sequence of small flashing lights is presented one at a time to the subjects. The lights are at known coordinates in the same system as the fixation data. An experimenter observes the output on the scene monitor and signals the computer to collect data when the infant appears to be fixating the reference light. The logic of the routine ultimately involves the provision of some "average" point of fixation for each reference light, but the routine is flexible so that each set of data potentially involving fixation of the reference point may also involve non-fixation data representing "wobble" in an attempt to maintain a steady fixation (which would probably be symmetric about a "true mean") or systematic movement toward or away from the reference point (which would probably not be symmetrical about the true mean). The calibration algorithm first estimates fixation coordinates for each reference point by calculating, separately for X and Y, a mean and variance of all the points in the set. Any points lying beyond a selectable number of standard deviations from the mean are rejected and a new mean and variance calculated, with outliers rejected again. This iterative procedure continues until the number of rejected points does not differ from one iteration to the next. This last mean is taken to be the most representative coordinate and can be used to find the calibration vector. The procedure makes two minimal assumptions—that the distribution of points which are true attempts to fixate the reference point is symmetrical, and that this distribution has a smaller variance than the distribution of non-fixation points.

Since the analysis is carried out in a two dimensional system, the X and Y coordinates can be treated separately, since means and variances are linear functions. However, in determining rejection limits for data points, the confidence interval, an area, is an ellipse with radii relating to the standard deviations of X and Y. Figure 3 illustrates how the process works. The data points are painted on a CRT screen and surrounded by a computer generated ellipse defined by the rejection interval and the standard deviations of X and Y. In this example, the rejection interval is two standard deviations on X and Y, so the larger ellipse has radii of two standard deviations from the original data, and the smaller ellipse of two standard deviations from the final solution set. This procedure is carried

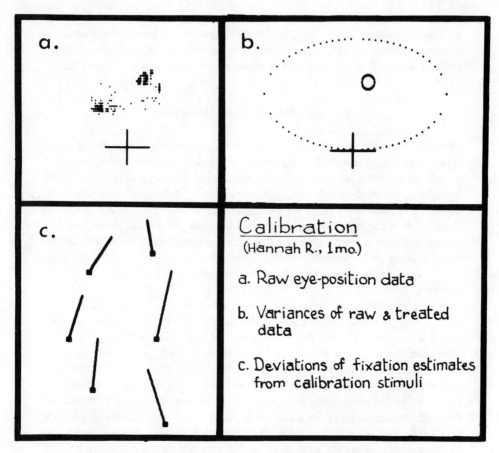

FIG. 3.   An example of output from the eye position calibration program. (a) The cross represents the location of the reference stimulus; the dots represent measured fixations to this point. (b) The larger dotted ellipse represents a criterion number of standard deviations on X and Y for the raw data, and the smaller solid ellipse represents these values for the data after treatment by the calibration algorithm (c) The result of the application of the calibration algorithm to obtained calibration data; the solid squares represent true position of reference points and the solid lines represent the direction and magnitude of the correction calculated for each point in the set.

out for all points for which there are data, although very large disparities between fixations and the point's true location may lead to the elimination of a particular point from future calculations. The problem then is to find the transformation that will simultaneously map all of the fixation estimates onto the original fixation points; the points can be weighted by their residual variance in obtaining a solution. The transformation is an Nth order polynomial whose actual order is determined by the number of fixation estimates obtained.

The power of the process is best illustrated by showing how it deals with large discrepancies. The correction for this subject, about 7°, is on the upper end of our distribution of error estimates. In Panel C, lines connect true fixation points to obtained points. For this subject, the correction is downward.

Figure 4 shows data from another subject and the results of applying the calibration corrections to obtained fixations. In Panel A are discrepancies from true fixation coordinates, in Panel B are uncorrected fixations to a small (5°) circle, and in Panel C, fixations to this stimulus after correction. The application of the calibration correction to the rest of this subject's data had the effect of placing fixations closer to all stimuli to approximately the same extent as shown in this example. Notice that for this infant, the correction was in the opposite direction to that of the previous example. This illustrates the variance in the type of correction required between subjects. Calibration information is not obtainable from all infants, and the variability in corrections found makes it unwise to apply an averaged correction to all subjects. We can, however, use this calibration information to estimate the magnitude of the error we are likely to find in uncorrected data—on the order of ± 3–4 degrees.

FORM SCANNING IN 1–3 MONTH OLD INFANTS

Existing research on infant scanning has focused mainly on simple geometric forms viewed by newborn infants. We are aware of only one set of data on the scanning of plane geometric forms in older infants (Salapatek, 1969; 1975). Based on the original 1969 scan plots, which were hand drawn by scorers viewing a videotape of the infant's eye, he reported a developmental difference in scanning between one and two month old subjects. The younger infants appeared to scan narrowly over a limited section of the figure's contour, while older infants scanned more broadly and into the interior of the forms. Salapatek (1975) presents computer plotted records, which appear to be quite different from the corresponding hand drawn records, but no further analyses are presented for the digitized, computer plotted records. Salapatek's conclusions about these data have been the basis for strong generalizations about developmental trends in scanning and have generated both psychological and physiological models as explanations (Bronson, 1974; Haith, 1978; Haith & Campos, 1977).

We decided that the question of developmental trends in form scanning merited a closer examination because Salapatek had a small and possibly nonrepresentative sample of infants, and because, as in many of the newborn studies, the forms used were very large.

It seemed likely that the size of the stimulus was probably related to how it was scanned, and, possibly, also to the developmental differences reported by Salapatek, so we initiated a study of size as a parameter of infant scanning in 1, 2, and 3 month old babies. The stimuli were 5°, 20°, and 30° circles, squares, and

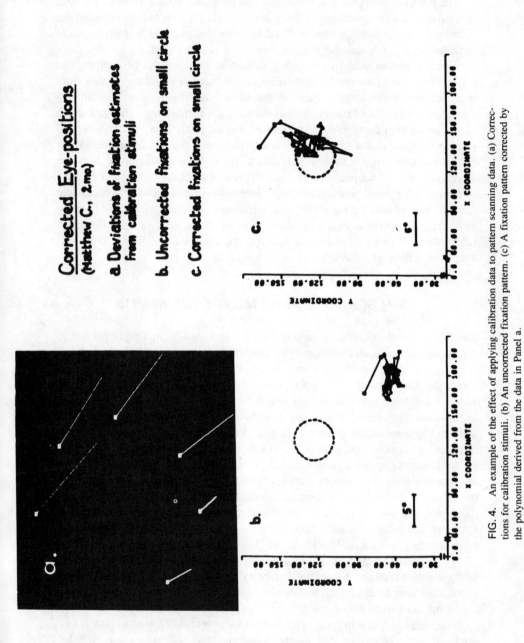

Corrected Eye-positions
(Matthew C., 2 mo.)

a. Deviations of fixation estimates from calibration stimuli

b. Uncorrected fixations on small circle

c. Corrected fixations on small circle

FIG. 4. An example of the effect of applying calibration data to pattern scanning data. (a) Corrections for calibration stimuli. (b) An uncorrected fixation pattern. (c) A fixation pattern corrected by the polynomial derived from the data in Panel a.

triangles, white on black background. The luminance was approximately 10 candles/m^2. Of this set of nine stimuli, each subject was presented with a subset of six, two of the shapes at all of the sizes. Stimuli were presented for 10 seconds with inter-stimulus intervals of 5 seconds.

One ineluctable conclusion quickly reached in research with infants is that they often don't or won't look at what you show them—our criterion for including an infant in the final sample was fixation data from at least four of the six stimulus periods. The data were obtained from 39 infants, 13 at each of 1, 2, and 3 months, out of a total of 118 tested. For 39 of these, we failed to collect data because the infant cried, fell asleep, moved too much, or because the characteristics of the eye did not allow measurement—usually too small or dim a pupil. Of the remaining 40 subjects, 7 met our criterion for inclusion in the study, but were longitudinal subjects who had already been included at another age. Of the remaining 33 subjects, we have partial data (1–3 stimuli); although we have not included these subjects in the final analyses, these data have been analyzed and do not appear to contradict any of what follows.

Before describing the results, our method for dividing the data into epochs of fixations and movements should be explained. Simplistically, a fixation is defined as relative stationarity of the eye while a movement involves rapid change in eye position. The algorithm defines fixations by analyzing the sizes and sequences of signs of successive differences between points for both X and Y, making it a kind of velocity measure. Eye movements are defined by large successive differences or by a string of smaller differences, all of the same sign (to catch slow drifts); fixations are small differences (on the order of half a degree) with no systematic pattern of signs.

The analyses of the scanning of these 39 infants are based on uncalibrated data. Analyses of variance have been performed on both the characteristics of the fixations, for example, where the fixations fall and what their durations (dwell times) are, and on the characteristics of the eye movements, for example, their lengths and velocities. Given the Salapatek (1975) results, the analyses of these data reveal surprisingly few significant age differences and the pattern they do suggest defies a simple linear developmental explanation.

For example, there were significant age effects for both duration and length of eye movements. In both cases, we found curvilinear relationships; length and duration of eye movements for three month olds were longer than those of one and two month olds, but eye movements of two month olds were shorter in both length and duration than those of one month olds. For the three month olds, eye movements were longer in both the horizontal and vertical dimensions, and the vertical components of their eye movements had greater variability than for the other age groups; this finding probably results from both changes in motor control of eye movements and in information processing capacity with age.

In order to analyze where infants looked and how extensively they scanned, we counted the number of fixations in certain regions of interest for the stimulus and the surround. The calibration data showed that an accuracy of ± 3° to 4° was possible; therefore 4° inner and outer zones around the stimulus were used to define contour looking. Analogously, we defined mutually exclusive zones of fixation in the central portion of each stimulus, and in regions at the edges of the visual display. We also divided the entire visual display into small subareas; extensiveness of scanning was assessed by counting how many subareas were fixated. On none of these analyses were there any significant age main effects. Younger infants did not scan less of a figure, or less of the internal portions of a figure or more of the contour compared with older infants. These results are clearly a disconfirmation of the developmental trends reported by Salapatek (1969, 1975).

In contrast, stimulus size clearly did influence scanning, independent of age, for both fixation and scan parameters. Eye movements to the small (5°) forms were significantly shorter in length than those to the medium (20°) and large (30°) forms. This effect resulted from a reduction in the horizontal component of eye movements to small forms. Vertical dispersion was not affected by size.

In terms of where the infants looked, we found that size of the stimulus reliably affected the distribution of fixations in the visual field. For all ages, more of the visual field was explored as the size of the form increased. However, if one controls for the area of the stimulus, small forms are scanned more extensively per unit area than large forms, another indication of the fact that infants modify their scanning as a function of stimulus parameters.

A closer look at scanning in relation to the specific stimulus revealed significant size effects as well. The rear projection screen on which the stimuli were shown subtended a visual angle of approximately 45°. We divided this area into two regions: "edge of screen", a ± 4° border around the actual edge of the screen, and "central visual field", the area inside this border. Across all stimuli, there were higher proportions of fixations to the central visual field, although the size of the stimulus did significantly affect the incidence of fixations in these regions. Infants were more likely to be looking in the central portions of the visual field when viewing a small (5°) stimulus than when viewing medium (20°) or large (30°) form. As compared with those to small stimuli, fixations to the larger stimuli were more likely to be near the edges of the screen, possibly because the edges of the screen, being near the contours of the stimuli, were salient contours in these cases. However, there were Age × Size interactions such that these findings were true for 2 and 3 month olds, but not for 1 month olds who were actually more likely to be looking in the central portions of the visual field for large forms and in the edges of the visual field for small and medium forms than were older infants. It should be emphasized that this finding does not imply that the youngest infants ignored all but the largest forms; the proportion of fixations in the central visual field was 50% or above for all ages and all sizes.

The forms themselves consisted of sets of contours—to what extent did these contours affect fixation patterns? Contour looking was defined as fixations within a $\pm$ 4° region of the figure's boundary. Once again, we found that the size of the stimulus, but not age of subject, influenced visual behavior. Fixations were more likely to be near the contour of a large figure than a small or medium form, but the contour zone in large forms had proportionately the largest area; when the proportion of fixations near the contour was divided by the area of the stimulus (to derive a measure of density of fixation per unit area), fixations were more likely to be near the contour of small forms. For the large and medium forms, subtracting the contour zone area leaves a central region; there were more fixations in this region for large forms than for medium forms. In this case, controlling for area equalized the density in this central region for large and medium forms.

Conclusions then, simply stated, are that size of stimulus appears to influence scanning behavior more than does age of subject. However, there is no one "style" of scanning that adequately charactizes the behavior of subjects toward these patterns. Variability is the order of the day and probably accounts for the lack of significant findings for age.

Why are these results so different from those of Salapatek? There were of course differences in the designs of the studies and in the methods. Salapatek's subjects were lying down, looking up at the stimuli, and were allowed to suck on pacifiers. Our subjects were upright and had no pacifiers. Details of the Salapatek procedures are somewhat sketchy in that no mention is made of how many subjects were tested to obtain the data presented. In Salapatek's study, the total time data were collected on each of the five stimuli was 50 seconds, although the data do not necessarily represent 50 seconds of uninterrupted scanning. If the picture of the eye was lost, the recording was stopped, so that one 50 second interval may have had several interruptions and would not indicate a continuous pattern of eye movements (Salapatek, personal communication). The present procedure involved showing each of the six stimuli for 10 seconds, separated by an ISI when data were not collected; the data for a stimulus represent a continuous, unbroken stretch of data collection.

Perhaps, most critically, the Salapatek study used a method of determining fixations based on an analysis of data sampled each quarter second; intervening data were not analysed and the data points sampled were called fixations even though there was no way of telling whether a particular point sampled occurred during a fixation or an eye movement. Our analysis, while admittedly a time sample at 60 times a second, ignores no data points in estimating fixations. On the chance that differences in the two definitions of "fixations" obscured age differences, we reanalysed all of our raw data at a 4 Hz sample rate and called each sample a fixation, thus mimicking Salapatek's analysis. On this reanalysis, we found even fewer age differences than in our original analysis. The time

Fixation Analysis vs. Simple Time Sampling

Sampled at 60 Hz; analyzed for fixations

Sampled at 4 Hz

Good Agreement

a.

(Megham W., 2 mo.)

X COORDINATE

Y COORDINATE

b.

(Megham W., 2 mo.)

X COORDINATE

Y COORDINATE

14

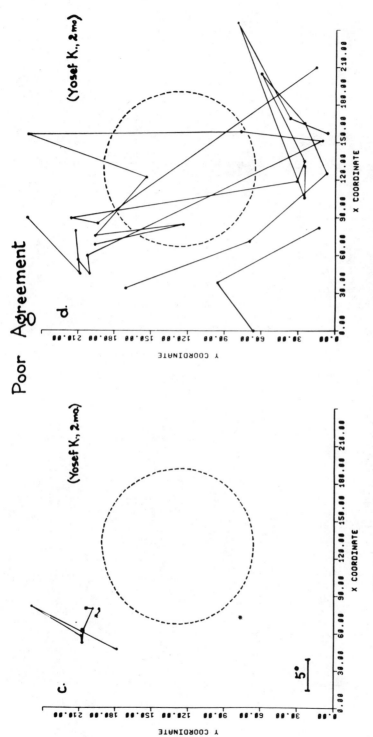

FIG. 5. A comparison of the results of two types of data analysis for the definition of fixations. Panels a and c illustrate the results of an algorithm defining fixations as regions of stationarity in data sampled at 60 Hz. Panels b and d illustrate the results of an algorithm that defines fixations as data frames sampled at a 4 Hz rate. Panels a and b illustrate a data set where the two methods agree reasonably well; panels c and d illustrate a data set with poor agreement between the measures.

15

Within-subject Variation in Scanning Patterns
"Narrow" vs. "Broad"

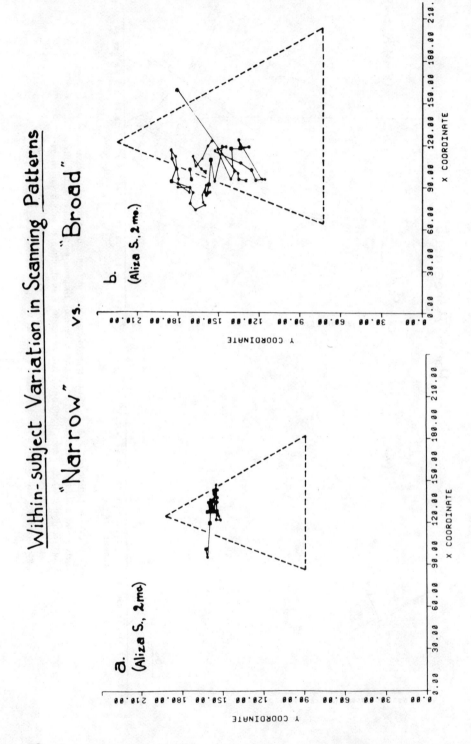

a.
(Aliza S., 2 mo.)

b.
(Aliza S., 2 mo.)

16

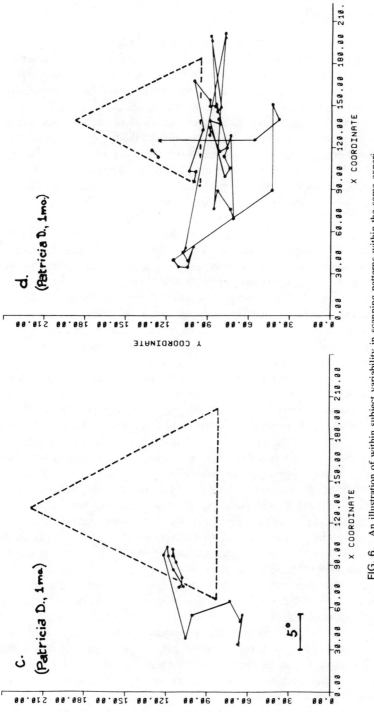

FIG. 6. An illustration of within subject variability in scanning patterns within the same experimental session. Panels a and b represent "narrow" and "broad" scanning from a 2 month old infant; panels c and d represent the same patterns of scanning from a 1 month old baby.

sample approach tended to make scanning appear broader, as defined by the number of zones entered, but the general effects of size of stimulus were essentially unchanged. In comparing the two methods, we sometimes found good agreement between the two methods and sometimes not. The two methods tended to give similar results when scanning was restricted to a small area or when dwell times were long since in the latter case the chances of "sampling" a fixation were greater. On the other hand, the two methods can give quite different results if scanning is very broad and dwell times are very brief, or if the data are noisy. Figure 5 shows computer plots of data analyzed by the two methods. In Panels A and B is an example of good agreement between the two methods, in Panels C and D, an example of poor agreement between the two methods.

The pattern of findings in these data, we believe, stems from the inherent variability of infant visual behavior across ages. To further illustrate this point, Fig. 6 shows examples of scanning records to support the claim that broad generalizations do not characterize these data well. The figure illustrates within subject variability on the "broad versus narrow" dimension. Salapatek (1975) has claimed that there is a developmental trend for one month olds to scan narrowly and for two month olds to scan more broadly. The subject in Panels A and B is a two month old who shows narrow scanning to a medium triangle and broader scanning to the large triangle in the same experimental session. Panels C and D show a one month old infant scanning narrowly to a large form and more broadly to a medium form. Although these data may suggest an age by size interaction, none were consistently found; the point is that these examples are not exceptional. All patterns of scanning occur at all ages and to all stimuli.

New techniques for studying infants have resulted in the discovery that the "twentieth century" infant is not nearly as incompetent as previous generations of psychologists had imagined. Past views of the young infant as locked into inflexible modes of data gathering seem counterintuitive if one regards the task of the infant as developing an understanding of the world around him/her through active visual exploration. The results of this study show that even the youngest babies can appropriately accommodate their visual behavior to fit the demands of the stimulus, and these infants appear not to be well characterized by a few generalizations about their visual exploration.

Such generalizations were proposed partly because earlier techniques for measuring infant visual behavior gave relatively gross measures of scanning that were not subjected to detailed analysis. There is a tendency to be seduced by the parsimony of simple explanations without awareness that the parsimony may result from limitations in methodology rather than from the characteristics of the thing being studied. Given the finer grained measures of infant visual behavior now provided by new techniques, further more subtle analytic techniques must be developed for dealing with the data. Previous discussions of infant visual behavior have stressed the characteristics of infant eye movements, although it is during fixation epochs that the infant is gathering information about the world. More attention needs to be given to the fixations, and how they are timed and sequenced if further understanding of how visual exploration yields information about a coherent world for the infant is to be gained.

In some ways, it is difficult to renounce the existing "rules" of infant visual behavior when nothing as coherent with which to replace them is available. In this case, however, the data allow us no alternative. Infants may simply be more complicated than previously believed.

ACKNOWLEDGMENTS

The research reported was supported by grant #GB43888 from the National Science Foundation, grant #HD08706 from the National Institutes of Health, grant #12-19, from the National Foundation-March of Dimes and grant #12220 from the PSC-BHE Faculty Research Awards Program of the City University of New York. I would like to thank Israel Abramov, Chris Harris, James Gordon, and Elizabeth Lemerise for their contributions to this research.

1.2 The Influence of Peripheral Stimuli on Infants' Eye Movements

Daphne Maurer and Terri L. Lewis
McMaster University

In 1825 Purkinje (cited in Zigler, Cook, Miller, & Wemple, 1930) demonstrated the important influence of peripheral stimuli on adults' vision. When wearing a pair of opaque spectacles with only a small central hole, he discovered he could no longer walk around the room satisfactorily and that fast activities like dancing were impossible. Subsequent studies confirmed that adults process and use information from peripheral vision. Even without previous scanning, they can identify the shape or orientation of stimuli far in the periphery (Collier, 1931; Johnson, Keltner, & Balestrery, 1978; Munn & Geil, 1931; Salaman, 1929; Whitmer, 1933). For example, Whitmer (1933) found that adults shown pairs of 3° figures drawn from a set consisting of a triangle, circle, diamond, hexagon, rectangle, and square could identify all figures out to 60° and all but the hexagon out to 90°. Moreover, adults use peripheral information to guide their eye movements toward parts of stimuli judged informative or salient (Antes & Penland, this volume; Bozkov, Bohdanecky, & Radil-Weiss, 1973; Cohen, this volume; Findlay, this volume; Friedman, this volume; Loftus, 1977; Mackworth & Bruner, 1970; O'Regan, this volume).

At first glance, these data seem to contradict perceptual learning theory. Both Hebb (1949, 1968) and Hochberg (1970a, 1971) argue that, except for gross features like brightness or contour, a stimulus can be seen only after it is scanned thoroughly with central vision; without scanning, the shape or orientation of a stimulus should be impossible to perceive. However, studies of peripheral vision in adults probably demonstrate what the "mind" reconstructs rather than what the eye sees. Indeed, subjects frequently name figures shown on previous trials, frequently draw more meaningful and symmetrical figures than shown, and accuracy depends on the number of available alternatives (Grindley, 1931; Haith,

21

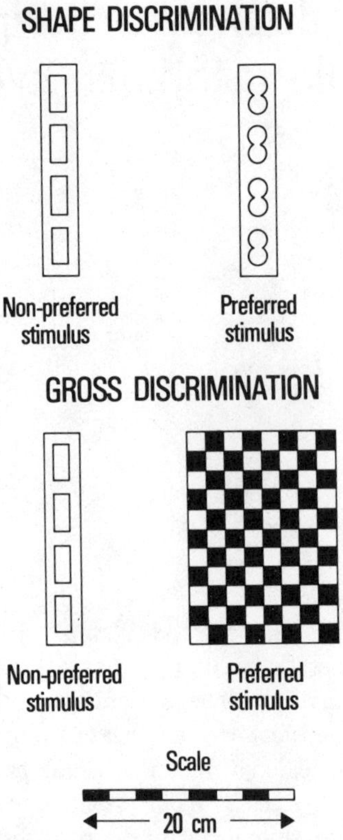

SHAPE DISCRIMINATION

Non-preferred
stimulus

Preferred
stimulus

GROSS DISCRIMINATION

Non-preferred
stimulus

Preferred
stimulus

Scale

← 20 cm →

FIG. 1. The discriminations tested. The checkerboard was black-and-white; the other stimuli contained white elements on a red background.

Morrison, & Sheingold, 1970; Kleitman & Blier, 1928; Miller, 1971; Salaman, 1929; Zigler et al., 1930). Since the perceptual learning theories allow for such reconstruction, any type of peripheral processing demonstrated by adults would not contradict the theories.

Peripheral discrimination in infants would be more likely to indicate what can actually be *seen* in the periphery as infants have little stored information from which to reconstruct a figure and it appears they do not fill in features missing from a highly familiar stimulus (Caron, Caron, Caldwell, & Weiss, 1973; Maurer, in preparation).

There are a few suggestions in the literature that infants can make peripheral discriminations and use them to guide their eye movements. Two-month-olds move their eyes first toward a region of greater contour 10° in the periphery (Salapatek, 1975); 3-month-olds look first toward a checkerboard 18° in the periphery rather than a picture of the mother with which it is paired (Maurer & Lewis, 1979); and the time it takes 4-month-olds to turn toward a checkerboard at 46° depends on the size of the checkerboard and the number of checks (Cohen, 1972).

We further examined the ability of 3-month-olds to make peripheral discriminations by presenting the two pairs of stimuli illustrated in Fig. 1 at 10°, 20°, and 30° along the horizontal meridian. One pair, a checkerboard and a pattern of rectangles, required a gross discrimination that could be based on size, shape, color, contour, etc.; the other pair, a pattern of circles and the same pattern of rectangles, required a finer discrimination that could be based on only the shape of internal elements. Preliminary research indicated that 3-month-old infants prefer to look at one member of each pair longer than the other. Specifically, infants looked significantly longer at the checkerboard and the pattern of circles than at the pattern of rectangles each was paired with. In the studies reported here we tested whether new samples of infants would move their eyes first toward the preferred member. (Three adults asked to name the side on which the infants' preferred member appeared were accurate at least 75% of the time for the gross discrimination out to 70° and for the shape discrimination out to 50°.)

In the first study, the subjects were 45 full-term, 3-month-old infants ($\bar{X}$ age = 91 days; range 84–98 days). Each infant sat in an infant seat inclined at 45° and faced a parallel display panel 33 cm away. Between trials a $16° \times 0.5°$ vertical strip of red lights was turned on in the center of the display panel. Then the central lights went off and a pair of stimuli were presented for 10 sec. During a sequence each discrimination was tested twice at 10°, at 20°, and at 30°, in random order and with the preferred member once on the left and once on the right at each distance. Since the sequence was repeated once, there were 24 trials.

Eye movements were recorded by corneal photography. Behind the display panel were a 16 mm movie camera and eight reference lamps, all trained on the infant's left eye. The reference lamps were filtered by Corning 7–69 and Wratten 87C filters so that they transmitted light mainly between 860 and 960 nm and were nearly invisible (to an adult). Kodak High Speed Infrared Film was used to photograph reflections of the reference lights to the infant's left eye four times a second at an exposure time of 100 msec.

Two naive scorers made three decisions on each trial: (1) whether the infant had in fact started the trial by fixating centrally (within 4° of the central red lights), and if so, (2) the direction of the first eye movement away from center, and (3) whether it was 10°, 20°, or 30° long. Scorers studied the film of an 8-year-old instructed to fixate specific points in the visual field and used the relationship between the center of the child's pupil and the reflections of the reference lamps as a template for each fixation point. Since that relationship will vary from individual to individual for any given fixation point (Hainline, this volume; Slater & Findlay, 1972, 1975b), the scorers also adjusted the templates to each infant. They noted the most frequent horizontal deviation of the reference lamps from the center of the infant's pupil just as the central lights went off at the beginning of each of the 24 trials, then changed the horizontal coordinates of the template for fixations on the center of the field accordingly so long as the change

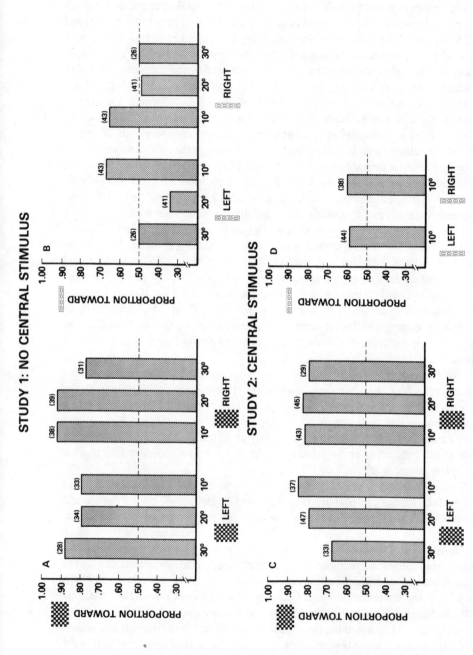

FIG. 2.   The proportion of infants who moved their eyes first toward the preferred member of a pair. The dotted line indicates the proportion expected by chance and the numbers in parentheses show the number of infants who contributed to each analysis. A and B refer to the first study; C and D, to the second study.

24

fell in the range of expected corrections. (The range corresponded to discrepancies between the visual and optic axes of 2° to 8°.) Corresponding adjustments were then made to all other templates.

The scorers agreed on 89% of the trials about whether the infant had begun by fixating centrally; on trials which they agreed began centrally, they agreed 84% of the time on both the direction and length of the first eye movement. Anytime the scorers disagreed, they rescored the trial together and reached an agreement.

Twenty infants were excluded from the analysis because more than 75% of their first eye movements were toward one side. For the 45 remaining subjects, trials were excluded if the infant had not begun by fixating centrally and/or did not look first toward one of the stimuli. (Multiple saccades to a stimulus were permitted so long as each saccade in the series followed the preceding one within 1 sec—see Aslin & Salapatek, 1975.) Some infants provided more than one usable trial for a stimulus and in those cases, only the first was included.

The results for the gross discrimination were striking. Figure 2A shows the proportion of infants whose first eye movements were toward the preferred stimulus, the checkerboard, at each distance. Binomial tests showed that the infants moved their eyes first toward the checkerboard significantly more often than expected by chance when the stimuli were 10°, 20°, and 30° in the periphery, both when the checkerboard was on the left and when it was on the right, all $ps \leqslant .025$. (Because the data were nominal, we used non-parametric statistics.) In other words, infants discriminated these stimuli in the periphery wherever tested.

The results for the shape discrimination were quite different (see Fig. 2B). Binomial tests showed that the infants moved their eyes first toward the preferred stimulus, the pattern of circles, when it was 10° to the left or right, both $ps \leqslant .05$, but not when it was at 20° or 30°, all $ps > .10$. Since slightly different combinations of infants had provided data for each of these analyses, we confirmed the results in subgroups that provided data at *both* 10° and 20°.

The first study shows that young infants can discriminate grossly different stimuli far in the periphery and use that information to direct their eye movements. They can also direct their eyes toward a particular shape 10° in the periphery. Unlike adults, the infants probably saw rather than inferred the stimuli: The stimuli were novel and the infant's performance was as good on the first two trials as on subsequent ones. Therefore, the data imply that infants can *perceive* shape in the periphery and contradict the perceptual learning theorists' assertion that the shape of a stimulus can be perceived only after thorough scanning. On the contrary, humans can perceive at least some aspects of shapes with peripheral vision.

Although the first study demonstrates that young infants can make peripheral discriminations, they might not be able to do so under more natural conditions, i.e. while fixating another object with central vision. Certainly neither infants nor adults localize objects as far in the periphery when they begin by fixating a central stimulus (Harris & MacFarlane, 1974; MacFarlane, Harris, & Barnes, 1976; Webster & Haslerud, 1946); nor under those circumstances do children or adults name peripheral objects as accurately (Holmes, Cohen, Haith, & Morrison, 1977).

In our second study we tested the ability of 70 3-month-old infants ($\bar{x}$ age = 93 days, range 87 to 98 days) to make the same peripheral discriminations while fixating a vertical white line (4.5° × 29°). An additional 58 infants were excluded because more than 75% of their first eye movements were toward one side. We tested the gross discrimination (checkerboard versus rectangles) at 10°, 20°, and 30°, and the shape discrimination (circles versus rectangles) at 10°, the only distance at which infants in the first study had shown they could make the discrimination without a central stimulus. During a sequence, the preferred member of a pair appeared on both the left and right, at each of the specified distances. The sequence was presented three times, so there were 24 trials.

The procedure and data reduction were the same as in the first study except that the length of trials was reduced from 10 to 5 sec. The two scorers agreed on 82% of the trials about whether an infant had begun the trial by fixating centrally; on trials they agreed had begun centrally, they agreed 81% of the time on the direction and length of the first eye movements away from center.

The results for the gross discrimination were similar to those of the first study (see Fig. 2C). Binomial tests showed that the infants moved their eyes first toward the preferred stimulus, the checkerboard, when it was on the left and when it was on the right at 10°, 20°, and 30°, all $ps \leq .05$. In contrast to the first study, there was no evidence for the discrimination of shape either when the circles were 10° to the left or 10° to the right, both $ps > .10$ (see Fig. 2D). Subgroups of infants with complete data at 10° confirmed that infants made the gross discrimination but showed no evidence of the shape discrimination. Thus, fixation of a central stimulus does not obliterate infants' processing of peripheral stimuli, but it does interfere with the processing of subtle peripheral information like the shape of a stimulus.

To learn more about peripheral discrimination, we examined the latencies of eye movements toward the preferred stimuli the infants had perceived peripherally. Studies of *detection* in infants, older children, and adults have shown that the latency of eye movements is longer for targets farther in the periphery (Aslin & Salapatek, 1975; Bartz, 1962; Cohen, this volume). To determine whether distance has a similar effect on peripheral *discrimination* we used Friedman analyses of variance to compare the latencies of eye movements toward the checkerboard as a function of its distance in the periphery, both when the central stimulus was absent (Fig. 3A) and when it was present (Fig. 3C). Infants were included only if their first eye movement was toward the checkerboard on at least one trial at each distance. There was a significant effect of distance when the central stimulus was present, $x^2 (2) = 6.02$, $p < .05$.

We also examined the latency of eye movements as a function of difficulty by comparing the two discriminations infants made at 10° in Study 1 (see Fig. 3B).

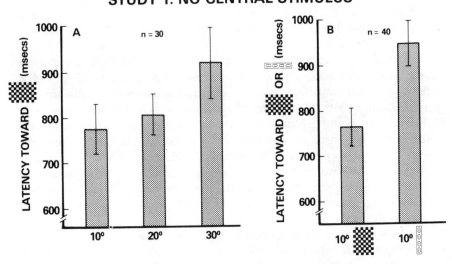

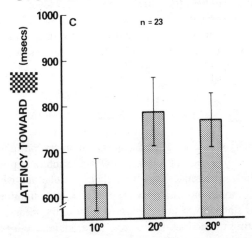

Fig. 3. The mean latencies of eye movements toward the preferred member of pairs discriminated in the periphery. The bars indicate standard errors. A and B refer to the first study; C, to the second study.

To be included infants had to have moved their eyes first toward the preferred stimulus on at least one trial for each discrimination. A Wilcoxon test of matched pairs showed that the latencies of eye movements toward the pattern of circles were significantly longer than the latencies of eye movements toward the checkerboard, $T(37) = 146.5$, $p < .01$, two-tailed.

These analyses suggest that infants take longer to move their eyes toward a particular stimulus in the periphery if the discrimination they are making is more difficult, either because the stimuli lie farther in the periphery or because the discrimination is a more subtle one. But the standard error bars in Fig. 3 also support the suggestion of Aslin and Salapatek (1975) that the latencies of infants' eye movements are too variable to be a promising research tool.

The results of a third study also provided lessons about not-so-promising research tools for studies of infants. In the first two studies, separate groups of infants were tested for shape discrimination in the presence and absence of a central stimulus. Only those infants who had nothing to look at centrally showed they could discriminate shape at 10°. The third study was designed to confirm those results in a single group of infants. On each trial infants were shown the pattern of rectangles paired with the pattern of circles, each 10° in the periphery. During a block of trials the preferred pattern, the circles, appeared on the left and on the right, with and without the central line. The order of trials within each block was randomized and the block of four trials was repeated until the infant ceased to cooperate.

Study 3 was appropriate psychophysically, but apparently not psychologically. Repetition of just two stimuli (this time there were no checkerboards), apparently bored the infants so that they provided no data. Of the 108 3-month-olds who began the procedure, 77 were excluded because more than 75% of their first eye movements were toward one side, and 7 because they provided incomplete data; the remaining 24 provided random data. This illustrates a common problem (see also Hainline, this volume) with eye movement studies: Many designs though intriguing are not feasible.

SUMMARY AND CONCLUSIONS

Adults can identify subtle details of objects far in the periphery; for example, adults could identify shape out to 50°. However, such data probably indicate as much about adults' inferences as about their peripheral vision. The data we collected from 3-month-old infants were probably uncontaminated by such cognitive inferences since the stimuli were novel, since the infants' performance did not improve during the course of the procedure, and since infants are likely too immature to make such inferences about stimuli. Thus, unlike previous reports on adults, our results probably indicate what can be *seen* with peripheral vision.

The results show that peripheral vision, unaided by cognitive inferences, can influence humans' eye movements. Those eye movements can be controlled by gross features of stimuli even far in the periphery and by the shapes of stimuli close to the fixation point. Although having a central stimulus to fixate interferes with peripheral processing, it by no means obliterates that processing or its influence on eye movements. Moreover, the speed of processing depends on the distance of the stimuli in the periphery and difficulty of differentiation.

Finally, the data point out the necessity of revising the fundamental premise of perceptual learning theories that, except for gross features like brightness and contour, stimuli can be perceived only after thorough scanning. Study 2 suggests that that is the case when a subject is fixating a central stimulus. However, Study 1 shows that in the absence of a central stimulus, shapes can be perceived 10° in the periphery. Unlike similar findings in adults, the results cannot be dismissed as the likely product of reconstruction. Thus, they suggest that perceptual learning theorists underestimated the processing possible with peripheral vision.

ACKNOWLEDGMENT

We would like to thank Deborah Kay, Mary Stire, Silvana DiPasquale, Wendy Debicki, Anne Lees, and Adrienne Richardson who helped collect and analyze these data. We would also like to thank Susan Crossgrove and Russ Adams for acting as adult subjects. This research was supported by Canadian National Research Council grant A9797. Some of the data from the first study were reported in Maurer and Lewis (1979).

I.3 Development of Smooth Pursuit in Human Infants

Richard N. Aslin
Indiana University

The oculomotor movements of human infants have fascinated scientists (and parents) for centuries, presumably because systematic changes in fixation indicate the presence of a functioning visual system. Although careful studies of infant eye movements were conducted 50 years ago (e.g., Beasley, 1933; Guersney, 1929) these early studies relied solely on simple observational techniques. In fact, even today the most commonly used method for assessing the young infant's visual abilities consists of a two-choice preference technique developed by Fantz (1958) and recently perfected by Teller (1979). This preferential looking procedure relies solely on observers who judge the infant's oculomotor behaviors. Although a skilled observer can reliably estimate the gross characteristics of an infant's eye fixations, judgments of the latency, accuracy, size and form of changes in fixation are clearly beyond the capability of a human observer.

It has been less than 20 years since a variety of objective recording techniques, originally developed for use with adults (see Young & Sheena, 1975, for a general review), were applied to the detailed study of oculomotor development in human infants (see Maurer, 1975, for a methodological review). The vast majority of these studies that used objective eye movement recording techniques were devoted to questions of pattern vision, and in particular how the young infant changes fixation from one region of a complex, stationary pattern to another (e.g., Salapatek & Kessen, 1966). Although such studies described the location on the pattern to which infants directed their fixation, they did not address basic questions of oculomotor control; for example, (1) the manner in which changes in fixation are accomplished, (2) the types of eye movements present at different developmental periods, and (3) the factors (neuromuscular,

31

sensory, and/or attentional) that influence the development of oculomotor control. These concerns have been a major focus of my research for the past five years. This research program began with an investigation of the infant's saccadic eye movement system (Aslin & Salapatek, 1975; Salapatek, Aslin, Simonson, & Pulos, in press) and was expanded to cover the vergence eye movement system (Aslin, 1977; Aslin & Jackson, 1979). The present chapter covers the development of the smooth pursuit eye movement system in 1- to 4-month-old infants.

SMOOTH PURSUIT: BACKGROUND AND RATIONALE

There can be little doubt that the smooth pursuit system—the oculomotor mechanism that maintains the image of a moving target on the fovea—is both complex and poorly understood. Despite the past decade of productive research, the following evaluation offered by Robinson (1971) still characterizes the state of our knowledge:

> of all the visually mediated eye movements, pursuit and fixation are the most elementary and the least understood and they represent a fertile field for investigation by both theoretical and empirical research [p. 537].

An even more intriguing corollary to Robinson's statement is the fact that there are *no* empirical investigations of the *development* of pursuit and fixation in animals. Although human infants are notoriously difficult to work with, there are several species of animals that would seem to be likely candidates for systematic studies of oculomotor development. This absence of research on oculomotor development is particularly curious in light of the vast literature accumulated during the past 20 years on the susceptibility of various structures and functions in the cat and monkey visual systems to environmental modifications received during the early postnatal period (see Grobstein & Chow, 1976; Hubel, Wiesel, & LeVay, 1977; and Pettigrew, 1978, for general reviews). The complex sensory-motor aspects of oculomotor control would seem to be a natural starting point for the investigation of early experiential influences (see Hein, Vital-Durand, Salinger, & Diamond, 1979 for a recent example). In fact, there are no known animal models of oculomotor development despite the accumulation of a wide variety of data on the neural mechanisms underlying oculomotor movements in adult animals (Baker & Berthoz, 1977).

Despite the absence of detailed descriptions of smooth pursuit in human infants, and the absence of animal models to provide a theoretical guide to the understanding of oculomotor development in humans, there are several qualitative findings on smooth pursuit in infants, as well as several systematic studies of smooth pursuit in human adults. Studies of human adults have provided a detailed characterization of smooth pursuit control, and several of these characteristics are relevant to the study of smooth pursuit in infants.

The pioneering work of Westheimer (1954), which was later clarified and updated with more sophisticated recording techniques (Rashbass, 1961; Robinson, 1965), illustrated that the smooth pursuit system is capable of accurately matching the velocity of a small moving target. Pursuit latency is typically 130 msec, significantly less than saccadic latency (200 msec), and maximum pursuit velocity is 30–40 deg/sec, considerably less than maximum saccadic velocity (600–900 deg/sec). As a result of the rather lengthy pursuit latency (compared, e.g., to the vestibular-ocular response latency of 10–20 msec), a stationary target that begins to move at a constant velocity will travel a considerable distance (dependent upon target velocity) before the eye begins to move. Since pursuit movements are velocity-limited, one or more saccadic movements are typically used to bring the fovea close to the position of the moving target.

In contrast to the saccadic system, the pursuit system appears to continuously update the estimated velocity of the moving target and program an appropriate acceleration or deceleration of the eye. Thus, target movements that contain changes in velocity are also responded to quite accurately (see Young, 1971 for a general summary). In fact, the typical control systems approach for characterizing the pursuit system consists of presenting a sinusoidal oscillation of the target, usually in the horizontal meridian of the fronto-parallel plane. This sinusoidal oscillation consists of a target that traverses a constant angular distance (the amplitude of the sine wave) while undergoing a continuous variation in velocity (maximum at midpoint; zero at two endpoints).

A quantitative characterization of the pursuit system, therefore, consists of specifying three functions: (1) the amplitude gain (ratio of the amplitude of eye excursion to the amplitude of target excursion), (2) the velocity gain (ratio of eye velocity to target velocity), and (3) the phase lag (temporal delay of the eye relative to the target). These parameters are plotted as a function of the frequency of the target oscillation, thus providing an input-output description of the pursuit system. As shown by several researchers (e.g., St. Cyr & Fender, 1969a,b), gain shows a significant decrease and phase lag shows a significant increase for oscillations greater than 1.0 Hz. In addition, at these higher frequencies of oscillation the pursuit system alone cannot keep the fovea on target, and saccadic movements become interspersed with smooth tracking. Thus, the amplitude gain of the overall tracking response (saccades plus pursuit) continues to approach unity even at high frequencies, and only the velocity gain (dropping out the intruding saccadic movements) is typically reported.

A variety of more complex forms of target movement have also been used to determine the limits of the adult's velocity matching (pursuit) system. These studies (e.g., Michael & Jones, 1966) have demonstrated quite clearly that a complex pattern of movement, e.g., a broadband or multi-frequency oscillation, results in a loss of gain and an increased phase lag, even if the highest frequency component in both the broadband and the narrowband (single frequency) oscillations is identical. One conclusion from these studies is that the pursuit system uses prediction information about the expected change in target velocity to more effectively program the smooth pursuit response. Thus, one could characterize this predictive operation as a bandwidth analyzer, such that the narrower the bandwidth (narrowest = single sine wave), the easier the prediction about changes in target velocity. However, as Rashbass (1971) has pointed out, a square wave oscillation in which the target jumps instantaneously between two positions, consists of a complex, broadband waveform which is nevertheless highly predictable. Thus, it appears that the pursuit system can accurately compute expected changes in target velocity, and that this prediction is not modeled very accurately by a processor that analyzes the bandwidth of the target oscillation. Finally, it is of interest to note that Fuchs (1967) found minimal evidence for predictive tracking in adult monkeys.

Given this background information on the adult smooth pursuit system, what is currently known about smooth pursuit in human infants? The first attempt at providing an objective description of pursuit movements in human infants was reported by McGinnis (1930). He filmed the eye movements of infants from birth to several months postnatally as they fixated a black vertically-oriented bar on a white background. The bar was moved laterally, but the rate of movement was not described. McGinnis reported that the infant's tracking movements were saccadic until approximately 6 weeks postnatally. Unfortunately, his data were based on global film records that included the infant's entire face. Therefore, he relied upon adult observers to judge from the film records whether the eye movements were smooth or saccadic. Nevertheless, this study was extremely thorough and the observers' judgments could be verified, at least qualitatively, from the film records. The accuracy of the tracking responses, however, could not be determined without a more detailed eye movement recording system.

After McGinnis' report, over 30 years passed before Dayton and Jones (1964) and Dayton, Jones, Steele, and Rose (1964) used electro-oculography (EOG) to record the tracking responses of young infants presented with a single moving target. In their two studies they presented a single 15 deg diameter black dot on a homogenous white background. The target traveled across the 180 deg stimulus field at a velocity of 16 deg/sec. The path of target movement was a simple ramp, i.e., the target was not oscillated back and forth, although the direction of target movement was randomized across trials. Like McGinnis, the Dayton, et al. studies demonstrated that the tracking movements of infants were totally saccadic until 6 to 8 weeks postnatally. After this initial postnatal period, smooth pursuit movements emerged, with saccades interspersed among the brief smooth components. The metric that Dayton, et al. used in their description of tracking movements during later infancy was the frequency of saccades. Unfortunately, this measure does not capture other quantitative aspects of smooth pursuit. In addition, their use of only a single target velocity restricted the conclusions they could draw. Nevertheless, their finding that tracking movements in the newborn are totally saccadic has been supported by numerous observational studies (e.g., Barten, Birns, & Ronch, 1971).

The most recent study of smooth pursuit was a report by Kremenitzer, Vaughan, Kurtzberg, and Dowling (1979) in which newborns (less than 1 week postnatal) were presented with a 12 deg diameter target that was moved at several different velocities. They recorded the infants' eye movements using EOG, and their results showed that even newborns exhibit some smooth pursuit movements. The gain of these smooth movements could not be calculated because the EOG records were uncalibrated. However, the relative velocity of the smooth components increased slightly as target velocity increased (from 9 to 19 deg/sec, but not beyond 19 deg/sec). The duration of the smooth components was quite brief, however, averaging only 300–400 msec. Moreover, the large size of the target raises the possibility that the optokinetic nystagmus (OKN) system may have mediated these smooth components via the peripheral retina. In fact, Kremenitzer et al. also recorded OKN in their newborn subjects and reported good evidence for the presence of the classic smooth and saccadic alternation shown in adults' OKN. The presence of smooth eye movements in an OKN task has also been reported by McGinnis (1930), Gorman, Cogan, and Gellis (1957), Fantz, Ordy, and Udelf (1962), Dayton, Jones, Aiu, Rawson, Steele, and Rose (1964), Doris and Cooper (1966), Tauber and Koffler (1966) and Atkinson and Braddick (this volume). Thus, it is apparent that smooth tracking eye movements can be elicited shortly after birth, but these smooth movements are quite brief, dependent upon target velocity and size, and typically interspersed with saccades. Moreover, it is not clear whether these smooth movements (before the 6th postnatal week) are mediated by central or peripheral retinal areas.

The purpose of the present investigation was to provide a detailed description of the smooth pursuit system in young human infants. Of particular interest were the following issues: (1) the age of onset for smooth pursuit movements to a small (2°) target that was moved through a sinusoidal trajectory, (2) the accuracy of infants' smooth pursuit at various target velocities (frequencies of oscillation), and (3) the search for possible prediction effects in the smooth tracking of young infants. These issues were investigated within the confines shared by past researchers, i.e., a basically uncooperative subject, but with the advantage of an unobtrusive and automated eye monitoring system and a well controlled stimulus display system. Before proceeding to a description of the methods and results, however, it is appropriate to briefly review the basic findings on the infant's saccadic system, since these findings may place the results on smooth pursuit in some perspective, and because they aided in generating a hypothesis for the mechanism underlying the development of smooth pursuit movements in early infancy.

SACCADIC EYE MOVEMENTS IN EARLY INFANCY

In 1975 Aslin and Salapatek reported the results of a study on the saccadic system in 1- and 2-month-old infants who were presented with small (4°) targets at various retinal eccentricities (10°, 20°, 30° and 40°). Their results, based on EOG recordings, provided three new pieces of data on the infant's saccadic system. First, young infants are highly motivated to localize peripheral targets, since the probability of a directionally-appropriate *first* saccade toward the target was very high (e.g., over 0.9 at 10 deg). Second, the latency to initiate a directionally-appropriate saccade is highly variable, with *median* latencies in the 500 to 800 msec range. However, the shortest latencies recorded, 240 msec, are quite similar to the performance of adults who are not specifically instructed to respond as quickly as possible. Third, the form of infants' localizing saccades is quite unlike the adult. Adults typically rotate the eyes approximately 90% of the angular distance to the target on the first saccade (Weber & Daroff, 1971). Infants, however, exhibit grossly hypometric saccades, rarely moving more than 50% of the angular distance to the peripheral target on the first saccade. More-over, saccades subsequent to the initial saccade are nearly identical in size to this first attempt at target localization (see Fig. 1A). Thus, it seems possible that the direction, but not the angular distance, of the peripheral target is available as input to the young infant's saccadic programming system. Apparently, a particu-lar saccadic step-size is selected and reapplied until the target is localized, pre-

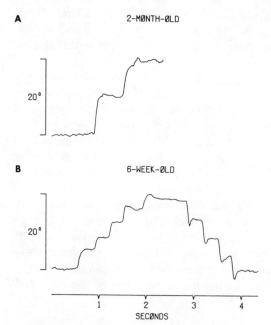

A   2-MØNTH-ØLD

20°

B   6-WEEK-ØLD

20°

1   2   3   4
SECØNDS

FIG. 1. Characteristic infant eye movement responses to a target that (A) jumps from one location to another and (B) moves smoothly from one location to another and back again.

sumably by the central retina (perhaps the fovea). Finally, the size of the saccadic step used to localize peripheral targets varies with target eccentricity, since a significantly larger initial (and subsequent) saccade size is used to localize more distant targets.

These findings on the infant saccadic system, particularly in light of the general conclusion that smooth pursuit does not emerge until several weeks postnatally, raised the possibility that smooth pursuit movements do not initially have a control mechanism independent of saccadic movements. In adults, there are several lines of evidence for the independence of the pursuit and saccadic controllers (e.g., Rashbass, 1961). However, for infants it seemed possible that smooth pursuit control emerges from the saccadic system via a reduction in the size of saccadic steps. This hypothesis seemed particularly appealing since a moving target, by the very nature of the continuous movement, translates over a very small region of extrafoveal retina compared to the large (10° or greater) displacements used in studies of saccadic localization. To preview the results of the present experiment on smooth pursuit, it is the case that infants' pursuit movements are not smooth at first; rather, they consist of a series of saccades whose size is, in general, inversely related to the velocity of the moving target (see Fig. 1B). Thus, the hypothesis that smooth pursuit emerges developmentally from a more basic saccadic system appears to be viable. Unfortunately, as we shall see in the more detailed results to follow, this hypothesis is in fact incorrect.

APPARATUS, METHOD AND ANALYSIS PROCEDURES

The preceding review of past attempts at describing the infant's smooth pursuit system has emphasized the need for more accurate and objective eye movement recording techniques. Currently, there are only two recording techniques that have been used successfully with young infants—EOG and corneal photography. The major problems with EOG are (1) the delays and frequent irritation caused by the placement of electrodes on the infant's face, and (2) the artifact introduced into the EOG signal by head movements. This latter problem is particularly troublesome because it is impossible to totally restrain the infant's head movements, and even a slight head rotation can result in a grossly inaccurate measure of eye position. The major advantages of corneal photography are (1) the absence of any attachments to the infant's head, and (2) the minimal confounding of head movements in the determination of eye position. This latter advantage holds true only if the camera and corneal reflection light source(s) remain fixed. Fixing the position of the camera necessitates the placement of the infant's eye within the camera's field of view. Unfortunately, this field of view is typically quite small to enhance the magnification of the picture of the eye. Thus, a major disadvantage of corneal photography is the restriction that the infant's eye must remain in the small (3 cm square) field of view of the recording camera.

In the past, corneal photography has used a movie camera and infrared film to unobtrusively record the position of the invisible corneal reflections with respect to the infant's pupil. However, the detailed measurement of the latency and form of eye movements would require a very high frame rate, which in turn would generate a tremendous amount of data to be scored by human observers (typically using a precise X-Y digitizer). Recent advances in integrated circuit technology have made the on-line analysis of corneal photographs possible. The system used for recording infants' eye movements in our laboratory is a commercially available automated corneal photography system (Applied Sciences Laboratory, Model 1994S). This system (Sheena, 1976) consists of a closed circuit television camera containing an infrared sensitive vidicon tube and a series of lenses that provide a close-up view of the eye. A near-infrared light source is collimated and aligned in parallel with the axis of the camera, thus creating a fundus reflex and its resultant bright pupil. This latter feature greatly enhances the contrast between the normally dark pupil and the slightly lighter iris. The light source also creates a corneal reflection that translates with respect to the center of the pupil as the eye rotates. The video signal from the camera is fed into analog and digital circuitry that analyzes the relationship between the pupil center and the corneal reflection and provides three separate voltages for horizontal eye position, vertical eye position and pupil size at a 60 Hz output rate.

Our application of this commercial system for use with infants involved a number of modifications. First, we built an enclosure containing two platforms. The lower platform consisted of a sliding table on which the infant was placed in the supine position, thus allowing us to locate the infant's eye within the field of view of the camera. Above the infant was a second platform that supported the camera and light source. A front surface mirror, oriented 45 deg from vertical, allowed the camera to view the infant's right eye. Above the infant's head was another mirror, in this case a large (20 by 25 cm) half-silvered "cold" mirror, which was also oriented at a 45° angle with respect to vertical. This cold mirror reflected 80% of the visible spectrum and transmitted 80% of the near-infrared spectrum. Thus, the camera viewed the infant's eye through this cold mirror with little attenuation of the video signal. The infant, then, viewed a stimulus display, actually located behind the infant's head, which was reflected in the cold mirror. The display device consisted of a standard 15 inch black and white video monitor that could present a target of variable size and intensity. The video monitor was interfaced to a PDP-11/34 computer which controlled the size, shape, brightness, and screen position of the target. The computer also recorded the horizontal eye position information from the eye monitoring system and stored this information on disk for later analysis.

In order to describe the onset of smooth pursuit we tested 35 infants ranging in age from 22 to 115 days postnatally. Most infants were tested at one week intervals during the 5 to 12 week age range, although several could not be tested at certain ages due to illness or scheduling conflicts. Only 3 infants failed to provide at least one session of scorable data because of fussiness, puffy eyelids or equipment failure. A total of 66 sessions were collected from the 32 infants who provided scorable data (absence of blinks and analysis system noise). Since our goal was to characterize each infant's optimum performance during different developmental periods, our data summaries will focus on the infants' most attentive tracking responses at a variety of target velocities, rather than the average performance of infants at different ages.

Each session consisted of a series of trials on which a black vertical bar (2° wide, 8° high) on a white background was moved through a 20° sinusoidal oscillation in the horizontal meridian. The black bar (2 ftL) and the white background (50 ftL) resulted in a stimulus of very high contrast (0.92). The frequency of the target oscillation was initially 0.5 Hz and subsequently varied by an experimenter to maintain the interest of the infant. Frequency values of 0.25, 0.33, 0.50, 0.67 and 1.00 Hz were used, which correspond to mean velocities of 10, 13.3, 20, 26.7, and 40 deg/sec. The target was positioned 10 deg to the right of the infant's midline at the start of each trial, and traveled leftward 20 deg on the first half-cycle before returning to the starting location. From 3 to 5 cycles of the target oscillation were presented on each trial.

Perhaps the most difficult problem facing any researcher who is attempting to accurately record eye movements from a non or preverbal subject is calibration. Obviously, it is impossible to instruct the infant to fixate several known points in the stimulus field. One could position small fixation lights in the stimulus field, but infants are only rarely interested in maintaining fixation for even a second or two. Moreover, one is usually forced to make some judgment as to when the infant is fixating the stimulus field; otherwise, calibration data will include periods of off-field looking, such as fixating the edge of the screen or the infant's own hands. We experimented with several calibration schemes, including very small spots of light (less than 1°) and whole field edges (the narrowest contour possible). Unfortunately, the most effective and reliable elicitor of the infants' fixation was a fairly large target, one that was also effective in eliciting smooth pursuit. Therefore, we made the assumption that the infants were in fact fixating the 2° target and used the actual eye movement records as within-session calibration trials.

This calibration procedure, of course, assumes that the infant fixates the same region of the target at all times during a trial. If this assumption is violated, then the error of measurement will be approximated by the width of the target. Since we used a target that was 2° wide, the data we will report may contain an error as great as 2°. However, this level of accuracy, especially since it is not confounded by head movement artifacts, is better than past studies of infant tracking movements. Moreover, the resolution of the recording system (smallest detectable eye movement) is approximately 5 minutes of arc. Finally, if the infants were inconsistent in fixating a particular region of the target at different times during a trial, then the position of the eye would vary at the endpoints of the target oscillation. This variable endpoint behavior, as will become apparent in the records to follow, was in fact quite rare. Thus, either infants were consistently fixating a particular region (e.g., the left edge of the bar) throughout a trial, or the shift in fixation from one region of the target to another during a trial was very systematic.

Each of the individual trials were displayed on a point-plot CRT and subsequently plotted on a digital hard-copy device. This plotting included the superposition of the target's location on each eye movement record, thereby illustrating the relationship between the target and eye positions. The position of the target was estimated by the position of the eye prior to the onset of target movement and the amplitude of eye excursion during the oscillation of the target. Although this target placement was based on a subjective judgment of the endpoints of target excursion, the consistency of the eye movement records appeared to justify such a procedure. The only significant error in this stimulus placement process occurred when the target velocity was high, since the eye rarely kept up with the target and the amplitude gain was typically diminished. However, at lower target velocities the endpoints of eye excursion during the sinusoidal oscillation were very consistent, and these same endpoints were used

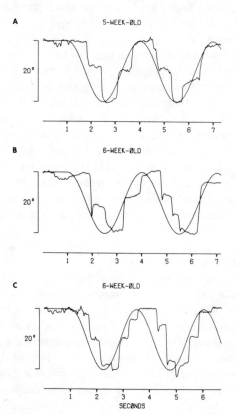

FIG. 2. Representative tracking responses by three infants who were presented with a target that moved smoothly through the indicated sinusoidal oscillation.

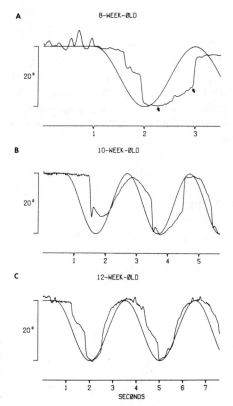

FIG. 3. Representative tracking responses by three infants who were presented with a target that moved smoothly through the indicated sinusoidal oscillation.

to estimate the location of the target on trials at the higher velocities within a particular session.

CHARACTERISTICS OF SMOOTH PURSUIT IN YOUNG INFANTS

The first aim of this investigation of smooth pursuit in human infants was to determine at what age instances of smooth tracking emerge. Figure 2 illustrates representative trials from three different 5- to 6-week-old infants. It is readily apparent that the tracking responses of these infants are totally saccadic. Moreover, the rate of target oscillation on these trials was quite low (0.33, 0.33, and 0.40 Hz, respectively). Thus, it would appear that smooth pursuit is not present prior to the sixth postnatal week, at least for a small target presented at the velocities used in this experiment.

Figure 3 illustrates the eye movement records of three different infants ranging in age from 8 to 12 weeks postnatally. The 8-week-old's record shows the first evidence of smooth pursuit (between the arrows), while several other infants showed evidence of smooth pursuit at slightly earlier ages. This 8-week-old's record also illustrates that the velocity gain of the smooth component is quite low (approximately 0.5). Thus, although smooth pursuit seems to emerge during the 6 to 8 week age range, as McGinnis (1930) stated half a century ago, the accuracy of these initial smooth pursuit movements is quite poor. As in the case of adults who are presented with high target velocities, infants program saccadic movements between the smooth components, presumably in an attempt to catch up to the moving target. These saccades are quite effective in maintaining a high amplitude gain and minimizing phase lag, particularly at the endpoints of the target excursion. The two remaining eye movement records in Fig. 3 show that by 12 weeks postnatally the smooth pursuit movements are quite effective in matching the velocity of the target, although the velocity gain is quite variable and rarely appears to reach unity. Finally, the records shown in Figs. 2 and 3, as well as all other recordings, demonstrate that the latency of smooth pursuit in young infants is *not* consistently shorter than saccadic latency. The initial eye movement is nearly always a saccade with a latency in the 500 to 800 msec range, as previously described by Aslin and Salapatek (1975).

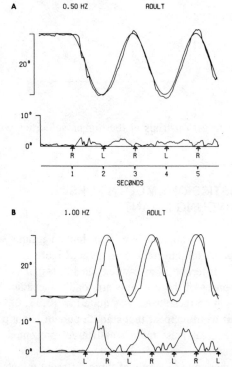

FIG. 4. Tracking responses by an adult presented with two frequencies of target oscillation. The lower portion of each panel represents the absolute error between the position of the eye and the target. R = target on right; L = target on left.

The second question of interest concerning the smooth pursuit movements of infants was the accuracy of tracking at different target velocities. In all of the eye movement records shown in Figs. 2 and 3 the frequency of target oscillation was low to moderate (0.33 to 0.50 Hz). Figure 4 illustrates the smooth pursuit responses of an adult presented with target oscillations of 0.50 and 1.00 Hz. In addition to the eye movement record the absolute error between eye and target position is also shown. It is quite apparent that tracking is very accurate at the lower frequency. However, at the higher frequency the accuracy of tracking is considerably poorer. Moreover, an asymmetry in tracking accuracy emerges at the higher frequency, with greater accuracy on the half-cycle, which returns the target to its starting position. This hysteresis effect was also evident in the records from several infants.

Figure 5 shows the general effect of target velocity on infants' tracking accuracy. Panels A and B are from a single infant and panels C and D are from another infant, both of whom were 10 weeks of age. At the lowest frequency, the accuracy of tracking was fairly good, with errors less than 10°. At the higher frequencies, however, the error increased quite dramatically, and in panel D the infant's smooth pursuit system has almost reached saturation, both in amplitude gain, velocity gain and phase lag. The error plot in panel D illustrates that at this high frequency of target oscillation the infant's eye position is approximately 180° out of phase with the target position.

At low frequencies of target oscillation (e.g., panel A in Fig. 5) there is a striking tendency for eye movements directed away from the target's starting position to contain more error than eye movements directed back toward the starting position. This hysteresis effect is shown even more clearly in the first three cycles of target oscillation in Fig. 6. This 10-week-old's tracking error exceeds 10° as the target moves from right to left (away from the starting location), but the error is 5° or less as the target moves from left to right (back toward the starting location). It is unlikely that this hysteresis effect is simply the result of a bias to return to the position of primary gaze (central orbital position), since the target's starting location was 10° to the right of midline. Rather, the hysteresis effect may reflect a bias (or memory) for returning to a previously steady fixation position.

The third question we hoped to address in this experiment was whether infants would show any evidence of predictive tracking. The previously described hysteresis effect could be interpreted as evidence of prediction, although it may only reflect a bias for returning to a previous muscle state. There were, however, several instances of error reduction over the course of the repetitions of the oscillation within a given trial. Figure 6 shows an example of this error reduction process. Initially, the hysteresis effect is quite evident, but by the fourth cycle the error in tracking the target does not differ between the two half-cycles. This record would seem to offer good evidence for the predictive control of tracking in young infants. In fact, this finding raises the intriguing possibility that the

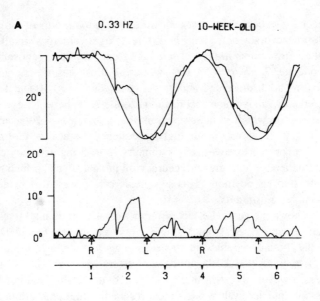

A   0.33 HZ   10-WEEK-OLD

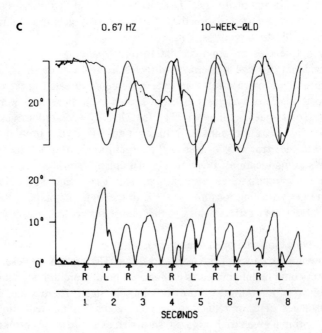

C   0.67 HZ   10-WEEK-OLD

SECONDS

44

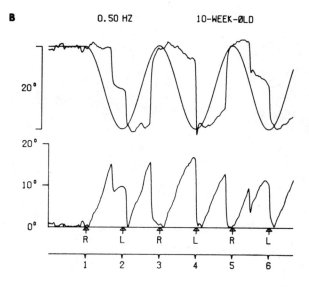

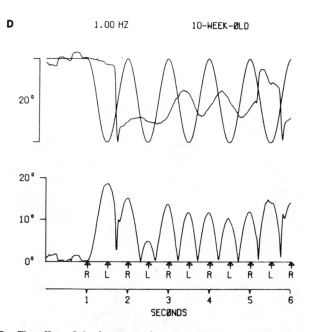

FIG. 5. The effect of the frequency of target oscillation on tracking by two 10-week-old infants. Panels (A) and (B) are records from a single infant, as are panels (C) and (D). The lower portion of each panel represents the absolute error between the position of the eye and the target. R = target on right; L = target on left.

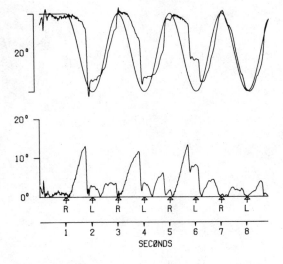

FIG. 6. The accuracy of tracking within different portions of a target cycle and across repeated cycles within a trial. The lower portion represents the tracking error. R = right; L = left.

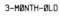

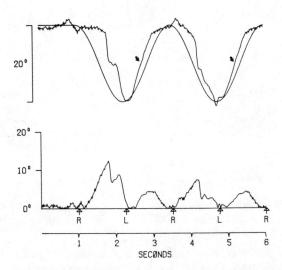

FIG. 7. The accuracy of tracking by a 3-month-old who shows smooth pursuit gain greater than 1.0 (indicated by the arrows). The lower portion represents the tracking error. R = right; L = left.

46

youngest infants may be capable of smooth pursuit if they are provided with a sufficient (i.e., very large) number of repetitions of the simple sinusoidal oscillation. This finding of predictive tracking in a 10-week-old raises the question as to whether predictive tracking would be found for less predictable patterns of movement (e.g., the sum of several sine waves).

Finally, a rather unexpected finding in several eye movement records concerned the velocity gain of the smooth pursuit system in infants. Although there has been some debate in the past as to whether the smooth pursuit system itself can catch up to a moving target, rather than relying on the saccadic system to correct positional errors, it is now clear that pursuit movements in adults can function in a position-correcting as well as a velocity-matching mode. The arrows in Fig. 7 illustrate a clear case of the smooth pursuit system exhibiting a velocity gain greater than 1.0 to catch up to, and in fact anticipate, the target's return to its starting position. Although this record may only be an extreme example of the hysteresis effect, it indicates that the saccadic system is not always needed to catch up to a target that is accelerating, provided that the peak velocity of the target does not exceed the maximum smooth pursuit velocity. In this particular infant's record the peak velocity of the smooth components is approximately 25 deg/sec.

THEORETICAL ISSUES IN OCULOMOTOR DEVELOPMENT

The results presented above on the development of smooth pursuit in young infants have clarified several questions while raising many more. Although these findings can only be considered part of a preliminary description of human oculomotor development, it seems quite clear that the original hypothesis that emerged from studies of the infant's saccadic system (see Fig. 1) must be rejected. That is, the smooth pursuit system does not appear to evolve from the saccadic system through a process of saccadic step-size reduction. Rather, smooth pursuit movements become evident as clear and discrete components of target tracking embedded within a background of saccadic steps. It is quite possible that the basic control system for smooth pursuit movements is present at birth, but that actual smooth tracking awaits the development of some other related mechanism or the elimination of one or more constraints on the programming of smooth movements. We can only conclude that under the present testing conditions smooth pursuit appears to be absent until 6 to 8 weeks after birth. Specifying the conditions under which smooth pursuit is exhibited by infants during the early postnatal period should be the goal of future more comprehensive investigations.

Although the gain and accuracy of the smooth pursuit system appears to improve markedly during the first three postnatal months, it remains unclear as to precisely the mechanism(s) underlying this improvement. Several researchers (e.g., Bronson, 1974) have proposed that smooth pursuit is mediated primarily by cortical structures, whereas developmentally immature saccadic movements are mediated primarily by subcortical structures (e.g., the superior colliculus). This theory of two visual systems (Schneider, 1969) is intrinsically appealing, but its applicability to humans is obscured by the absence of animal data on the functional development of visual structures and pathways that mediate specific oculomotor responses. Moreover, the cortical-subcortical distinction is undoubtedly too simplistic since many cortical, thalamic, cerebellar, and brain stem areas are known to be capable of influencing oculomotor responding. For example, cerebellar lesions in adult monkeys result in gross deficiencies in smooth pursuit and reduced gain in the slow phase of OKN (see Dichgans & Jung, 1975 for a general review). Thus, it seems reasonable to delay speculations about the anatomical and physiological mechanisms underlying the development of smooth pursuit until more data on these issues of structure and function have been collected. The approach which will guide the remainder of our discussion of oculomotor development, therefore, is to focus on those general abilities that we believe to be necessary for the control of smooth pursuit in early infancy, without recourse to detailed speculations about the specific physiological mechanisms underlying these abilities.

Table 1 lists several possible factors that may provide an explanation for the absence of smooth pursuit in the early postnatal period and the emergence and improving accuracy of smooth pursuit during the second and third postnatal months. The first type of explanation, and perhaps the most intuitively appealing, is to claim that infants are drowsy, inattentive, and basically unmotivated to perform up to capacity under arbitrary laboratory testing conditions. Although both the duration of waking time and general activity level increase during

TABLE 1
Possible Explanations for the Absence
of Smooth Pursuit in Early Infancy

A. Attentional/Motivational Factors
B. Anatomical and Neuromuscular Factors
    1. Damping Characteristics
    2. Frequency Response
C. Sensory Mechanisms
    1. Acuity and Contrast Sensitivity
    2. Temporal Resolution
    3. Velocity Analysis
D. Sensory-Motor Control Mechanisms
    1. Muscle Programming Based on Velocity Information
    2. Binocular Interference (Diplopia)
    3. Peripheral Field Interference
    4. Motion Perception

postnatal development, even newborns exhibit brief periods of alertness. Moreover, inspection of the eye movement recordings in the younger infants who did not show smooth pursuit indicates a very striking consistency in their tracking responses. Thus, it is unlikely that a simple attentional or motivational explanation can fully account for the absence of smooth pursuit in young infants. Unfortunately, it may be impossible to rule out the partial contribution of attentional factors in the poor smooth tracking of very young infants.

The second type of explanation involves several potential anatomical and neuromuscular developments in the early postnatal period that could enable smooth pursuit to emerge. The data on OKN in newborns indicate that slow, smooth movements are present. Thus, the extraocular muscles are capable of smooth eye rotations. However, characteristics of the eyeball, the orbital tissues, the extraocular muscle fibers and the neuromuscular signals may undergo considerable change postnatally. A given neuromotor command may not be as effective in rotating the eyeball in young infants. In addition, overcoming inertia, reaching a steady-state velocity, returning to and maintaining a steady orbital position, and the sequencing of agonist and antagonist firings may be quite different in early infancy. Thus, the damping characteristics of the eye within the orbit and the frequency response of the oculomotor system in general may change significantly during early development. These changes may in turn allow the oculomotor commands to more effectively rotate the eyes to smoothly follow a moving target.

The third type of explanation for the absence of smooth pursuit in early infancy centers on the various sensory mechanisms required for accurate oculomotor control. Both acuity and contrast sensitivity are relatively poor in young infants compared to adults (see Dobson & Teller, 1978, and Banks & Salapatek, in press, for general reviews). During the first six postnatal months, acuity and contrast sensitivity undergo very large improvements. Thus, although the targets used in studies of the infants' pursuit system have been suprathreshold, the newborn may be incapable of the fine resolution required for detecting small changes in the target's spatial location. In fact, the relatively wide dispersion of fixations around a small stationary target may also reflect the young infant's poor spatial resolving powers. Unfortunately, all studies of acuity in human infants have used grating patterns. Perhaps a measure of vernier acuity in infants would provide an index of improvements in spatial resolution that was more relevant to the control of smooth pursuit movements.

A second aspect of sensory development relevant to smooth pursuit is temporal resolution. The presence of increased myelination and more selective synaptic connections during the first few postnatal months may allow spatial information to be processed more quickly and with less interference. Moreover, the continuous updating of changes in spatial location required to smoothly pursue an accelerating or decelerating target would seem to require good temporal resolution. Unfortunately, only one recent study of sensitivity to flicker

(Regal, 1979) has provided data relevant to temporal resolution, and only infants of a single age (2-month-olds) were tested. Thus, any changes in temporal resolution during the first two postnatal months when smooth pursuit emerges are as yet unknown. We do know, however, that the developmental decrease in response latency shown by the saccadic system (Aslin & Salapatek, 1975) does not appear to explain the emergence of smooth pursuit, since smooth pursuit latencies were longer than saccadic latencies, even in infants who showed smooth tracking.

A third sensory factor relevant to smooth pursuit is the analysis of the relative spatial location of the target over time, i.e., target velocity. Although either spatial or temporal resolution could limit the accuracy of velocity analysis, good spatial and temporal resolution are not necessarily *sufficient* for good velocity resolution. Young infants may have an ineffective system for integrating changes in spatial location over short time periods, thus providing inaccurate estimates of target velocity. However, this assumption of inaccurate estimates of target velocity cannot explain why pursuit velocity always has a gain less than 1.0, since a random error in the computation of target velocity would predict eye velocities both higher and lower than target velocities.

Taken together, these three sensory factors offer a reasonable and comprehensive hypothesis for explaining the absence of smooth pursuit in the first few postnatal weeks. The newborn's spatial resolution may be very poor, thus diminishing the ability to detect small changes in the location of the target relative to the current fixation position. In other words, newborns may have a relatively large "functional fovea" within which spatial resolution is more or less equivalent. This poor spatial resolution would require a relatively large retinal area to calculate target velocity. If this retinal area required to estimate target velocity exceeded the minimum displacement needed for initiating a saccade (the saccadic "dead-zone"), then a saccade would be initiated before the velocity calculation had been completed. Obviously, this is only a tentative working hypothesis, and it requires extensive empirical tests in the future.

The fourth and final class of explanations for the absence of smooth pursuit in young infants relates neither to purely sensory nor to purely motor issues. Rather, there are several aspects of oculomotor control that are dependent upon the link between accurate sensory information and appropriate motor programming. First, one can imagine a system provided with precise spatial, temporal, and velocity information about the target that, nevertheless, is uncalibrated, i.e., the system cannot program an appropriate eye movement to capture and maintain foveation. Second, very young infants are known to have deficiencies in binocular alignment (Aslin, 1977; Ling, 1942; Slater & Findlay, 1975a). Binocular misalignment may result in conflicting information concerning the spatial location of the target, which in turn may interfere with the programming of accurate oculomotor movements (both saccadic and smooth pursuit). Third, very young infants may be incapable of suppressing information from the peripheral retina.

Thus, while rotating their eyes to catch up to the target, the visual frame surrounding the target may provide a signal opposite in direction to the eye movement. This peripheral retinal signal may (as suggested by Morgan, this volume) induce an OKN response, thereby shutting off the initial tracking response and creating step-like saccadic movements. If one assumed a developmental improvement in the ability to suppress peripheral information, then this theory could account for the subsequent emergence of smooth pursuit in the second postnatal month. Pilot testing in our lab using a white on black display (thus eliminating the peripheral frame surrounding the target) has shown little difference in infants' tracking responses compared to the black on white display used in the present experiment. Nevertheless, this theory of peripheral competition merits further study.

Finally, a fourth sensory-motor factor relates to the signal that actually elicits smooth pursuit movements. Young (1977) has argued that the signal for pursuit is any stimulus that leads to the perception of target motion, even if that perception of motion is non-veridical (e.g., afterimage tracking). This motion percept must, in simplest form, arise from a combination of information about the translation of the target across the retina and the velocity of eye rotation. For example, a moving target is judged to be moving whether the eye is stationary or traveling at the same velocity as the target. At the retinal level, these two situations result in grossly different forms of stimulation. It is possible that young infants have inaccurate or uncalibrated information about the state of their eye position and about the velocity of eye rotation. Under such circumstances, an inaccurate perception of target motion would be likely, and the absence of smooth pursuit would not be surprising.

In summary, this chapter has attempted to provide new findings on the developmental onset, accuracy, and control system characteristics of smooth pursuit tracking in young human infants. In addition, a wide variety of possible explanations for the qualitative and quantitative developmental differences in tracking have been discussed. The task of future research is to determine which of these explanations, in isolation or in combination, provides the best account of human oculomotor development.

ACKNOWLEDGMENTS

This research was supported by grants from NSF (BNS 77-04580) and NICHD (HD-00309). I am grateful to Jerry C. Forshee and David Link for their technical assistance in the design and implementation of all software and hardware systems. I am also indebted to Rick Jackson, Wendy Crawford, and Susan Dumais for their assistance in the scheduling and testing of the infants. The helpful critical comments offered by Conrad Mueller are also gratefully acknowledged.

1.4 Development of Optokinetic Nystagmus in Infants: An Indicator of Cortical Binocularity?

Janette Atkinson and Oliver Braddick
University of Cambridge
England

One long term effect on kittens of monocular or binocular deprivation is an asymmetry in the ease of eliciting optokinetic nystagmus (OKN) if the stimulus is presented monocularly (Van Hof-van Duin, 1976a,b, 1978). When viewing monocularly these animals only give OKN if the stimulus field moves horizontally in front of them in a temporal to nasal direction; if the stimulus moves in the opposite horizontal direction very little, if any, OKN is elicited. This difference in ease of eliciting OKN will be called "asymmetrical OKN" throughout this chapter. Asymmetrical OKN is also found in very young kittens (Van Hof-van Duin, 1978), and in mature cats with bilateral cortical lesions (Wood, Spear, & Braun, 1973). Species with little or no cortical binocularity show very weak, if any, OKN to nasal to temporal stimulation. These include pigeons (Mowrer, 1936), chickens (Fukuda, 1959), guinea pigs (Smith & Bridgman, 1943) and rabbits (Braun & Gault, 1969; Collewijn, 1969).

Directionally selective units in the nucleus of the optic tract in the pretectum have properties that make it likely that they are involved in the control of OKN (Hoffmann, 1979). Similar units have been found in the pretectum of rabbit (Collewijn, 1975). In cats these units receive a direct input from the contralateral eye that responds only to temporal-to-nasal stimulus motion, and a binocular input from cortex that permits a response to nasal-to-temporal motion in the ipsilateral eye (Hoffmann, 1977; Hoffmann & Schoppmann, 1975). A diagram of the hypothetical pathways is shown in Fig. 1. This suggests that a functioning binocular cortex is necessary for the nasal-to-temporal OKN response. This is consistent with the absence of the response in visually deprived cats and in animals with little binocular field. The appearance of symmetrical OKN in development may indicate the development of cortical binocularity, or at least of a binocular pathway from cortex to pretectum.

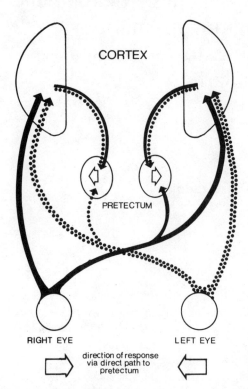

CORTEX

PRETECTUM

RIGHT EYE   LEFT EYE

direction of response
via direct path to
pretectum

FIG. 1. Schematic diagram of the hypothetical connections between the eyes, pretectum and cortex to control OKN.

The rationale behind the present set of experiments, which grew out of discussions with those involved in the animal experiments just mentioned, is to use the likely connection between asymmetry of OKN and lack of binocularity to gauge the development of visual cortex in the human infant.

In describing the following experiments, OKN will be examined relating to development (Experiments 1 & 2), abnormal visual development (Experiment 3), and its relationship to smooth pursuit movements (Experiment 4). The details of Experiments 1 and 2 have already been published (Atkinson, 1979), so they will only be briefly stated here.

EXPERIMENT 1

The OKN eliciting stimulus was a cine film, viewed monocularly by the infants, showing a moving panorama of newspaper print and brightly colored paint spots, some individual spots subtending up to 10° at the viewing distance of 40 cm. The stimulus covered approximately 180° of visual field and passed in front of the infants' eyes at an average speed of 36 deg/sec. As the film was projected on a translucent hemisphere, the velocity was higher at the outer edges than in the center.

A stop watch was used to time the total duration of the infants following eye movements in a series of 15 second trials. The direction of movement (temporally or nasally) was randomized from trial to trial with the observer being "blind" as to the direction of movement.

The time spent following included bursts of classical high-frequency OKN, long OKN cycles in which the slow phase consisted of a traverse for a large fraction of the distance between extreme positions of the eye and irregular sequences of saccades in the direction of the motion (these were seen only for the nasal to temporal movement).

The mean total time of following movements was calculated for each infant and the sample divided into three age groups, with mean ages close to 1, 2, and 3 months. These means are plotted in Fig. 2. Younger infants showed very little OKN or following if the stimulus moved nasal to temporal. One- and two-

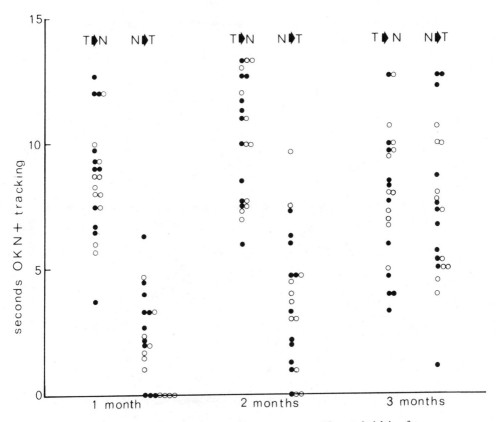

FIG. 2.   Mean total time of following eye movements per 15-second trial time for human infants in 3 age groups in Experiment 1. T → N = temporal to nasal movement of the stimulus field, N → T = nasal to temporal movement of the stimulus field. Filled circles: right eye; open circles: left eye. *From Atkinson (1979) by permission.

month-olds tended to stare at the pattern and occasionally give a short burst of saccades or short OKN following the stimulus movement. They sometimes gave very brief periods of OKN whose slow phase was opposite to the stimulus motion. In the 3-month group there is very little difference in the times for following movements in the two directions, although small differences in gain and/or frequency of the OKN were apparent to the observer.

A small number of EOG records were made, one of which is shown in Fig. 3 to illustrate asymmetrical OKN in a 2-month-old. However, for the main data collection direct observation of eye movements yielded satisfactory results and was preferred to EOG recording for practical and theortical reasons. Young infants tend to become fussy when one eye is occluded and this problem is intensified when facial electrodes are worn and the head is restrained to give an artifact-free EOG record. In consequence, fewer infants would have completed

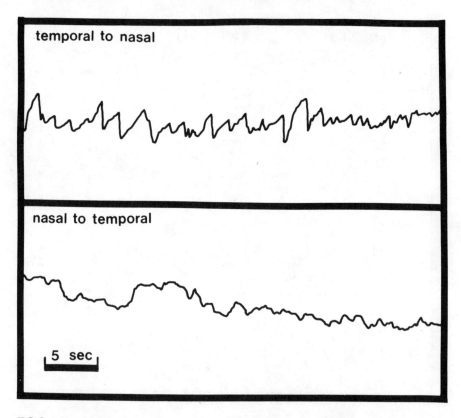

EOG records of asymmetrical monocular OKN

FIG. 3.   EOG record showing asymmetrical OKN in a 2 month old human infant. Note both long and short OKN in the record for temporal to nasal movement. Stimulus as in Experiment 1.

testing with EOG recording and those would have been a sample biased towards less active infants. With the method employed, only two out of 33 subjects failed to complete the test.

Smooth pursuit is usually distinguished from OKN as the response to follow a small moving target rather than a large moving field. In the stimulus of Experiment 1 portions of the pattern could possibly have been isolated and treated as targets for pursuit. Experiment 2 was conducted to test whether the results could be maintained with a purer OKN stimulus.

EXPERIMENT 2

The stimulus was a projected moving loop of film covered with a finely textured black and white pattern that appeared as a sea of maggots moving smoothly in a horizontal direction. It proved to be powerful in eliciting short high-frequency OKN in adults and infants, and subjectively it was impossible to track a single element over any distance.

Other than the fact that the subjects in Experiment 1 were from Cambridge, England, and those in Experiment 2 were from Cambridge, Massachusetts, there were three other small differences between experiments. In Experiment 2 a slightly lower speed was used (30 deg/sec), the stimulus was projected on a flat screen subtending about 120° and the observer was not "blind" as to the direction of the pattern movement.

The results of Experiment 2 were very similar to those for Experiment 1 except that the response observed was predominantly short high-frequency OKN, with little of the long slow phase or saccadic following. Figure 4 shows the mean times of OKN in 15-second trials for individual infants in the three age groups. A marked asymmetry is present in the 1- and 2-month groups but is no longer apparent at 3 months. Therefore, neither stimuli nor populations for the two experiments can be the source for OKN differences in development.

EXPERIMENT 3

A clear developmental trend in human infants, who were assumed to have normal visual development, was found in Experiments 1 and 2. In Experiment 3, we looked at monocular OKN in a number of infants, children and adults who were known or expected to have abnormal visual development in terms of binocularity, to identify possible associations with asymmetrical monocular OKN. The results of previous studies of adults (Crone, 1977; Nicolai, 1959) showed that strabismic amblyopia is frequently associated with asymmetrical OKN.

The clinical cases tested in the present study have been categorized in Table 1, along with their OKN responses. In general these cases were tested using the same stimuli as in Experiment 1, but with trials of approximately 5 seconds duration. OKN was not timed; it was simply noted whether it had occurred. Binocular and monocular eye movements were observed. For most of the infants accurate clinical histories were available, whereas for the adults there was sometimes doubt as to the exact age of onset of visual problems. For the infants there were no tests carried out of stereoscopic vision; for young children and adults the presence of stereopsis was tested using random dot stereograms in a synoptophore (set at the angle of deviation in strabismic cases).

Although the numbers are small and the cases are varied it seems that, in cases of early strabismus, OKN remains asymmetrical (even though the strabismus may have been corrected very early in life). There may be some congenital defect of binocular cortex in these cases. Alternatively it is possible that if their strabismus had been corrected in the first 3 months of life, then cortical binocularity and symmetrical OKN would have developed normally. It will not be possible to

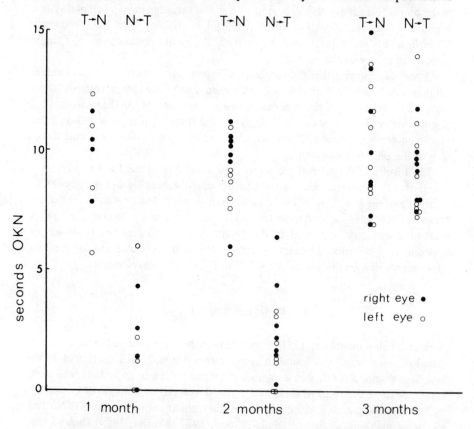

FIG. 4.   Mean total time of OKN in stimulus direction per 15-second trial time for human infants in 3 age groups of Experiment 2. T → N = temporal to nasal movement of the stimulus field; N → T = nasal to temporal movement of the stimulus field. Filled circles: right eye; open circles; left eye. *From Atkinson (1979) by permission.

TABLE 1
OKN in Subjects Tested in Experiment 3. Asymmetrical OKN: Very Little
Nasal to Temporal OKN. Stereo: Showed Positive Evidence of Stereopsis;
?: Not Tested for Stereopsis. N: Number of Individuals in the Group.

Visual Disorder	N	Asymmetrical OKN	Stereo
1. Congenital Strabismus (with/without amblyopia)			
Infants (3 mon → 2 yrs.)	6	6	?
Children (2 yrs. → 5 yrs.)	3	3 (2 in strab. eye only)	1
Adults - (onset ?): Conv.	1	1	0
Div.	2	0	1
Alternator Div.	1	0	1
2. Amblyopia (no strab.)			
Infant (4 months)	1	1	?
Adult (onset ?)	3	0	3
3. Family history of strabismus but no obvious deviation			
Infants (3 mon. → 1 yr.)	9	0	?
Children (2 yrs. → 5 yrs.)	3	0	3
4. Congenital occlusion in 1 eye			
Infants (3 mon. → 1 yr.)	3	1	?
Infant (3 months, mild psotis birth → 6 weeks)	1	0	?
5. Cataract			
Bilateral (6 months)	1	? (congenital nystagmus)	?
Unilateral (6 months)	1	0	?

decide between these theories until a substantial number of very early strabismus
corrections have been performed with subsequent testing of binocularity and
OKN.

EXPERIMENT 4

When a large field of moving pattern is viewed the result is generally OKN;
when a single moving target is presented it may be followed either by a series of
saccades or by a smooth pursuit movement. Smooth pursuit movements and the

slow phase of OKN have similar velocity ranges and are both serving to stabilize a moving target on the retina, but it has widely been supposed that they represent the operation of two different mechanisms (see, for example, Robinson, 1976). This view gains support from the course of development. OKN is effective at birth (Dayton, Jones, Aiu, Steele, & Rose, 1964). The literature shows some disagreement over the age of onset of smooth pursuit but it appears to develop over the first few months of life (see review by Salapatek & Banks, 1977). However, there does not seem to have been any direct developmental comparison of pursuit and OKN.

The present experiment had two aims: first, to examine whether, when the same infants were tested, with stimulus properties and velocities as comparable as possible, OKN and pursuit movements would indeed be dissociated in development; second, to discover whether smooth pursuit, when present, showed any asymmetries analogous to that of monocular OKN.

Stimuli were digitally generated by a microprocessor system with analog output and displayed on a large CRT display (subtending 62° at the infant's viewing distance of 25 cm) with a mean luminance of 105 cd/m^2. The screen was surrounded by featureless black material and the general level of room illumination was low.

The OKN stimulus consisted of a high-contrast vertical square-wave grating of spatial frequency 0.19 c/deg which filled the screen and steadily drifted in either direction at 12 deg/sec. A trial consisted of 11 seconds observation of this stimulus. The pursuit stimulus consisted of a single cycle of the same grating, with the rest of the screen uniform at the same mean luminance. A trial began with the single-cycle target flashing at 2 Hz for 3.5 seconds in the center of the screen, to attract the infant's attention. It then moved off at 12 deg/sec to either side of the screen.

The rather low velocity was selected after pilot trials as a compromise that could elicit both OKN and smooth pursuit in infants. However, it may be that a different stimulus velocity would produce a different pattern of results.

Seventeen infants between 4 and 18 weeks of age, whose parents were volunteers from the Cambridge, England, area acted as subjects. Testing of each infant was completed in either one or two sessions within 7 days.

All testing was monocular, with the other eye occluded by an adhesive orthoptic patch. The order of testing eyes and conditions was randomized across subjects: Trials with one eye and one stimulus were blocked together but the two directions of motion were randomized from trial to trial. Between 5 and 8 trials for each condition in each direction were run with each eye, making a total of about 50 trials for each infant.

Observations with the OKN stimulus were made by an observer positioned below the display, reporting for each trial, the presence of eye movements in one or more of four categories: (1) "long" OKN, i.e., with an excursion in the slow phase across at least half the screen; (2) "short" OKN (in which the slow phase

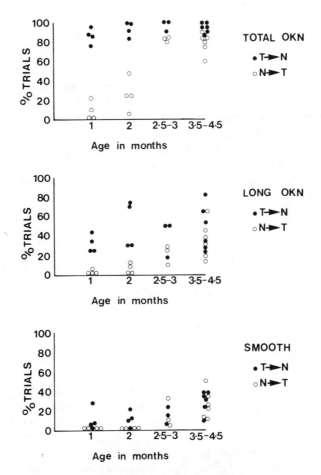

FIG. 5. Experimental results for Experiment 4. Top graph shows asymmetrical OKN in infants under 3 months of age. T → N = temporal to nasal field movement, N → T = nasal to temporal field movement. (Results from the L & R eye have been combined). Middle graph shows the % of trials on which long OKN was present as a function of age, for the 2 directions of stimulus movement. Bottom graph shows the % of trials on which smooth pursuit eye movements were made for the 2 directions of stimulus movement.

is of short excursion and the fast phases are much more frequent and therefore more conspicuous than in "long" OKN); (3) saccadic eye movements; (4) maintenance of a static eye position throughout the trial.

Observations with the pursuit stimulus were made using a procedure similar to that for the OKN stimulus, with the categories reported being: (1) smooth pursuit of the target; (2) saccadic eye movements following the target: (3) saccadic movements unrelated to the target's motion; (4) static eye position.

Trials were only initiated when the infant was looking toward the screen; trials in which the infant's eyes were shut or turned away from the screen for a substantial proportion of the trials were discounted. Data were scored as percentages of trials in the various categories. If more than one category was reported for a given trial, the trial was taken to be divided equally among the categories reported. The infants were separated into 4–6 week, 8–10 week, 11–14 week, and 16–18 week age groups.

The OKN stimulus data shown in Fig. 5A are the percentage of trials showing OKN ("long" and "short" combined) for nasal-temporal and temporal-nasal directions of stimulus motion (data from the two eyes of each infant being combined). The asymmetry between these two directions is striking for infants under 3 months of age, as was the case in Experiments 1 and 2. In fact, using this stimulus, a small asymmetry seems to persist for some of the infants in the older groups, but it is clearly much less than in the two youngest groups. We are not sure why this occurs.

Figure 5B plots "long OKN" as a separate category. The asymmetry between the two directions for the younger age groups is striking: Long OKN is effectively absent in the nasotemporal direction in infants of 2 months or less. Long OKN in fact accounts for the majority of the asymmetry observed in total OKN. OKN is a mixture of long and short at all ages for temporal-nasal motion, but only for the older groups for the reverse direction.

The occurrence of long OKN may be very stimulus dependent: It was rare with the finely textured stimulus of Experiment 2. It is possible that long OKN occurs when an isolatable element (like a single bar of a low-spatial-frequency grating) fills the fovea and can be tracked. This hypothesis could be tested by varying the spatial frequency; it would predict less long OKN for higher-frequency gratings.

It should be emphasized that while in this experiment directional asymmetry was manifest mostly in the long OKN, it is not a property of long OKN alone. In Experiment 2, OKN was almost entirely of the classic short form and a clear asymmetry occurred.

Figure 5C plots the percentage of trials on which smooth pursuit occurred. Smooth pursuit was not very reliably elicited by the single cycle stimulus in any of the age groups: The highest figure for any individual infant is 50% of trials. However, the change with age is clear: There is considerably more pursuit made by the older infants. There is also an asymmetry in onset, similar though lesser in degree to that for OKN. Infants under 3 months show more smooth pursuit for targets moving temporal-nasal than for those moving nasal-temporal. Whether this asymmetry would be enlarged or diminished by use of a more effective elicitor of smooth pursuit remains an open question only to be answered by future experiments. The age trend and asymmetry are properties of smooth pursuit specifically: If smooth pursuit and saccadic following are combined, then the proportion of trials showing following is about 70% for all age groups in both directions, with perhaps a slightly higher incidence of random eye movements or lack of movements in the 1-month-olds.

Comparison of nasal-to-temporal OKN with smooth pursuit shows that both increase over the age range studied and it may be that these developments have a common origin. Correlations across infants were calculated for each of the percentages of trials showing long OKN, short OKN, and total OKN with the percentages for smooth pursuit, for nasotemporal motion in each case. The highest correlation (r = .71) was between long OKN and pursuit.

The experiment supports the idea that temporal-to-nasal OKN occurs at ages when pursuit is rare, and therefore that these involve separate mechanisms. The onset of nasotemporal OKN and the increase of smooth pursuit are correlated, implying that these may share common (cortical?) mechanisms. However, this account leaves unexplained the early asymmetry of smooth pursuit, which suggests that the subcortical pathways responsible for the asymmetry of OKN are also involved in pursuit of a single target. It is also unclear at what point a stimulus ceases to be an isolated target that may be pursued and starts to elicit more or less compulsory OKN. Possibly the critical factor is not target size, but the presence of static contour in the field of view. The development of smooth pursuit may depend on development of a mechanism that can gate out the influence of such contours (e.g., our screen edges) on the mechanisms that drive OKN slow phase. If so, pursuit might be produced even in young infants if the screen edges were invisible.

GENERAL DISCUSSION

A clear developmental change has been observed in the ability of young infants to give monocular OKN responses to stimulus movement in the nasotemporal direction. We have found an analogus result in infant monkeys (Atkinson, 1979). The period of asymmetry extends to about 3 months, though it may be apparent for different periods with different stimuli. Although at 3 months the amount of time spent in OKN is approximately equal for the two directions, it is possible that more detailed measures (e.g., of gain or frequency) might show up asymmetries at later ages. The occurrence of what we have called "long OKN" is particularly striking in the temporal-to-nasal direction and it is possible that this also might show up a more persistent asymmetry. Indeed there has been no investigation of monocular OKN in normal adults and it is conceivable that permanent detailed asymmetries could be demonstrated.

A different but related measure would be the comparison of monocular with binocular OKN. Braun and Gault (1969) found that in the rabbit (for temporal-to-nasal motion), the frequency of OKN was identical for monocular and binocular stimulation, while for the cat, binocularly driven OKN was of higher frequency than monocular. They took this as evidence for binocular interactions in the cat's oculomotor control that were not present for the rabbit. It would be interesting to see whether the binocular/monocular comparison changed for infants over the first few months of life, either for frequency or for gain.

How do the results of these experiments relate to binocularity? The species differences, effects of deprivation on animals, and results with amblyopes, suggest that binocular cortex is a necessary condition for symmetrical OKN. However, we do not yet have direct evidence that the development of cortical binocularity, rather than any other part of the pathway, is the critical factor in the onset of symmetrical OKN in infancy.

The ability to detect binocular disparity is a clear criterion of cortical binocularity. On the evidence presently available (Appel & Campos, 1977; Atkinson & Braddick, 1976; Fox, Aslin, Shea, & Dumais, 1980) this ability is present by 2–4 months; the best behavioral data, from Fox et al., suggest about 3½ months as the earliest age at which disparity discriminations can be reliably elicited. A review by Aslin and Dumais (in press) also considers other aspects of binocularity, such as convergence control. The problem with inferences in this field is that many visual functions are rapidly developing in the first few months of life and it is difficult to argue from this that any particular group of visual functions are associated.

Recently we have used a rather direct means of assessing cortical binocularity in infants. This is the recording of evoked potentials that are time-locked to the appearance and disappearance of binocular correlation in a dynamic random-dot pattern. In a preliminary study (Braddick, Atkinson, Julesz, Kropfl, Bodis-Wollner, & Raab, in preparation) we found positive evidence of binocularity in most infants over 3 months, and in some younger infants also. A direct test comparing this or an allied behavioral measure with symmetry of monocular OKN in the same subjects would be valuable and is planned in our laboratory. The two techniques, separately and in comparison, promise to be of clinical value in detecting disorders of binocular development and also to advance our understanding of the coupled development of eye movement control and binocular vision.

ACKNOWLEDGMENTS

We would like to thank Jennifer French for assistance in Experiment 1, Joseph Bauer for assistance in Experiment 2, Elizabeth Pimm-Smith, Lesley Ayling, and Kim Davis for assistance in Experiment 4, and all the parents and infants who took part in this study.

This work was supported in the main part by the Medical Research Council and in part by research grants from the National Eye Institute (NIHE 01191) and Core Grant (NIH-1-P30-EY0261-01) to Prof. R. Held.

II | ILLUSIONS AND AFTEREFFECTS

What can illusions and aftereffects tell us about the visual system in perception? How much do eye movements contribute to the sensory "foul-ups" responsible for misperception of movement, distance, size and shape? Can illusions and aftereffects of direction be facilitators of performance, e.g., in sport and aviation?

In Chapter II.1 Coren describes historic evidence for a motor theory explanation of visual illusions and new insights into their cause, like the compelling aspects of the length of the wings on the familiar Mueller-Lyer illusion. By taking an atypical back door approach Coren and his associates first isolated stimulus patterns that biased saccadic sequencing and then rearranged those elements to "redirect" the eye movements. In so doing not only were new illusions created but the magnitude of those affects were made predictable. Although Coren is not ready to admit that the eye movement to percept approach can explain all illusory affects, his notion strongly suggests that illusory distortions can be expected under those conditions where the eye movements do not match up to the physical stimulus relationships.

In Chapter II.2, Ebenholtz describes a distance aftereffect model in which slow fusional vergence is accompanied by tonic innervation, the resulting phoria (change in resting level) represents a lag in the vergence posture from its previous position and results in a distortion in distance perception. Induction and adaptation experimental paradigms are discussed. Data are fit to the model and Ebenholtz concludes that those conditions which alter steady state levels of muscular tonus may therefore be expected also to produce changes in apparent distance.

Shebilske describes sensorimotor and ecological implications of visual direction illusions to everyday life in Chapter II.3. He details how Minor Motor Anomalies (errors in registered eye and limb position) frequently affect performance in nonlaboratory situations like batting in baseball. Compensatory techniques are used to dramatize these effects in an attempt to increase batting performance. The capability of sensorimotor and ecological theories to account for these data are described along with other practical implications for aftereffects in usual environments.

Chapter II.4 presents Morgan's account of the pursuit system's contribution in converting temporal to spatial visual information. He provides a new twist to the classic anorthoscopic effect or visual persistence where successive portions of a display contribute to the painting on the retina of the entire visual image. Morgan describes experiments with an intriguing design in an attempt to resolve the issue of smooth pursuit's contribution to space perception using intermittent right-to-left and left-to-right going stimuli to paint the retina. The effect is not easily explained unless it can be assumed that some sort of tracking of the stimulus is being made as portions of it move between slits. Morgan concludes that without smooth pursuit, perception of shape is severely restricted but also acknowledges that lower level analyses are still possible.

II.1 The Interaction Between Eye Movements and Visual Illusions

Stanley Coren
University of British Columbia

When Bain (1855) published the first English text book on the psychology of perception, there already existed a theoretical tradition that maintained that sensory and motor functions are part of a unified system that operate together to form the conscious percept. The nature of this sensory-motor interaction has never been completely specified, however, since eye movements are clearly made in response to perceptually relevant inputs, it was only natural that they should be singled out as the motoric response most likely to interact with the conscious visual percept. Thus Bain proposed that "by a horizontal sweep, we take in a horizontal line; by a circular sweep, we derive the muscular impression of a circle. . . ." In synthesizing the work that had gone before him, Bain concluded that the "muscular consciousness" is an indispensable element in any percept. In this context "a circle is a series of ocular movements" and "naked outlines, as the diagrams of Euclid and the alphabetical characters, are to say the least of it, three parts muscular and one part optical. . . ." In this early motor theory all of visual perception is reduced to a set of eye movements.

When Wundt (1898) began his psychological research program, he extended these ideas, and applied them to a number of visual-geometric illusions. His premise was quite simple. He noted that since it takes a longer eye movement to traverse a long line in the visual field than to traverse a shorter line, the amount of effort expended in making eye movements should be proportional to the length of the stimulus. He argued that feedback indicating the amount of effort actually expended could be used as part of the estimate of the length of a given element. The cleverness of this approach is, perhaps, best seen by recognizing that anything that alters the effort needed to make an eye movement should then alter the estimate of the size of the target. Wundt's introspections convinced him that horizontal movements of the eye were apparently more freely and easily made (with less of a subjective feeling of effort) than were the vertical movements that must fight the force of gravity. If such is the case, it might explain why vertical lines are seen as longer than horizontal lines of equal length, as in the horizontal-vertical illusion shown in Fig. 1A. A vertical extent of the same physical length as a horizontal extent would be perceived as being longer simply because it elicits eye movements requiring more effort. In a similar fashion, Wundt went on to explain the Oppel-Kundt illusion (Fig. 1B). Here he argued a divided space induces a tendency in the eye to stop occasionally on the elements which divide the space. This stopping and starting requires more effort than does a free single movement across the open extent, hence the divided space is seen as longer.

Such theoretical conjectures stimulated a desire to obtain measurements of eye movement patterns over various stimulus configurations. One class of stimulus arrays which were singled out for special attention were those in which the observers' conscious percept differed from what might be expected on the basis of actual physical measurements. The simplest of these stimuli are the visual-geometric illusions. Numerous investigators argued that these distortions might be accompanied by, or even explained by, systematic eye movement errors.

Such reasoning was applied to the Mueller-Lyer illusion (Fig. 1C) in which the upper horizontal line, with out-turned wings, appears to be longer than the lower horizontal line with in-turned wings. Some of Wundt's contemporaries maintained that proprioception from erroneous eye movements enters into, and distorts the conscious percept in this array. Van Biervliet (1896) and Binet (1895) in France, Lipps (1897) in Germany, and Judd (1905) in the United States, each separately proposed that the Mueller-Lyer illusion (Fig. 1C) could be explained

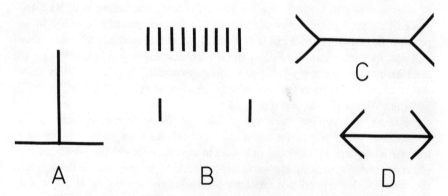

FIG. 1.   (A) The horizontal-vertical illusion; (B) The filled space-open space illusion; The overestimated (C) and underestimated (D) segments of the Mueller-Lyer illusion.

by the fact that the eyes tend to be drawn outward into the wings of the perceptually longer segment of the figure causing an inappropriately long eye movement. On the other hand, in the perceptually shorter segment the eye tends to be arrested by the in-turned wings before it reaches the end of the line. Proprioception from such erroneous eye movements, if incorporated into the percept, could easily explain the illusory distortion.

Empirical confirmation was soon provided. The existence of such a pattern of erroneous eye movements was first confirmed by DeLaBarre (1897). He heroically attached a plaster cap to his eye and thence to a set of levers. This system mechanically recorded his eye movements while viewing the Mueller-Lyer illusion. His results (and those of later workers using photographic and bioelectrical methods of recording) indicated that the eye movements emitted while scanning the apparently longer segment, in fact, are longer than those over the apparently shorter segment (De Sisto & Moses, 1968; Judd, 1905; Stratton, 1906; Yarbus, 1967). Festinger, White, and Allyn (1968) even reported that the *perceptual* over and underestimations in the Mueller-Lyer were correlated to the size of the over and under shootings of the eye within individuals.

Although these data seemed to confirm the original hypothesis, some disturbing points were hard to explain. For instance, Judd (1905) observed that the eye shows a tendency to immediately correct its initially erroneous movement. Thus, for instance, if the eye movement is too long, there is a corrective flick backwards to center the fovea on the vertex. If the percept is simply based upon feedback from the actual eye movements emmitted, the extents traversed by these corrective flicks should be added into the estimate of length. Since the eye eventually accurately centers upon the vertex, no illusion should be seen.

Some investigators adopted an alternative mode of investigating the effects of eye movement on illusions. In essence, they attempted to eliminate the effects of eye movements by flashing the illusion stimuli too briefly for eye movements to be made over the pattern (Hicks & Rivers, 1908; Lewis, 1908). More recently the stabilized retinal image technique (Ditchburn & Ginsborg, 1952) where an optical system is used to fix an image on the retina, regardless of eye movements, has been used (Pritchard, 1958) as has an afterimage method of decorrelating the eye movements from image change (Evans & Marsden, 1966). For both techniques (briefly flashed and stabilized arrays) the expected classical illusory distortions are still found. While these data would seem to sound the death nell for eye movement involvement in the formation of visual illusions, it should be noted that, while these procedures do disrupt the normal relationship between eye movements and retinal image changes, they do not actually stop the eye from moving. Eye movements may still occur in the same direction and to the same extent that they would occur under normal scanning conditions. There is some evidence that, even after a briefly presented image has disappeared, saccadic eye movements are emitted on the basis of information extracted from the pattern

(Crovitz & Davies, 1962). Theoretically, as long as such movements occur, whether or not they are effective in the actual scanning of the stimulus, their extent could be entered into the final computation of perceived distances.

There is another version of a motor theory of visual illusions, which might be called the underground theory. This position was originally propounded by Washburn (1916). She maintained that, although overt eye movements were indeed necessary for the developing young organism to establish spatial and directional percepts, in the mature individual the overt eye movements need no longer be made. Instead, the percept is supported by implicit or partial components of the movement. These are, of course, the same implicit movement components that Watson's *behaviorism* adopted as the basis of thinking (Watson, 1930). In this formulation the percept depends upon feedback from covert muscle twitches, rather than over movements. An even more underground version of this theory has achieved some recent popularity. It proposes that eye movements are computed and held in readiness to be emitted across the array, and it is these eye movement tendencies, not the actual eye movements, or even partial eye movements, that are used in the synthesis of the conscious percept. While this theory has existed for quite some time (Heymans, 1896; Muensterberg, 1899), Festinger, Burnham, Ono, and Bamber (1967) and Sperry (1952) have offered more contemporary versions. Eye movements held in readiness have been used to explain several illusory distortions (Burnham, 1968; Coren & Festinger, 1967; Festinger, White, & Allyn, 1968; Virsu, 1971).

The research strategy used in investigating implicit movement theories are the same that one uses to investigate overt eye movement theories. Since the best index of the eye movement held in readiness is the actual eye movement emitted, researchers simply resorted to measuring eye movement patterns across illusion configurations, while looking for systematic biases that might be correlated with the percept. Coren, Bradley, Hoenig, and Girgus (1975) have also used this as the method of choice. Several years ago, we noted an interesting illusory phenomenon. If a spot of light was rotated in a circular path in a totally darkened room, the apparent diameter of the circle seemed to vary as a function of the speed of the target's movement. At slow speeds, subjects accurately estimated the path diameter. However, as the speed of the rotation increased the diameter of the circular path apparently began to contract. As the speed of the rotation was further increased, the circle again seemed to expand back to its normal size. It was the illusory perceptual phenomenon that caught our attention. Using the customary approach, we proceeded to measure eye movements as a subject attempted to follow the target in its circular path. The results we obtained were consistent with an eye movement explanation. At the intermediate speeds subjects tended to track in a circular path with a reduced diameter, and the perceptual underestimates were correlated highly with the obtained eye movements. As the speed of the target increased, more saccadic eye movements began to intrude, and the proportion of saccadic eye movements to the outer limits of the target path correlated with the expansion of the circle diameter toward veridicality. Following the tradition of the motor theories of perception, outlined earlier, we concluded that the perceptual distortion was, at least in part, *caused* by the systematic mistracking of the stimulus, and boldly proclaimed this in print. Unfortunately, in so doing, we may have been falling into a methodological and philosophical trap.

As I shall describe, our study was characteristic of most studies investigating the influences of eye movements on perception. Yet, let me carefully analyze our procedures for a moment. First we discovered an illusory distortion. Next we measured eye movements during the occurrence of that perceptual distortion. Finally, we established that the eye movements correlated in direction and magnitude with that illusory effect. In essence all we had was that correlation. It is certainly presumptuous for us to say anything about causal relationships with such data. While it may well be the case, that the eye movements do, in fact, provide some source of information that is incorporated into the percept, it is also possible that the perceptual distortion preceded the eye movements. In other words, the perceived distortion could have elicited the erroneous eye movements. The same argument could be used to explain many of the results that seem to support the interaction between eye movements and illusions. Thus, in the Mueller-Lyer illusion, it may well be the case that, rather than the overly long eye movements causing an overestimation of the shaft in the apparently longer segment, it is the perception of an apparently longer line that serves as the basis for emitting the longer eye movement. Unfortunately the only data we have is the correlation between the eye movement and the percept. What is even more disturbing is the fact that the eye movements usually are only measured *after* some perceptual distortion is found. It seems as if no one ever goes from the eye movement to the percept. Certainly, if there is any casual interaction this ought to be possible.

Suppose that we could find a set of conditions under which we know that the eye movements emitted over a pattern of stimuli differ systematically from what would be expected on the basis of accurate scanning of the stimulus array. If it is the case that the eye movements, or the information extracted to guide the eye movements, interacts in the formation of the phenomenal percept, we ought to be able to predict that the systematic differences in the eye movement patterns would be reflected in the subjective percept. Furthermore, we would expect that the subjective percept would vary as a function of the same parameters that cause the eye movement pattern to vary. Finally, we would expect that any stimulus array that could, in turn, trigger the same systematically biased pattern of eye movements, should also be accompanied by a systematic distortion in the subject's conscious representation of that stimulus. More directly stated, if there is a casual interaction between eye movements and perception in any situation where the eye movements are biased, we would expect this to be accompanied by a predictable illusory distortion.

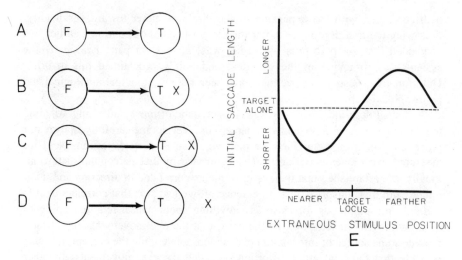

FIG. 2.   Figures A through D show the alteration in foveal length in the presence of an extraneous stimulus (X) placed beyond the target. E shows an idealized version of the over and under shooting of the eye in the presence of an extraneous stimulus as found by Coren and Hoenig (1972).

This line of reasoning led me to reconsider a series of studies on the accuracy of voluntary fixations that we conducted several years ago (Coren & Hoenig, 1972b). In these studies we encountered a class of conditions where the pattern of eye movements, expressed as the length of an initial saccade to a target, was systematically distorted. The conditions eliciting these biased eye movements are actually quite simple. Suppose that the observer is viewing a central fixation point. Randomly, to either side of the fixation, a target appears. If the observer attempts to fixate this target he tends to be fairly accurate. If, however, there is an extraneous stimulus in the field (for instance a second target clearly distinguishable from the first in terms of either color or form, which is located beyond the target) there is a tendency for the initial saccade to be longer. Thus, the eye tends to be "pulled" in the direction of the extraneous stimulus. If, on the other hand, the extraneous stimulus was between the initial fixation point in the target, there is a tendency for the saccade to be shorter. Following the suggestions of Bruell and Albee (1955) and Kaufman and Richards (Kaufman & Richards, 1969; Richards & Kaufman, 1969), we reasoned that the spatial information controlling the length of the saccade was not solely the locus of the target, but rather some estimate of the center of gravity of the stimuli in the immediate vicinity. Such motoric behavior is actually quite sensible, if one recognizes that the fovea is not punctate but is extended over several degrees. Within a 2 to 4 degree circle around the fovea, visual acuity is best. Since the eye functions as an information gatherer, it seems reasonable to suppose that it would be generally directed toward regions of space that contain the most stimuli, and hence, the most information.

Consider Fig. 2A in which the functional fovea is depicted as a circle. If the eye movement begins at the point marked F and is directed toward the stimulus marked T, it seems reasonable to suppose that the saccade would be programmed to center the image of the stimulus on the fovea. Now, suppose that an additional stimulus X was near T. With merely a slight increase of length in the saccade, both stimuli could be placed on the fovea, as shown in Fig. 2B. This means that clear vision of both the target T and the extraneous stimulus X can now be obtained. If we move stimulus X further away, as in Fig. 2C, a longer saccade still places the image of both targets in the fovea. Beyond this range, however, further increases in saccade length would not be functional. Thus in Fig. 2D, if the saccade were made long enough to bring X onto the functional fovea, T would no longer be adequately centered in clear vision. Since T was the original target of intent, rather than losing accurate vision of it, one would expect that the strategy of lenthening the initial saccade to pick up information from nearby extraneous stimuli would gradually be abandoned, as the distance between the target and the extraneous stimuli increased. A similar effect, causing shortening of the initial saccade length, might be expected if the extraneous stimuli were between the fixation point F and the target T. Figure 2E shows an idealized version of the shape of the eye movement pattern that one might expect on the basis of such considerations. In general these were the results we obtained. We found that the presence of extraneous stimuli did alter saccade length such that the eye was pulled toward extraneous stimuli. The saccade length did vary as the position of the non-target stimuli varied in a pattern similar to 2E. Furthermore, our experiments showed that these effects were not ascribable to poor discriminability between the target and the extraneous stimuli. Even when task demands were placed upon the observers to be as accurate as possible, similar error patterns still emerged (Coren & Hoenig, 1972b).

Now, these data provide a simple set of stimulus conditions by which the patterns of eye movement emitted over a stimulus array can be systematically biased. We ought to be able to create many different stimulus configurations, by merely introducing extraneous stimuli and altering their location relative to the target elements, which we know will produce systematic eye movement errors. If eye movements interact with the percept, these same arrays ought to produce systematic perceptual errors. Notice that we are now in a situation where we have enough eye movement data to make predictions, but now the test of the theory requires there should be perceptual distortions present, and these should be predictable on the basis of these eye movement errors.

Let us see if we can find the "illusions" predicted by the eye movements. Figure 3A shows the basic component we will use to create a series of stimuli that should be misjudged. This component consists of a target (a dot), and a clearly

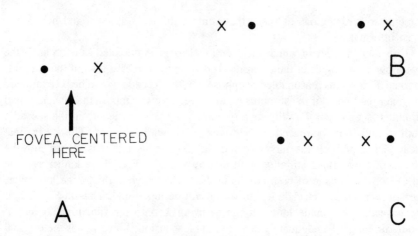

FIG. 3.   (A) Shows the target stimulus (dot) and the extraneous stimulus (X) and the hypothesized foveal center between them. An overestimation (B) and an underestimation (C) created using the elements in (A).

discriminable extraneous stimulus (an X). Now, if the observer were asked to fixate the dot, on the basis of the Coren and Hoenig (1972b) data, we would expect the fovea to be centered not symetrically around the dot, but rather displaced toward the extraneous X. In other words, the fovea would be centered at approximately the position indicated by the arrow. It is easy to concatenate these target and extraneous stimulus units to produce an array in which we would expect a measurable perceptual distortion. Consider Figs. 3B and 3C. Notice that in 3B, we have two dots with the extraneous stimuli placed in a position such that, if the observer were asked to look at the left-most dot and then shift his gaze to the right-most dot, the resultant saccade would be longer than if the observer were asked to look at the left-most dot in Fig. 3C and shift his gaze to the right-most dot in Fig. 3C. This occurs because the length of the saccade is biased toward the center of gravity indicated in 3A. If it is the case that the eye movement system interacts with the perceptual system, one might expect that the different pattern of eye movements elicited would result in the apparent overestimation of the distance between the dots in Fig. 3B relative to the dots in Fig. 3C. You can probably detect this distortion in the array for yourself.

In a more formal experiment, a set of twenty student volunteers were presented with Figs. 3B and 3C. The dots were separated by 8 cm, the extraneous X was 1 cm from the dot, and viewing distance was 40 cm. Subjects were asked to adjust a variable distance so that it appeared to be equal to the distance between the two dots in each of the arrays. As expected, they overestimated the distance in 3B by 4.1 mm while they underestimated the distance in 3C by 3.2 mm. Both of these differences are statistically reliable with $t(19) = 4.17$, $p<.01$ and $t(19) = 3.96$, $<.01$, respectively. While this finding is heartening, one must recognize that we simply have shown that a distortion exists, not that it parametrically varies as would be expected on the basis of the known eye movement biases. In order to do that another experiment was conducted.

In this next experiment we sought to see if the magnitude of the distortion varied as the distance between the extraneous stimulus and the target varied. On the basis of the eye movement results we might expect that the illusory effect would increase as we increased the distance between the extraneous stimulus and the target, but only to some point. When the extraneous stimulus was far enough away from the target, the distortion should then decrease. To test this prediction, the configuration shown as in the inset of Fig. 4 was used. Using an adjustable tongue and groove arrangement, eleven subjects were required to set the distance between the center- and right-hand dots so that it appeared to be equal to the distance between the center- and left-hand dots. Notice, that on the basis of the preceding experiment and the eye movement data, one would expect that the extent on the left side would be overestimated relative to the extent on the right. The extraneous stimulus was located at one of seven distances from the left-hand dot, 0.25, 0.5, 1, 2, 4, 6, or 8 cm beyond the test stimulus. There was also a

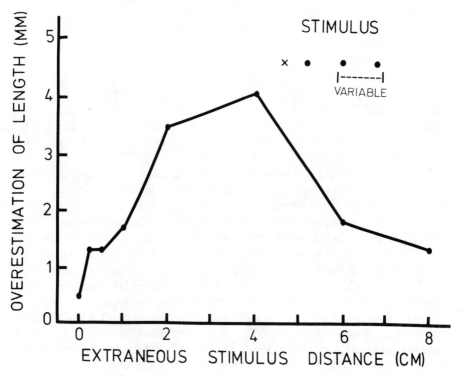

FIG. 4.   The change in the overestimation of an extent as a function of varying position of an extraneous stimulus. Inset shows the stimulus configuration used.

control configuration in which there was no extraneous stimulus. The results are also shown in Fig. 4. It is clear that the inducer distance does affect the magnitude of the illusion, and in the direction predicted. The illusion increases in magnitude up to a maximum and then decreases as the distance to the extraneous stimulus varies. This exactly parallels the eye movement data schematically presented in Fig. 2. The effect of extraneous stimulus distance is significant with $F(7,77) = 2.38$, $p < 0.05$, and the predicted quadratic trend also significant with $F(1,77) = 5.53$, $p < 0.05$.

The second experiment indicates that we can predict a set of perceptual distortions on the basis of knowledge of some simple biases in the eye movement system. In essence, the eye movement data suggested a new set of illusions. One might ask whether this analysis can now be turned back to some of the classical visual-geometric illusions. In this context it is interesting to note that many of the more familiar visual-geometric illusions may be analyzed in terms of the presence and locus of extraneous stimuli. It is easy to see how the outwardly turned wings in the Mueller-Lyer figure (Fig. 1C) might serve as extraneous stimuli that shift the center of gravity outward from the vertex, which demarcates the end of the line, thus producing a stimulus array where we would expect (on the basis of the eye movement data) an overly long saccade and corresponding an overestimation of the extent. Conversely, the inwardly turned wings (Fig. 1D) would shift the center of gravity inward, thus producing conditions for underestimation of length. Such reasoning suggests that we could simply degrade this stimulus such that we demarcate the extent to be judged and the wing tips with dots, and we should still get the classical illusion. This is done in Fig. 5A. Coren (1970a) has shown that the classical illusion, albeit somewhat reduced in magnitude, is still obtained in such figures. In fact, in a number of illusory configurations it is possible to remove most of the line segments, leaving only the end points, and still obtain the expected illusory effect (Coren, 1970a,b; White, 1972).

If the wing tips of the Mueller-Lyer illusion simply serve as extraneous stimuli, the eye movement data predict that the magnitude of this classical illusion should vary as a function of varying wing length. On the basis of the preceding experiment we could predict that as the wing length increases the illusion magnitude will increase up to some maximum and then will decrease. As we can see in Fig. 5B, such seems to be the case. The center version of the apparently longer Mueller-Lyer, has an intermediate wing length and appears to be longer than either the version with very short wings of the varient with very long wings. This impress was experimentally confirmed using the apparently longer half of the Mueller-Lyer figure, with a shaft length of 6 cm and an angle between the wings of 90 degrees. The wing length was either 0.5, 1, 2, 4, or 8 cm in length. Estimates of shaft length were made by eight subjects who adjusted a variable line length until it appeared to be equal to the shaft length. The results are shown in Fig. 5C. Notice the inverted "U" shaped function predicted from the eye movement pattern predicted. The effect of wing length is significant with

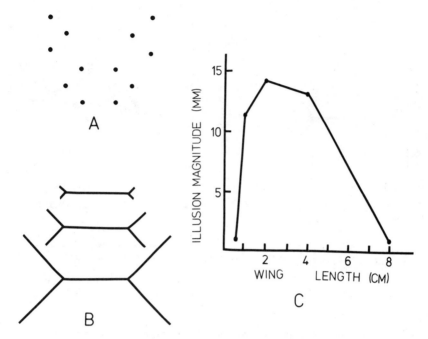

FIG. 5.   (A) A dot version of the Mueller-Lyer illusion; (B) Demonstration of the effect of wing length on the magnitude of the Mueller-Lyer illusions; (C) Experimental data showing variation in the magnitude of the Mueller-Lyer illusion as a function of wing length.

$F(4,34) = 4.31, p < .01$ as is the quadratic component $F(1,34) = 8.14, p < .01$. Notice that this represents a prediction made on the basis of our simpler arrays and the eye movement data, which has now been confirmed in a standard illusion configuration.

The preceding experiment involved a redefinition of the function of the wings in the Mueller-Lyer configuration. Notice, that for the purpose of our analysis the presence of angles was not the critical variable, rather, it was the relative horizontal distance of the wing tips of the line end. This shift in viewpoint allows us to address ourselves to a long standing conflict in the illusion literature. It has long been known that the magnitude of the Mueller-Lyer illusion varies as a function of its angle. The specific pattern variation is somewhat more ambiguous. Some investigators report that as the angle between the wings become smaller and smaller, the magnitude of the illusion increases in a monotomic fashion (Dewar, 1967; Heymans, 1896; Lewis, 1909). On the other hand, other investigators report that the magnitude of illusion increases up to some maximum at an intermediate level and then decreases as the angle becomes yet smaller (Auerbach, 1894, Brentano, 1892; Nakagawa, 1958; Restle & Decker, 1977). The simple resolution to the apparent contradictories of results is suggested by

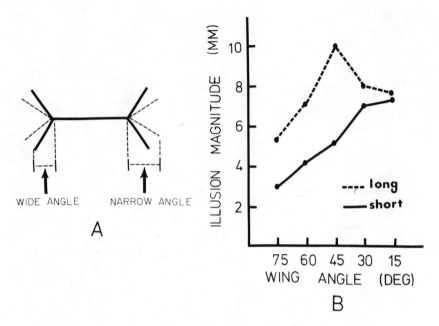

FIG. 6. (A) Shows variation in horizontal distance (vertex to wing tip) as the angle becomes more acute; (B) Experimental data showing variation in the magnitude of the Mueller-Lyer illusion as a function of angle, for two wing lengths.

our foregoing analysis. Since the horizontal extent between the test element (the end of the line) and the extraneous element (the wing tip) is, according to this theory, the critical feature, it is important to note that as the angles between the wings become more acute, the effect is to increase the horizontal distance between the line end and the wing tip, as can be seen in Fig. 6A. Clearly, if the wing is long then as the angle is made more acute there is a greater change in the horizontal distance than if the wing is short. If we remember that the magnitude of the illusion predicted on the basis of the eye movements, increases as the horizontal distance increases up to some maximum, and then decreases, we might then suggest that if the wing of the Mueller-Lyer is long, as the angle is made more acute we will obtain the inverted "U" function for illusion magnitude, whereas if the wing is shorter, variations in angle might merely increase the distance toward the maximum without ever passing the flexion point. To test this prediction, the apparently longer half of the Mueller-Lyer figure was again used. Shaft length was 8 cm and wing length was either 2 or 6 cm. The angle between the wings and the horizontal could be 75, 60, 45, 30, or 15 degrees. Twelve observers adjusted a variable line length to match the apparent length of each configuration.

The results of this experiment are shown in Fig. 6B. Notice, that as the angle between the wings is made more acute, there is a gradual increase in the overestimation of the figure when the wings are short, which shows only a significant linear trend with F (1,54) = 8.63, $p < .01$. With the long wings, however, where the horizontal distance between line and wing tip varies over a considerable distance, we obtain the inverted "U" shaped function as predicted, which is reflected in the significant quadratic component with F (1,54) = 9.60, $p < .01$. The striking aspect of these results are that we are able to predict an interaction between the wing length and the angle size in this classical illusion figure, solely on the basis of reanalysis of the array based upon eye movement considerations.

Up to now we have shown that a new set of illusions can be predicted on the basis of simple eye movement data, and that some parametric variation of classical illusions can also be predicted on this basis. It is possible to extend this process and to use it to create some rather striking illusory effects. Let us consider Fig. 7. Our eye movement data would indicate that if asked to look at the ends of the horizontal shaft, observers will tend to have their eyes pulled in the direction of the wing tips, here rightward into the body of the angle. Thus when scanning, this horizontal shaft the saccadic eye movements should be biased too far to the right, when looking at both ends. If our hypothesis is correct, and the eye movement tendencies will alter or distort the percept, then this leads to an interesting prediction. Although we would not expect the length of this shaft to be distorted, we would expect the entire shaft (and perhaps the entire figure) to be mislocalized in space. Since the eye movements used in scanning such a figure will be biased toward the right side (away from the direction in which the arrow is pointed) we would expect the entire figure to be perceptually located too far to the right. Methodologically this could be measured by asking

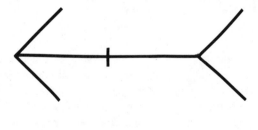

FIG. 7.   An illusion of direction, in which the arrow-head figure is seen too far to the right, relative to the hatch marks on the horizontal line which actually delineate the location of the vertices. A similar shift in the apparent location of the bisector of the shaft is also seen.

an observer to indicate the position of the line ends. Furthermore, one could predict that if the observer is asked to bisect the figure, he should bisect the apparent figure since the percept is apparently shifted toward the right, he should place the bisector too far to the right. Both of these effects can be seen by looking at Fig. 7. The mark on the horizontal shaft accurately bisects the figure, yet it appears to be too far to the left. On the horizontal line below the figure there are two hatch marks that are perpendicularly aligned with the vertices of the configuration, yet they appear to be also too far to the left, again suggesting that the entire figure is seen as too far to the right.

An experiment was conducted to verify these observations, using fifteen observers. The shaft was 8 cm long, wings were 4 cm in length, and the angle between the wings was 90 degrees. Eight cm above and below the figure was a horizontal line parallel to the shaft of the illusion figure. Over a series of eight measurements each observer was required either to place a pencil mark at the apparent midpoint of the shaft, or to indicate the apparent locus of the two end points of the line on the horizontal line beneath the figure. The figures were alternately oriented pointing right and left. The mean displacement of the apparent bisector of the shaft of the figure was, in fact, displaced away from the arrow head of the configuration an average of 3.6 mm, which is statistically significant with $t(14) = 3.11$, $p < .01$. The mean displacement of the figure was also in the direction away from the arrow head and was 2.3 mm, which was also significant with $t(14) = 2.93$, $p < .025$. Since both of these displacements are in the same direction, and we are assuming that they are both due to the mislocation of the figure as a consequence of an interaction with the eye movement biases, we would expect that for any given subject the magnitude of displacement of the bisector and the apparent displacement of the figure as measured by the locus of the line ends, should be correlated. In fact they are quite highly correlated with $r_s = 0.62$, $p < 0.01$.

The five experiments described above have approached the interaction between illusions and eye movements from an atypical direction. Rather than beginning with a series of illusory distortions, and then measuring eye movement patterns across those distortions, we began with some simple eye movement data. We then isolated those stimulus parameters that would systematically bias the saccadic eye movement pattern. By arranging the stimulus elements we could create a set of configurations that should produce eye movements that manifest particular constant errors. If there is an interaction between eye movements and the conscious percept, these same arrays should also manifest predictable apparent distortions. In effect we created a new set of illusions. Further analysis of the stimulus parameters that affect the eye movements then permitted some predictions about some classical illusion varients. Finally, extrapolating from the eye movement data, we were able to predict an illusory effect in which an object is veridically seen, at least as far as its size and shape is concerned, however, it is apparently displaced in space. An interesting aspect of this approach is that once we had the data pertaining to the biases in the eye movement control system we did not have to resort to additional eye movement measurements. Since we were predicting that the pattern of movements would interact with the conscious percept, all of the succeeding measurements had to be geared toward the measurement of what the observer actually saw, rather than how he moved his eyes.

Has this method of attack, from eye movement to percept, rather than from percept to eye movement, allowed us to make causal rather than correctional statements? Perhaps not completely, since, of course, we are still dealing with data that simply represent a covariation between eye movements and perception. However, it does seem more convincing to be able to predict what will be perceived especially if those percepts will embody illusory distortions or hithertofore unexpected perceptual errors. The fact that we can predict several classes of distortion, namely distortions in length and distortions in locus, suggest that there may be some generality to the underlying principle. Furthermore, such data suggest an interesting research strategy. We know many factors that selectively affect eye movement accuracy or cause predictable constant errors. Perhaps our approach should be, not to simply continue to measure the eye movements, but to now go back and look at what the observer perceives under conditions where the eye movement patterns are atypical. If the theory holds, then we would expect illusory distortions under *all* conditions where the eye movements themselves do not accurately reflect the physical stimulus relationships.

Bain (1855) proposed that the conscious representation of a stimulus might be affected by the pattern of eye movements across that stimulus. This triggered an era of scientific investigation into eye movement patterns. The technology has become more sophisticated since then, and our data base has grown by leaps and bounds. We now know much more about conditions under which eye movement patterns are accurately correlated with, or biased relative to the stimulus being viewed. Bain knew much about the percept, but little about the eye movements themselves. Now that we know much more about eye movements, perhaps it is time to go back and look at the percepts.

Hysteresis Effects in the Vergence Control System: Perceptual Implications

II.2

Sheldon M. Ebenholtz
University of Wisconsin-Madison

Fusional or disparity vergence serves the purpose of binocular single vision. This is accomplished through the action of a negative feedback loop that reduces disparate visual stimulation by the control of disjunctive eye movements. The response is relatively rapid with typical latencies to the onset of disparity on the order of 200 ms (Rashbass & Westheimer, 1961). Singleness of vision is also promoted on the basis of feedforward control, by a second system operating through the synkinesis between the stimulus to accommodation and convergence.

It has been known for some time, at least in the case of fusional vergence, that removal of the disparity stimulus, by either covering one eye or eliminating visual stimulation entirely, does not bring with it the immediate relaxation of the vergence posture (Alpern, 1946; Bielschowsky, 1938; Krishnan & Stark, 1977; Ogle & Prangen, 1953). Rather, the time period of relaxation varies from a few seconds (Krishnan & Stark, 1977) to several hours (Carter, 1965) depending, apparently, upon the length of time during which vergence was in force. Further evidence for a slow component to the vergence response is provided by the gradual reduction in fixation disparity with maintained fusion over periods in excess of 15 min (Carter, 1965; Ogle & Prangen, 1953; Ogle, Martens, & Dyer, 1967). It has been proposed (Ogle & Prangen, 1953; Schor, 1979a) that the slow fusional component of the disparity vergence system serves the purpose of releasing stress on the fast fusional component, thereby reducing fixation disparity and perhaps facilitating the response to subsequent stimulus disparities.

Whatever additional functions it may have, slow fusional vergence represents an adaptive response to maintained disparity-vergence stimuli. It is accompanied by an increase in normal tonic innervation as evidenced by a shift in resting level or phoria, measured in the fusion-free position, and therefore, it is a hysteresis effect in the sense that the induced phoria represents a lag in vergence posture in the direction in which the eyes were last held.

Insofar as vergence magnitude acts as a cue to perceived distance, it is of interest to speculate on the premise that the signal governing the level of tonic innervation has utility beyond the vergence control system itself, in the perceptual representation of vergence-mediated distance. Accordingly, the studies reported below represent an exploration of the effects on distance perception of factors that also condition hysteresis effects in the vergence control system.

But before proceeding it is important to be explicit about the possible relation between hysteresis effects in the vergence control system and the perception of distance. How might the two be related? Let us assume that there exists a tonus control mechanism responsible for the maintenance of normal tonic levels of the extra-ocular muscles. The reference input to such a control system would, in the absence of visual stimulation, cause the eyes to fall to some position of physiological rest, representing a tonic balance between medial and lateral muscle tension. A call from the disparity-vergence system to produce a disjunctive eye movement would then be added algebraically to the reference level and tonic adjustments would be made as negative or positive increments to the reference level, the latter serving the function of reducing steady-state error (Milhorn, 1966; Schor, 1979b). As an analog of the reference tonus level, one should expect to find associated with it a reference *distance* (in the absence of other distance cues) in comparison to which vergence nearer or beyond the reference distance would correspond, respectively, to nearer or farther increments in perceived distance. It follows that if hysteresis effects can be modeled as changes in the tonus-control reference signal, then changes in perceived distance would be a necessary consequence, since the additional tonus needed to verge on a particular point in space will vary with the level of the reference signal. Thus moving the tonic balance in favor of the medial recti would shift the reference distance inward (toward the subject) and cause a given target to be seen as farther away, while the opposite shift in favor of the lateral recti would cause targets to be seen as nearer than usual.

As a heuristic device, Fig. 1 represents a flow chart model of the accommoda- • tion and vergence feedback systems and of their interrelationships (Krishnan & Stark, 1977; Schor, 1979b; Toates, 1974). In the model the tonus control mechanism of each system is assumed to be the source of hysteresis effects that act by producing a lag in the relaxation either of the extra-ocular muscles in vergence or the ciliary muscle in accommodation. The hypothetical "distance operator" is given the function of assigning some value of apparent distance to the tonus signal and of determining the weighting function required when integrating common information from the two systems. In the studies to be reported here the focus of attention will be on the vergence system.

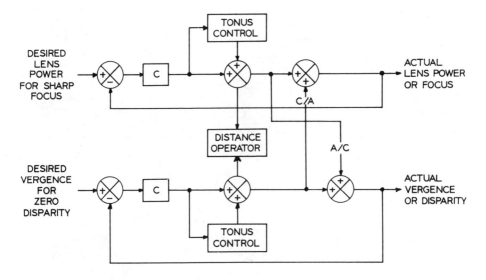

FIG. 1.   Block diagram of accommodation and vergence control systems. C/A represents convergence-produced accommodation and A/C accommodative convergence. The boxes labeled C represents the respective controllers for each system.

METHODOLOGY

Distance Perception.   The technique for measuring distance perception is represented in Fig. 2 and consists essentially of matching the unseen position of the index finger with the fixed visual position of the target. Presumably the manual system ''reads out'' the convergence distance and uses this information to position the limb proprioceptively. Although studies have shown the converse operation, i.e., matching a visible target to a fixed limb position, to be equally feasible, only the former method was used in the present studies. The target used in the first two studies is shown in the inset in Fig. 2. It was composed of six pinholes, about 1 mm in diameter, arranged in a circular pattern 17 mm in diameter around a central point. Nothing else was visible to the subjects. In all conditions, the subject's match was taken as the average of two settings, one from a starting position 10 cm beyond, the other 10 cm nearer the actual target position.

Phoria Measures.   Phoria represents the degree to which the ocular axes verge in front of, at, or beyond a given target in the absence of fusional stimuli.

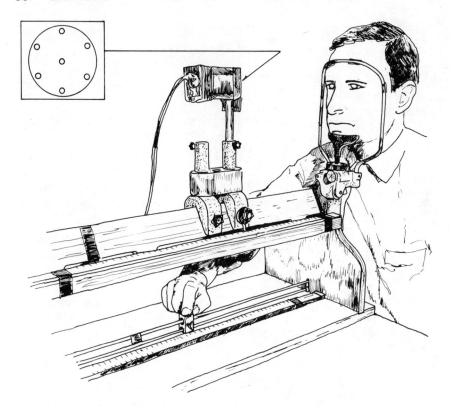

FIG. 2.   Apparatus for measuring apparent distance of target (inset) with unseen hand.

Two methods were used for measurement. In one case the near slides (optically at 33.3 cm) of the Bausch and Lomb Master Orthorater presented a vertical arrow to one eye and a horizontal series of numbered dots to the other. The reported position of the dot conforming to the location of the arrow tip established the phoria in 1.5 diopter steps. In the second method the right eye position was measured with an Eye-trac (Model 200) infra-red monitor. Pen recordings were made over a 20 sec fixation period, once with the right eye occluded while the left eye fixated the target (viz., the fusion free position) and again with both eyes fixated, in that order. Measurements of the trace were taken at 5, 10, 15, and 20 sec and then averaged. The phoria was defined as the difference in mean position of the right eye under the two conditions. The target used to assess distance perception and that used to measure the phoria both were set at identical distances.

THE CALIBRATION OF CONVERGENCE DISTANCE
AGAINST MANUAL SETTINGS

In order to examine the validity of the distance measurement technique, 8 subjects made 2 manual settings under binocular viewing at each of six target distances, vis., 28.4, 30.0, 34.4, 38.5, 44.4, and 50.0 cm. Four different sequences selected from a balanced latin square were used but in no case was there an orderly increase or decrease in target distance.

Figure 3 represents the mean settings as a function of actual target distance. The linear function was fit by a least squares procedure applied to the data with the exception of the 50 cm point where the settings were spuriously low since many subjects reported not being able to reach far enough for this target. Several results of this study are worth noting: first, the excellent fit provided by the linear function ($r = .998$). It is thus clear that vergence and/or accommodation pro-

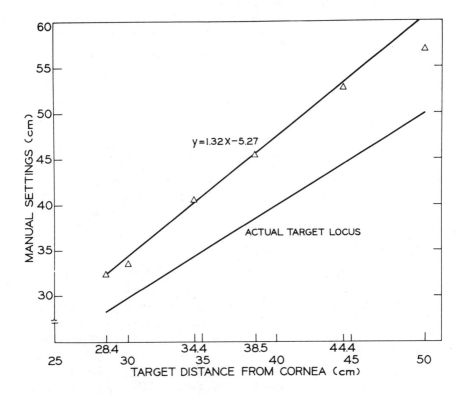

FIG. 3.   Manual setting as a function of target distance. Least square function fitted to data points.

vides a linear signal to the manual system that faithfully encodes distance. Second, there was a consistent over-reaching that ranged from 3.4 to 8.4 cm in the range of target distances examined. This may be functional rather than maladaptive since overreaching would ensure contact and utlimate grasping of the target. Third, the positive slope (1.32) of the fitted function indicates that as target distance increases there will be an increasing departure of manual settings from actual target positions. This probably reflects a constant error in the vergence signal since the addition of a constant number of degrees of convergence represents increasing increments in distance, as observation distance increases.

Generally, the first two characteristics are consistent with the results of Foley and Held (1972) and Foley (1975) who also examined the manual response to visual targets. However, the increasing pointing error with target distance represents a trend exactly opposite to that found by Foley (1975), although in that study only targets that were 12 deg to the left and right of the median plane were used. Furthermore, in these studies the pointing response was not constrained to any single lateral direction and hence their data exhibited considerably larger constant errors than those of the present study. It is not known to what extent this, together with the use of equivalent optical distances (as opposed to changes in actual target distance) and additional procedural differences may be responsible for the opposed trends.

The data shown in Fig. 3 indicate quite clearly that at least within the range of distances from 28.4 to 44.4 cm vergence and accommodation are linearly related to manual distance settings. To some extent relative retinal size may have contributed to the correct ordering of the target distances, but it is doubtful that this played a significant role since it is less effective in binocular than in monocular viewing (Gogel & Sturm, 1972) and furthermore the very first manual settings of the subjects also exhibited an order appropriate to the target distances. Hence it may be concluded that changes in vergence-mediated distance also will be reflected in the pointing response.

ADAPTATION AND INDUCTION PARADIGMS

Two methods were used to investigate hysteresis effects in the form of an induced phoria and to examine their effects on distance perception. In the case of the adaptation paradigm spectacles that contained pairs of 5^Δ base out prisms together with -1.5 D lenses were worn by subjects for periods of 10 to 15 min. Wearing these spectacles while walking in lighted, normal environments reliably causes an increase in apparent distance to visual targets. They first were used in perceptual adaptation studies by Wallach and Frey (1972) who interpreted the resulting aftereffects as a recalibration of the distance signal normally provided by the oculomotor system (von Hofsten, 1979; Wallach, Frey, & Bode, 1972).

Presumably monocular distance cues like linear perspective and motion parallax, which remain unaltered through the spectacles, served to "reeducate" the oculomotor cues of vergence and accommodation, the latter being systematically increased by the conbination of base out prisms and negative lenses. These studies supporting the recalibration theory did not, however, examine the possibility that the spectacles induced hysteresis effects (phoria), which in turn may have served to mediate the obtained changes in distance perception.

The second method, referred to as the *induction paradigm*, simply requires that subjects fixate targets at various optical distances for periods ranging from 6 to 15 min. The targets may be viewed directly, through prisms, or with the aid of a haploscope (Ebenholtz & Wolfson, 1975; Paap & Ebenholtz, 1977) but in all events viewing is in the absence of secondary cues to distance. As in the case of the adaptation paradigm fixation on near targets, within about 30 cm, causes an increase in apparent distance. The magnitude of the distance aftereffect however has been considerably lower than that obtained under the adaptation paradigm. Hence, although secondary cues cannot be credited with a role in the induction paradigm, recalibration has been thought to account for most of the aftereffect under the adaptation paradigm (Wallach & Halperin, 1977). Although the induction paradigm is known to produce hysteresis effects in the vergence system (Schor, 1979a) they have not been measured comcomitantly with the distance aftereffects. Thus the role of the induced phoria in distance perception remains to be explicated in both the induction and adaptation paradigms.

The results of an experiment comparing the two paradigms with the same set of 11 subjects is represented in Fig. 4. In the induction paradigm the fixation target was set at 20 cm. Distance settings to a target at 34 cm were made before exposure and then every 3 min during the 15 min exposure period. They were continued for 15 additional min with the subjects in the dark, to examine decay rates. The data plotted in Fig. 4 are the differences between the manual settings at any given time period and those taken prior to the exposure period.

A number of important differences and similarities result from the comparison of the two paradigms. First, both paradigms produced statistically significant ($p < .05$) levels of aftereffect as measured by the pointing procedure, and in both cases the aftereffect was asymptotic within about 15 min. For the adaptation condition this level of aftereffect was well below that expected from complete perceptual adaptation to the prism and lens system. This would entail "undoing" the optical effects by perceptually subtracting a full 10^Δ from any given convergence distance. For an interocular axis of 6.20 cm a target at 34.4 cm would be seen as though it had an optical distance of 75.24 cm. Applying the function described in Fig. 2 to obtain the corresponding pointing response, complete adaptation would require a pre to post shift of 53.91 cm. Thus the effect of 10.43 cm was only 19.3% complete. A limit to the growth in adaptation aftereffect has been previously noted (Ebenholtz, 1974) when increasing levels of prism power

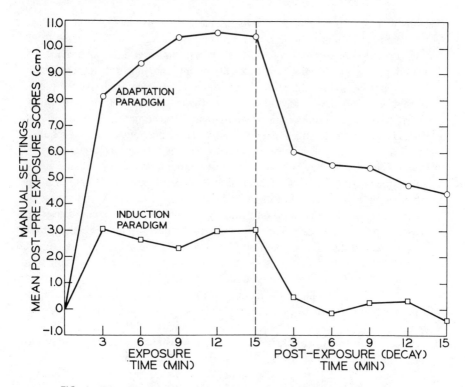

FIG. 4. Distance aftereffect and decay as a function of exposure time, under adaptation and induction paradigms.

from 6 to 10$^\Delta$ per eye produced insignificant increases in aftereffect. Hofsten (1979) also has observed the asymptotic limit with exposure time beyond about 8 min and suggested a limiting magnitude comparable to a 4° shift in convergence angle. It is an important theoretical question to consider why the aftereffect magnitude should be constrained. Learning theories of the type on which the notion of recalibration is predicated, would seem to be quite inadequate to account for such limited learning. Deducing the constraints from the underlying mechanism would seem to be more promising.

A second issue concerns the relative magnitudes of aftereffect in the induction and adaptation paradigms. The ratio of induction to adaptation post-pre difference scores after 15 min of exposure showed the former to be 29.1% of the latter. Does this imply that the two paradigms represent fundamentally different underlying processes? Not at all. Analysis of the optical inputs in the two paradigms suggests an essential reason for the different aftereffect magnitudes that is compatible with a single mechanism, viz, the slow relaxation of the fusional response after a period of maintained disparity vergence. Since vergence movements are elicited by disparate stimuli distributed over foveal, parafoveal, as well as peripheral regions (Burian, 1939; von Noorden, 1980) it would seem likely that the greater the number of such regions implicated, the greater the magnitude of the aftereffect. In physiologic terms, one might consider a large population of disparity detectors distributed over the superior colliculus and striate regions of the brain. As more detectors are triggered, precision of eye position control exerted by the vergence system in the closed loop mode improves. In fact the number of disparity detectors active at any given time might represent an important gain control in the system.

When comparing the induction and adaptation paradigms it is necessary to consider that in the former case only foveal stimulation by a target of about 1.8 deg was present whereas, in the latter case a large array of stimuli was available over the entire retina to control vergence movements and to stabilize eye position. It is possible then that the greater number of fusional stimuli that are presumed to be present in casual viewing was responsible for the larger aftereffect in the adaptation condition. Pilot studies now in progress support this interpretation and show an increase in the induction aftereffect, by a factor of 2, simply by increasing the number of vertical fusional stimuli present during the exposure period.

A third point, essential to the position taken, is the question of whether there is evidence for the presence of hysteresis effects in such magnitudes and proportions as to account for the obtained differences in pointing response in the adaptation and induction paradigms. To this end phoria measurements on the Orthorater were taken before and again after the exposure period (at 15 min). The changes in phoria are represented in Table 1 along with the difference scores associated with the distance settings. In both conditions a statistically significant shift in phoria (at $p < .05$) occurred in the direction of esophoria clearly reflecting the hysteresis in the disparity vergence system. Furthermore a close relationship between phoria and distance aftereffects is suggested by the virtual identity in the ratios of induction to adaptation between the two measures. Thus, in both cases the induction condition produced only about 30% of the aftereffect obtained under adaptation.

TABLE 1
Changes in Pointing Response and in Phoria as a
Result of a 15 Min Exposure Period[a]

	Distance Settings (cm)		Phoria (Δ)	
	M	σM	M	σM
Adaptation (A)	10.43	1.37	5.16	.62
Induction (I)	3.03	1.43	1.57	.84
Ratio: I/A	.29		.30	

[a] Positive numbers indicate increased distance and esophoria.

A separate question concerns how much of the induced phoria was manifest in the changes in apparent distance. To answer this it was necessary to convert the distance settings and phoria measures into common units of degrees of convergence angle. This is straightforward in the case of phoria measures but it required several steps to convert the distance settings since the target distance and hence actual convergence angle remained fixed before and after exposure. It was reasoned, however, that the change in distance setting could be interpreted *as though* the subject were viewing the target with vergence cues appropriate to a farther distance after exposure than before. The next step was to estimate this distance from the pointing response data. The function represented in Fig. 3 was used to determine the increment in target distance that corresponded with the obtained increment in the pointing response. This "apparent" target distance was then used to calculate an *effective* increment ($\Delta\gamma$) to the convergence angle (γ) associated with the actual target distance. For example, a pointing-response increment of 10 cm, because of the slope of 1.32 of the calibration function, corresponded to a change in target distance of only 7.58 cm. This value was added to the actual target distance of 34.4 cm and the effective convergence angle for a distance of 42.0 cm calculated. Subtracting the actual convergence angle for the true target distance then yielded the desired increment ($\Delta\gamma$). Given the mean changes in pointing distance represented in Table 1, these calculations yielded $\Delta\gamma$ values of 1.92 deg for the adaptation condition and .64 deg for the induction paradigm. The ratios of $\Delta\gamma$ to the change in phoria (in degrees) were .653 and .719 for adaptation and induction respectively. Thus it can be concluded that only 65 to 70% of the phoria was expressed in the illusory target distance.

A final observation on the data represented in Fig. 4 concerns the decay of the aftereffect in the post-exposure period. For the induction condition, the low level of aftereffect decayed to zero within about 6 min, with only slight oscillation thereafter. The pattern of decay after adaptation, however, was quite different. After 15 min the aftereffect reached 4.5 cm and was 42.9 percent complete. This suggests a time constant of about 27 min, which would lead one to expect complete decay in somewhat over 1 hr and 47 min. It is interesting that although the adaptation paradigm produced about 3.4 times the level of aftereffect as the induction condition, the rate of decay after adaptation was about $^1/_{18}$ that after induction (i.e., 6 min/107 min). Thus decay rates are not linearly related to the levels of aftereffect achieved. Furthermore, although the computation of the time constant presumes an exponential decay eventually reaching a zero level, in fact one cannot be sure that the function for the adaptation paradigm will ever decay completely without additional disparate stimulation. Since "leaky integrator" models (Krishnan & Stark, 1977) require complete dissipation, it is important to establish whether decay levels stabilize at non-zero values. If so it would support the premise that such long-lasting hysteresis effects represent a change in the muscle tonus reference signal.

TABLE 2
Changes in Pointing Distance and Phoria after
Binocular and Monocular Exposure[a]

		Distance Settings (cm)		Phoria (Δ)	
		M	σM	M	σM
Exposure Condition	Monocular	2.43	1.02	−0.83	2.19
	Binocular	10.84	1.70	4.82	0.96

[a] Positive numbers indicate increased distance and esophoria.

MONOCULAR VS. BINOCULAR EXPOSURE

Another examination of the relation between hysteresis effects in the vergence system and distance aftereffects is provided by a comparison of binocular and monocular exposure conditions in the adaptation paradigm. Under monocular exposure, the disparity-vergence system is in the open loop mode, but increased vergence is maintained through the accommodation-convergence link due to the presence of the −1.5 D lens in the spectacles. If the pairing of altered oculomotor with veridical monocular distance cues is responsible for the changes in perceived distance through a process of recalibration, then monocular and binocular viewing should be equally effective. On the other hand, if disparity vergence is essential to the effect, then monocular viewing should produce no aftereffect.

Results after a 15 min exposure period under binocular or monocular viewing are shown in Table 2. Data are for 8 subjects and are post-pre difference scores. Pointer settings were made with binocular vision and phoria was determined either by an infra-red monitor or the Orthorater. Clearly, disparity vergence is critically implicated in the distance aftereffect as evidenced by the large induced esophoria after binocular exposure. On the other hand monocular viewing led to a slight exophoria and little support for the recalibration theory since the distance aftereffect was only about one-fifth that of the binocular condition. The presence of a slight aftereffect of monocular exposure may be explained as resulting from accommodative hysteresis but other possibilities remain to be tested.

CONCLUSIONS

Experiments have shown that hysteresis effects in the disparity vergence or slow vergence system are manifest in the form of an induced phoria as well as in changes in apparent distance. Thus roughly parallel effects in esophoria magnitude and distance overestimation were found in comparing the adaptation and induction paradigms, and in the relative effects of monocular and binocular exposure conditions. Only about 70% of the phoria was manifest as a change in distance.

After monocular viewing through adapting spectacles an aftereffect of one-fifth that under binocular viewing was obtained. This strongly implicates the disparity vergence system and runs contrary to the recalibration theory that a mere pairing of oculomotor and monocular distance cues is sufficient to alter the visual perception of vergence mediated distance.

Distance perception seems to be intimately related to the properties of the disparity vergence control system that characterize its *steady state,* and probably does not have a corresponding relation to the transient states associated with the control of disjunctive eye movements. Conditions like hysteresis effects that alter steady state levels of muscle tonus may therefore be expected also to produce changes in apparent distance.

ACKNOWLEDGMENT

The chapter was prepared while the author was on Research Leave awarded by the Graduate School Research Committee from funds provided by the Wisconsin Alumni Research Foundation.

The author thanks Sherry Fisher for her aid in conducting the experiments and analyzing the data.

Visual Direction Illusions in Everyday Situations: Implications for Sensorimotor and Ecological Theories

II.3

Wayne L. Shebilske
University of Virginia

The crash of Pan American Flight 707 at Pago Pago International Airport illustrates the high cost of visual illusions. Near the end of a routine flight, the captain started an instrument approach, which he had not done for 132 days. He intercepted the glide path too high and was about 100 ft above the glideslope when the runway came in sight eight miles out. At 700 ft the captain went visual to complete the landing. Within 3 sec after that, the first officer said, "You're a little high." Four seconds later, the captain increased the rate of decent from 690 feet per minute to 1,470 feet per minute and continued at that until impact. About half of the passengers and some of the crew survived the crash. The possibility that a visual illusion contributed to the accident is suggested by the third officer's statement that "just prior to impact everything looked normal." This example, is not unique. Kraft and Elworth (1969) provided data supporting the possibility that illusions account for about 16% of air transport accidents. With a night visual approach simulator, Kraft and Elworth found that under certain conditions a descent path can null out information in the optical flow pattern leading to illusions, causing incorrect interpretations of altitude and distance.

Althetes too are plagued by illusions. While the consequences are less disastrous, deceiving eyes are probably the cause, on some occasions, when tennis players miss an easy shot, baseball players misjudge a fly ball, or basketball players shoot an air ball. The present chapter investigates a particular kind of visual direction illusion, an illusion that is caused by misjudging the direction of gaze. It will argue that such illusions are induced by everyday manipulations and occur in everyday situations.

Although people can adjust their direction of gaze to see the direction of a light in an otherwise dark environment, the mechanism that makes this possible is not identified (Shebilske, 1978). But, there is general agreement that errors in registering eye position can lead to misjudgments of the direction of objects (Shebilske, 1977a). Under unusual conditions like eye muscle paralysis or externally produced eye movements, visual direction illusions can be observed. One such illusion is demonstrated by closing one eye and gently pushing the other eye with your finger through your eye lid. The externally produced eye movement is not accurately registered centrally, but the error in registered eye position causes a corresponding error in the perceived direction of objects. Turn your head away from your desk while you push your eye down with one hand. Turn back and try to reach quickly for some object on your desk with the other hand. I think you will be convinced that your eyes can play tricks on you under these unnatural conditions, but, do similar illusions occur in everyday situations?

It is not obvious that everyday conditions disturb the registration of eye position. After all, the neuromuscular system is designed to perform accurately in the face of highly variable conditions imposed by abnormal body temperatures, illness, inadequate diet, lack of sleep, over work, etc. The focal issue for most neuroscientists is the way the neuromuscular system achieves its high fidelity. This has overshadowed the fact that the neuromuscular system is not completely reliable. For example, when people maintain unequal tension in antagonistic skeletal muscle pairs, they make small errors in various psychophysical tasks including estimates of weight and tension (Hughes, 1958). A growing body of research shows that similar aftereffects in the oculomotor control system disturb visuomotor coordination. Five kinds of aftereffects have been studied:

1. When the eyes maintain an eccentric direction of gaze for about 30 sec. or longer, people make errors in judgments of direction of gaze and visual direction (Craske, Crawshaw, & Heron, 1975; Ebenholtz, 1976; Levy, 1973; Paap & Ebenholtz, 1976; Park, 1969).

2. When the head is tilted back for about 2 minutes and then returned to upright, people misjudge their line of sight causing illusions of visual direction (Fogelgren & Shebilske, 1979; Shebilske & Fogelgren, 1977; Shebilske & Karmiohl, 1978).

3. After maintaining convergence of more or less than about 30 cm, people misjudge their degree of convergence causing them to misperceive visual distance (Craske & Crawshaw, 1978; Ebenholtz & Wolfson, 1975; Ebenholtz, this volume).

4. When people scan in one direction as in reading, they develop erroneous shifts in registered eye position causing illusions of visual direction (Shebilske, 1977b).

5. When a wedge prism is placed in front of one eye, people make fusional eye movements, which lead to unregistered shifts in eye position that persist after the prism is removed (Alpern, 1969; Ellerbrock & Fry, 1941).

In discussing these effects, I find it helpful to use the term "Minor Motor Anomalie" to refer to errors in registered eye or limb position occurring in healthy neuromuscular systems as the result of disturbances caused by naturalistic conditions.

Minor Motor Anomalies have many possible physiological determinants. They could be caused by fluctuations in intramuscular temperature as the result of changes in local circulation and metabolic levels (Hayes, 1975). They could also be caused by electrophysiological phenomenon common to all cholinergic transmission: depression, facilitation, and post-tetanic potentiation (Barrett & Magleby, 1976). All of these merit further investigation because they have undertermined roles in normal synaptic integration. However, only post-tetanic potentiation has a time course that is consistent with the perceptual illusions mentioned above (Hughes, 1958). Potentiation is a long lasting effect. For example, Barrett and Magleby (1976) found about a two-fold potentiation over a baseline response at a frog neuromuscular junction. It developed within seconds of a tetanic train delivered for 90 seconds, and it decayed gradually back to baseline over a 20 minute period. Potentiation has other properties that are consistent with the above illusions. For example, some experiments have found phasic decay of eye position aftereffects (Craske & Templeton, 1968) while others have found linear decay (Craske et. al., 1975). Paap (1975) noted that these results are consistent with influences of intensity and duration of a tetanic train on potentiation in a wide variety of preparations as follows: sympathetic ganglion (Larrabee & Bronk, 1938; 1947), spinal cord (Lloyd, 1949), neuromuscular systems (Bagust, Lewis, & Luck, 1974; Brown & von Euler, 1938; Hughes & Morrell, 1957) and muscle afferents (Hughes & Morrell, 1957; Hutton, Smith, & Eldred, 1973). Nevertheless, we will not be sure of the physiological determinants until we take physiological measures during well defined psychophysical tasks.

We can expect this major undertaking only after physiologists are convinced that the perceptual illusions caused by Minor Motor Anomalies are something more than artificial laboratory phenomena. Toward this end, this chapter will:

1. describe the relevant illusions in more detail;
2. describe everyday conditions that induce the illusions;
3. investigate the illusions with the environment dark or fully structured; and
4. consider the practical and theoretical implications especially for sensorimotor and ecological theories.

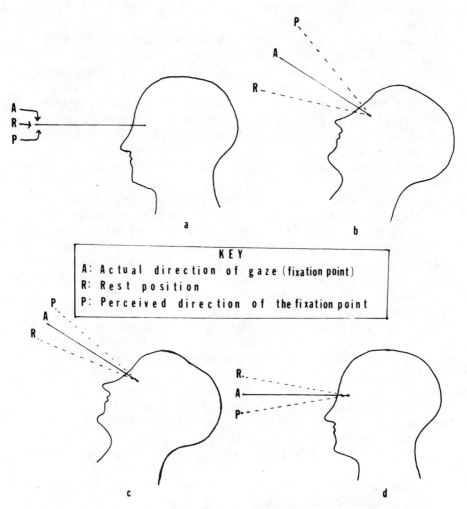

FIG. 1. Illusions of visual direction associated with head tilts actual direction of gaze (A), the rest position of the eyes (R), and the perceived direction of the fixation point (P), are shown. See text for detail. (From Fogelgren and Shebilske (1979) with permission).

ILLUSIONS OF VISUAL DIRECTION
INDUCED BY MINOR MOTOR ANOMALIES

Figure 1 (from Fogelgren & Shebilske, 1979) shows the relationships between the actual direction of gaze, which is determined by a fixation point, the rest position of the eyes, which is operationally defined by the position chosen when a subject is asked to put his or her eyes in the normal straight-ahead position with respect to the head, and the perceived direction of the fixation points.

Figure 1a shows a person whose head is upright and whose eyes are uninfluenced by any aftereffects of head tilts. The fixation point is placed in line with the rest position, and the perceived direction of the fixation point corresponds to its actual direction. Notice that the fixation point is in the same location with respect to the head in Figs. 1a, 1b, 1c, and 1d; therefore, the actual direction of gaze is in the same place with respect to the head in all diagrams.

Figure 1b shows a person whose head has been tilted back for about 2 min and whose eyes are therefore under the influence of the doll reflex. The doll reflex is compensatory eye movements driven by the gravity receptors in the vestibular system. Like the toy dolls with counterweighted eyes, a person's eyes rotate down when he or she is tilted back. It is possible to prevent doll-eye movements simply by looking at a fixation point. However, even when this is done, an extra component of innervation from the gravity receptors is added to the muscles that move the eyes downward. As a result of this, the rest position of the eyes is lower (Ebenholtz & Shebilske, 1975) and the perceived direction of the fixation point is higher (Ebenholtz & Shebilske, 1973). This is called the elevation illusion.

Figure 1c shows a person who has been tilted back for about 5 min and whose eyes have therefore adapted partially to the doll reflex (Shebilske & Karmiohl, 1978). Consequently, the rest position is lowered less than it is in Figure 1b, and the elevation illusion is smaller.

Figure 1d shows a person who has been returned to upright after partially adapting to the doll reflex. The result is a negative aftereffect; the rest position of the eyes is raised and the perceived direction of the fixation point is lowered (Shebilske & Fogelgren, 1977). The elevation illusion is about 6° for a 40° head and body tilt; it is reduced to about 4° after 5 minutes. The negative aftereffect after 5 minutes at 40° is about 3°.

Figure 2 illustrates a visual direction illusion induced by maintaining an upward direction of gaze. In Figure 2a the fixation point is placed in line with the rest position, and the perceived direction of the fixation point corresponds to its actual direction. In Figure 2b, the person is fixating a point above the eye's rest position. Figure 2c shows the aftereffect of holding the eyes upward. The rest position of the eyes is raised and the perceived direction of the target is lowered. A comparable sideward illusion is obtained when the eyes are held to the left or right. The magnitude of this illusion is about 4° after the eyes are held about 40°

100

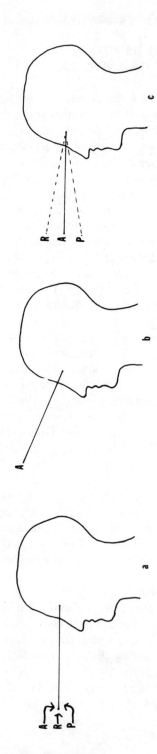

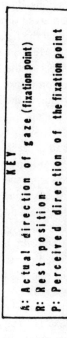

KEY

A: Actual direction of gaze (fixation point)
R: Rest position
P: Perceived direction of the fixation point

FIG. 2. Illusions of visual direction associated with eccentric directions of gaze actual direction of gaze (A), the rest position of the eyes (R), and the perceived direction of the fixation point (P). The three diagrams show a person in the following conditions: (a) before eyes are held up, (b) during upward direction of gaze, and (c) after eyes are held up.

off center for 2 minutes and about 1° after the eyes are held about 10° off center for 30 seconds (Paap & Ebenholtz, 1976).

The important thing to remember regarding the experiments to be reported is that after being tilted back, or after holding an upward direction of gaze, people judge their line of sight to be lower than it actually is and as a result they see objects as lower than they actually are.

EVERYDAY CONDITIONS INDUCE
MINOR MOTOR ANOMALIES

The head tilts and eccentric directions of gaze used to induce the above illusions are common in everyday situations. For example, people generally read or watch TV with their head tilted back and tilt their head forward for long periods during handwork. Figure 3 shows a common eye position during conversations.

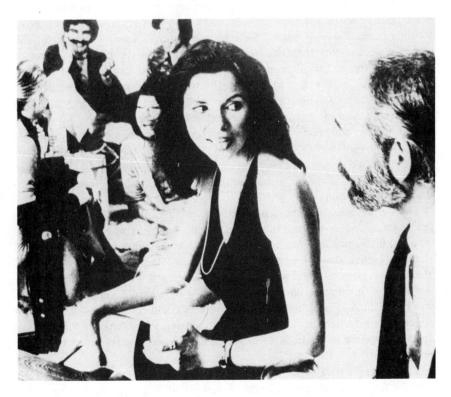

FIG. 3. Eccentric direction of gaze (45 degrees or greater) is common during conversations.

During casual conversations people usually hold their head at about 45° angles with respect to one another. Thus, they hold their eyes at about 45° angles whenever they make eye contact (Argyle, 1969). Pilots, on the other hand, spend a good deal of time looking down at their instruments and then must raise their head and eyes to look out the windshield. These conditions are sufficient for inducing the described illusions. Why then have the illusions not been noticed? Perhaps they do not occur in a fully structured illuminated environment. The following experiments were designed to find out.

ILLUSIONS OF VISUAL DIRECTION IN FULLY STRUCTURED ILLUMINATED ENVIRONMENTS

Experiment 1

Three subjects chosen for these experiments were baseball players on an American Legion team in Jamestown, N.D. and seven played on the University of Virginia team. Figure 4 shows the response measure used. I thought of the bat as a pointer that indicated where the batter saw the ball. If the batter swung over the ball or hit a ground ball I took this as evidence that the batter saw the ball higher than what it actually was; if the batter hit a line drive, I assumed the batter saw the ball where it actually was; and if the batter hit a pop up or swung under the ball I took this as evidence that he saw the ball lower than what it actually was, realizing that other things could cause a batter to swing off target. Even skilled players cannot always put the bat where they want it; in fact, they do well to get a hit once out of every three trips to the plate. Nevertheless, I proceeded in the hope that the illusion would be large enough to overshadow the variability.

During two sessions, subjects rested one minute, hit 6 pitches thrown by a pitching machine, rested one minute and then hit another 6 pitches and so on until they had hit 30 pitches in each test period. While the subjects batted, they used whatever batting stance they were accustomed to using. During the rest periods of session 1, subjects stood with their head upright and their eyes in their normal rest position. In contrast, during the rest periods on session 2, subjects layed back on a board tilted 45° and looked up as far as they could comfortably. Recall from our earlier discussion that the effect of both manipulations, the head tilt and the upward direction of gaze, is to cause people to see objects lower than they actually are.

I analyzed the data for each subject by comparing the first swing in session 1 with the first swing of session 2 and so on until all 30 swings were compared. I classified each swing into one of five categories: swing over, ground ball, line drive, pop up, or swing under. When swings fell into different categories on the

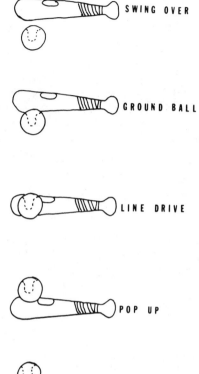

SWING OVER

GROUND BALL

LINE DRIVE

POP UP

FIG. 4. Baseball bat used as pointer. Errors in pointing are indicated by the effect on the ball. Results can be categorized into at least five categories.

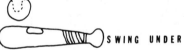

SWING UNDER

pretest and posttest, I recorded whether the difference indicated that the batter saw the ball higher or lower in session 2. This permitted a simple binomial test. Each batter was scored as "plus" if he saw the ball lower more frequently in session 2 and as "minus" if he saw the ball higher more frequently in session 2, understanding that there should have been an equal number of pluses and minus if there was no tendency to see the ball lower. In fact, 9 out of 10 batters saw the ball lower in session 2, which was statistically significant, $p < .05$.

The effect was most dramatic on the first 3 swings of each block of 6 swings. On the first 3 swings, 9 out of 10 batters showed the predicted effect. On the second 3 swings only 7 out of 10 batters showed the effect. Furthermore, I found that on the first 3 swings, 4 out of the 9 who went in the predicted direction did so strongly enough to show significant trends in their own data (9 out of 9, 9 out of 10, 10 out of 11, and 12 out of 15). This was never the case on the second 3 swings (the highest was 10 out of 14).

Experiment 2

Before concluding that batters swung lower because they saw the ball lower, I ran a control experiment to check the possibility that the batters swung lower because the manipulation had somehow altered their ability to swing. Before the experiment, subjects practiced hitting a target position on a 2" × 2" wooden stake until they could hit it consistently with their eyes closed. Then the two sessions proceeded as above except that subjects did not swing at a ball. Instead they swung with their eyes closed at the remembered target position on the 2" × 2" wooden stake. Session 2 minus session 1 shift on this test should have been downward if the eye and head manipulation caused people to swing lower. In fact, there was no shift.

Experiment 3

Since swinging at the stake was not as difficult as swinging at the ball, would similar effects occur? I repeated the control experiment with the difference that subjects opened their eyes briefly before each swing at the stake. They saw one of five target positions spaced equally within 2 inches of each side of the original remembered target position. They closed their eyes before swinging so they could not visually guide the bat, and they attempted to hit the target they had seen. In this experiment, there was a significant downward shift of 0.56 inches, $p < .01$. Taken together, the experiments 1 and 3 suggest that being tilted back and holding an upward direction of gaze for 1 minute before batting causes batters to swing low because they see the ball as lower than it actually is.

Experiment 4

Having shown that Minor Motor Anomalies disturb vision against a homogeneous background of darkness and against a fully structured environment, comparisons between the two situations were not possible. Using the everyday structured environment of my laboratory, I had subjects perform a simple eye-hand coordination task either in the structured environment or in a homogeneous dark environment. Figure 5 shows the backgrounds that subjects saw when they faced each of the four walls of the lab, which was decorated like an office.

If you look carefully, you can also see a small luminescent target mounted on top of a box in the foreground. Tests of eye-hand coordination were given by having subjects slide a pointer directly under the target. During the test subjects' heads were free to move and the box hid their hand and arm from view. A prettest was given with the lights on and with the lights off; then a series of 1 min exposure periods were given with a posttest after each. During the exposure periods, subjects held their eyes 60° to the right or left while their heads were supported by a chin rest. On half the posttest the lights were on; on the other half

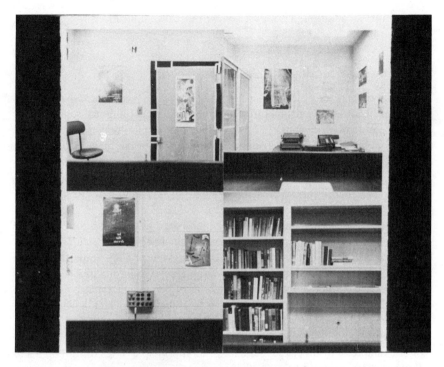

FIG. 5.   Background that subjects saw when they faced each of the four walls of a lab decorated like an office. Upper left is south wall. Upper right is north wall. Lower left is west wall. Lower right is east wall.

the lights were out. The order of testing in the light and dark was counterbalanced across subjects. On the posttest, subjects always faced the wall that was toward their back on the pretest. The foreground was also changed to a different contact paper pattern.

The dependent measure was the degree of posttest minus pretest shifts in pointing at targets after the exposure periods as a function of the lighting during the pointing test. An analysis of variance showed that Minor Motor Anomalies cause significant pointing errors in a fully structured visual environment (2.52 cm; $p < .01$) and that these errors are signficantly smaller than those obtained in the dark (4.83 cm; $p < .01$).

THEORETICAL AND PRACTICAL IMPLICATIONS

Most of the remaining discussion will focus on theoretical implications with a few words at the end reserved for practical implications. The emphasis will be on implications for sensorimotor theories and ecological theories of visuomotor coordination. In addition, a brief section will discuss implications for theories of visual learning.

Sensorimotor Theories and Ecological Theories

These experiments may allow discrimination between sensorimotor theories and ecological theories of visuomotor coordination. According to sensorimotor theories, a critical process in seeing direction is the central registration of direction of gaze by means of nonvisual information within the oculomotor system (e.g., von Holtst & Mitelstaedt, 1950; Matin, 1976; Shebilske, 1977b; Skavenski, 1976). According to ecological theories, visual information is sufficient for, and motor information is irrelevant to, the perception of direction (e.g., Gibson, 1966, 1979; Turvey, 1977, 1979).

Most experiments on the functional significance of visual information use moving environments to simulate observer movement or use actual head and body movement (see Shebilske, 1977a, for a review). They show that visual motion information completely preempts proprioceptive information. These experiments have not only contributed to theories of perception but also to safety in aviation. They tell us little, however, about the situation in which a nonlocomoting observer explores his or her environment with eye movements. On this topic, ecological theories have many hypotheses, but little data.

For example, Gibson (1966) stated a general principle of ecological optics as follows: "the perception of a unitary constant object over time, or of a unitary visual world over time, might be explained by the assumption that unchanging [visual] information underlies the changing sequence of obtained stimulation, and that it gets attended to" [p. 251]. This principle can be applied to all the perceptual constancies including visual direction constancy for which Gibson stated a more specific hypothesis: "any two successive samples have a large overlap since the maximum excursion of an eye movement cannot approach the angular field of the eye, and the same is true of a head movement. The amount of overlap is the amount of structure common to the two samples. It is permanence in change or, in mathematical terms, the invariance under transformation" [Gibson, 1966, p. 261-262]. Tacit in this hypothesis is a device that samples the structure of the ambient array and, based on invariance, directly gives a constant perception of egocentric direction despite changes in oculocentric direction.

Gibson (1950) also recognized that an observer who is asked to judge the direction of an object relative to himself can see both the object and himself. He speculated, along with others before him that the perception of body parts, including the nose, is an important source of visual information for seeing direction (cf. Fick, 1905; Mach, 1885). The most recent rendition of this hypothesis was stated by Bower (1974) as follows: "the location of objects relative to the observer is possible only if the observer can see himself and the object to be located. We are saying that the retinal position of the nose and orbit specify the observer's position to himself. If this information is available, position perception will be accurate. If it is not available, position perception will be innaccurate" [p. 51]. Shebilske and Nice (1976) tested this hypothesis and found that direction judgments were not improved by nose visibility suggesting that Bower's strong claim must be qualified. But the importance of seeing body parts for making direction judgments remains a possibility.

A third hypothesis was proposed by Linksz (1952) who suggested that static perspective information may be critical in seeing direction. He illustrated his idea with a lamp shade. At the horizon, the base of the shade would project a single horizontal line on the retina; above the horizon, the bottom of the shade image would be elliptical. The shape of the ellipse would indicate the direction of the shade with respect to the horizon. Hidden in this example is the importance of using an object with a familiar orientation like the horizontal orientation of a lamp shade; the object's egocentric orientation would have to be known before static perspective could indicate direction. Therefore, this is the least parsimonious model considered so far. It bears an uncanny resemblance to modern artificial intelligence models that are notorious for their disregard for parsimony. For example, in Minsky's (1975) framework model he states that the constancies depend on "the confirmation of expectations which in turn depends on rapid access to remembered knowledge about the visual world" [p. 221]. Applying this to direction constancy, Minsky notes that we have considerable knowledge and expectations about the orientations and directions of contours in most environments. For instance, in a room, we know that the floor-wall texture boundary is horizontal and that it is below eye level; in outdoor scenes, we know that the horizon is horizontal on flat ground and so on. In familiar rooms and landscapes, even richer landmarks would be available to build an internal representation of where things are located. In Minsky's model, expectations serve as null hypotheses for perceptions, and, in that sense, the model is like MacKay's (1973) model of direction constancy.

In summary, there are potential sources of visual information about direction that could operate for nonlocomoting observers who are exploring their environment with eye movements. These can be grouped into three classes according to the hypothesized source of information as follows:

1. structural overlap,
2. visibility of body parts, and
3. static perspective plus expectations.

Prior to the present experiments, there were no observations that proved that any of the three alleged sources of information are actually used. However, there were some relevant, albeit inconclusive, results. When observers attempt to point to targets with their unseen hand, they are much more variable when the targets are viewed against a homogenous background of darkness (von Kries, 1962).

Similarly, when one watches a single light in an otherwise dark environment, its apparent location is highly variable. The light appears to glid, jerk, and swoop through space in what has been called autokinetic movement. These results are consistent with the claim that visual structure contributes metric information about direction. However, reduction of variability can be explained without assuming that higher-order visual information is directly processed for seeing direction. In principle, visual localization in this task could depend on proprioceptive information about eye-in-head position and the proprioceptive information could be less variable in a structured environment. For instance, Skavenski and Steinman (1970) and Matin, Matin, and Pearce (1969) argue that eye position maintenance depends on two separate control systems, one based on visual feedback and another based on proprioception. The visual feedback system is more stable and dominates in a structured setting. In darkness, the proprioceptive system takes over but with much less precision. This effect has been implicated in explanations of the autokinetic effect (e.g., Matin & MacKinnon, 1964) and could be responsible for the difference in the variability of pointing in a structured environment and in darkness.

This alternative explanation is consistent with another observation that raises doubt about all the hypotheses about the contribution of static visual information. People with paralyzed eye muscles see the world move in the direction of intended eye movements that in turn cause pointing errors (e.g., Stevens, Emerson, Gerstein, Neufeld, Nichols, & Rosenquist, 1976). These errors are contrary to all the above hypotheses because the errors happen in the presence of all three alleged sources of visual information: structural overlap, visible body parts, and static perspective plus expectations.

Although none of the authors of the visual information hypotheses have commented on these results, it would be possible for them to speculate that visual information dominates except in extreme cases like paralysis (or externally caused eye movements) where there is a large difference between retinal and extraretinal information. This kind of argument has some precedence. For example, Gibson (1966, p. 262) made a similar point in relation to another observation. He stated that "the anatomical fact of an approximate 'wiring system' from retina to brain has nothing to do with perception. It is evidenced on occasion, as when an after-sensation burned into the retina persists at the photochemical level. This illusion then seems to sweep across the structure of the optic array when the eye is turned; it 'moves with the eye' as we say. But the nervous system surely did not evolve to pick up these subjective sensations. They are incidental." This kind of argument must be taken seriously because all commonly used perceptual mechanisms may have boundary conditions, beyond which qualitatively different process take over. The two eye position maintenance systems are examples. This argument also applies to all experiments showing that motor information influences the perception of direction in the dark.

There are two problems with previous observations about the contribution of visual information: (1) the positive evidence involves the reduction of *random error* and therefore can be explained by the assumption that visual stimulation merely stabalizes proprioceptive information, and (2) the negative evidence can be ignored because it involves *extreme conditions* that may lie outside the boundary conditions of the commonly used perceptual mechanisms. The experiments reported in this chapter overcome both of these problems.

Minor Motor Anomalies induce *constant errors* rather than random errors and they are induced by *common conditions,* which have been available to pressure the evolution of perceptual mechanisms. According to sensorimotor theories, the constant error induced by Minor Motor Anomalies should have been manifested equally in dark and light conditions. According to ecological theories, the visual direction illusion observed in the dark should be eliminated in the lighted condition that provided structural overlap, visible body parts, and static perspective, plus expectations.

The results contradicted both these predictions. On the one hand, visual direction illusions were significant in fully structured, well illuminated environments. This is contrary to the view that oculomotor information is irrelevant to the perception of direction. The baseball experiment, which allowed batters to hit the way they normally do, is the best evidence to date that oculomotor information is taken into account in seeing direction even when higher-order visual information is available. Thus, while I agree with Turvey's (1977, 1979) argument that at present there is no apparent evolutionary or logical reason for oculomotor information to be taken into account when higher-order visual information is present, I conclude that oculomotor information is taken into account nevertheless. On the other hand, the illusion was significantly smaller in the light. This is the best evidence to date that higher-order visual information is used to see direction even when people are not locomoting. Future experiments, will have to isolate the relevant source or sources of higher-order visual information. Future experiments will also have to clarify how people intergrate visual and nonvisual sources of direction information. If the present conclusions are on track, then out of these future experiments will emerge logical and evolutionary reasons why both kinds of information are used.

Minor Motor Anomalies and Visual Learning

The illusions studied here can be compared to similar illusions induced by visual rearrangements through the use of prisms and other devices. Traditionally, rearrangement illusions have been explained in terms of central visual learning (e.g., Epstein, 1975; Craske & Crawshaw, 1978; Howard, 1968; Rock, 1966; Wallach & Halperin, 1977). Recently, Ebenholtz and others have pointed out that most, if not all, the results in rearrangement experiments can be explained in terms of peripheral muscle physiology without assumptions about central learning (e.g., Ebenholtz, 1974, this volume; Paap & Ebenholtz, 1976; Willey, Gyr, & Henry, 1978). We now know that many rearrangement experiments confound opportunity for learning with conditions that produce Minor Motor Anomalies without the opportunity for learning. But we cannot conclude with certainty that visual learning contributes nothing to temporary alterations in space perception.

I want to consider the possibility that visual learning does contribute to sensory-motor recalibration. If so, Minor Motor Anomalies are much more than an artifact to be avoided in tests of recalibration theories. They could be the principle reason for the evolution of learning mechanism that make temporary sensory-motor recalibrations. One can explain why such adjustments would be adaptive if one assumes, as above, that there is some evolutionary reason for attending to oculomotor information, and that this information is subject to transitory disturbances from Minor Motor Anomalies.

Practical Applications

One application that has not been considered so far is in ophthalmology. Future experiments should explore the relationship between Minor Motor Anomalies and major motor disorders. Are the factors used to cope with Minor Motor Anomalies (e.g. higher-order visual information) also important in coping with major motor disorders? Could patients be trained to take better advantage of higher-order visual information?

More immediate applications are in sports and aviation. For pilots, the direction of locomotion is usually specified by the center of the outflow of optical texture. This information is either not available, or only minimally available, to baseball batters depending upon when, and to what extent they stride forward during their swing. Therefore, it is not safe to generalize from the above experiments to pilots who have unambiguous direction information from outflowing optical texture. However, as mentioned earlier, visual motion information is sometimes ambiguous during night approaches. In this situation, pilots may have even less visual information about direction then did the baseball players in the present experiments. Thus, existing research seems to justify examining whether or not pilots suffer illusory visual direction caused by Minor Motor Anomalies. This should be investigated under actual or realistically simulated flight conditions because the effect of the illusion is likely to interact with work load, terrain slope, and the specific visual information attended to by different pilots. If the visual direction illusion proves to be an important factor, we should be able to find ways to reduce or avoid the conditions that induce the illusions.

ACKNOWLEDGMENT

The preparation of this chapter was supported by NIE Grant R01-EY02291-01.

How Pursuit Eye Movements can Convert Temporal into Spatial Information

II.4

M. J. Morgan
University of Durham, England

I would like to describe a class of visual phenomena that occurs when we attempt to pursue a moving target with our eyes. These phenomena arise because during smooth pursuit there is little or no compensation for changes in retinal position caused by the eye movements themselves (cf. Festinger, Sedgwick, & Holtzman, 1976). However, it would be incorrect to think of these effects as "illusions." On the contrary, as we shall see, they allow us to perceive objects veridically in some rather surprising circumstances.

An early report of this phenomenon was by Mach in the well-known paper on the Mach-Dvorak effect (Mach, 1872). This described the effect of looking at a horizontally moving target through an episcotister, which is simply a rapidly revolving disc with a slit that gives the observer periodic brief glimpses of the target. If both eyes are used, the slit exposes the two eyes successively, so that there is an inter-ocular delay in viewing the moving target. Since the target moves during the delay, a retinal disparity is induced, which causes the target to appear shifted in depth, exactly as in the Pulfrich stereophenomenon (where the delay is caused by reducing the intensity of the stimulus in one eye.) This is the much-quoted conclusion of the Mach-Dvorak paper, and it is not very surprising. However, Mach further noted that the effect was seen only if the eyes were kept steadily fixated; if they were permitted to track the moving target, the depth effect was either substantially reduced, or even disappeared. This latter finding, which is easy to replicate, has interesting implications. Presumably the eyes must have moved during the inter-ocular delay so as to parallel the movement of the target, thus removing the retinal disparity. Moreover, there was evidently no compensation of visual direction for the movement of the eye during the inter-ocular delay. If ther had been such compensation, the visual direction of the target in

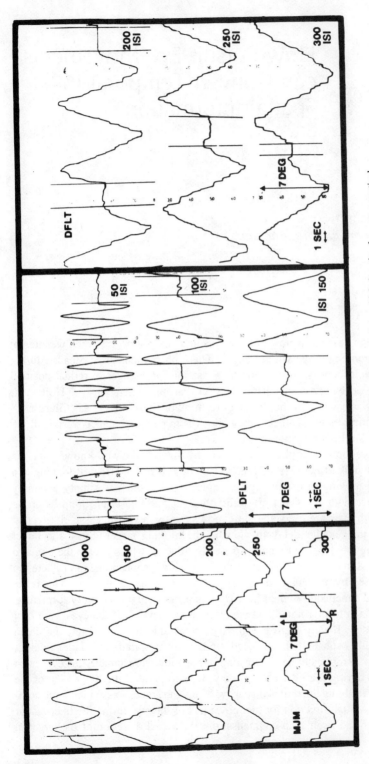

FIG. 1. Horizontal eye movement records from a tracking task in which the stimulus was a vertical bar in discontinuous (apparent) motion with a range of different ISI's: Left panel: subject MJM, ISI's 100–300 msec. Middle panel: subject DFLT, ISI's 50–150 msec. Right panel: subject DFLT, ISI's 200–300 msec. In each panel the ISI increases from top to bottom.

the two eyes would have been different, even though the retinal positions were in correspondence, and the depth effect would not have been abolished by tracking.

The first implication, that the eyes can smoothly track an object even when it is visible only intermittently, has abundant supporting evidence (Westheimer, 1954). In a recent study (Morgan & Turnbull, 1978), we looked at the temporal limits of such tracking. If the interval between target presentations (the ISI) is lengthened, at what point will smooth pursuit be replaced by a series of saccadic eye movements? We found that ISI's up to about 150 msec supported nearly pure pursuit with a target velocity up to 9 deg/sec. Above 150 msec saccades began to intrude progressively, but it is not possible to establish a definite point at which pursuit could be said to have broken down. One interesting finding was that in all the subjects, saccades were much more likely to intrude in one direction of tracking (i.e., left to right) than the other. This is clear in the records shown in Fig. 1. We thought at first that there might be a systematic asymmetry favouring smoother pursuit in the right-left direction, but further testing proved otherwise. The asymmetry appears to be idiosynchratic, and uncorrelated with the subject's preferred hand for writing.

Thus smooth pursuit of a moving target is possible, even when the image of the target is not moving smoothly on the retina. In the situation described by Mach (1872), it may be assumed that both eyes were engaged in such pursuit with a temporal phase lag between their respective targets. To keep the image of the target on the foveas of both eyes, it would suffice to pursue the target with the eyes converged on the real depth plane of the motion. Thus the target will be seen at its correct depth. If this is the case, however, it is clear that there is no compensation for movement of the eyes during the interocular delay. Suppose the leading eye in some way "remembered" the direction in space in which it was pointing when it was presented with the target, and retained this information until the lagging eye was presented with its target. Then target depth could be computed from the vergence angle between this remembered direction and the current direction of the lagging eye. This would result in the target's being localized at a virtual position in front or behind the real depth plane. It is just as well that this clever mechanism is not actually used, for if it were, the target would be mislocalized in depth! The simpler mechanism, which takes no account of the relative temporal delay between the eyes at all, is actually the more effective.

The explanation of these effects is not particularly controversial, but I turn to another kind of phenomenon where the role of eye movements is much less clear. This is the celebrated "neue Art anorthoskopischer Zerrbilder" described by Zöllner (1862), and the subject of numerous conflicting accounts up to the present day. Zöllner reported that if a line drawing were moved backwards and forwards behind a narrow slit observers saw the whole shape represented by the drawing, even if the slit was considerably more narrow than the figure itself. The important point here is that it was the figure that was moved, not the slit. It was well known before Zöllner's experiment that a shape could be perceived behind a rapidly moving slit, as in Plateau's (1850) Anorthoscopic machine: And this was not too surprising, since it demonstrates nothing more than persistence of vision. But when the figure rather than the slit moved, all the successively exposed parts of the figure should fall on top of one another, so even with persistence of vision there would be no spatially extended shape on the retina. This is why Zöllner called it a "new kind of Anorthoscopic figure," and why it has been claimed by other investigators of the phenomenon, e.g., Cattell (1900), that it demonstrates the inadequacy of the retinal-picture theory of shape perception.

It was pointed out by Helmholtz (1909/1962), however, that the effect could be explained equally well by assuming that the eyes tracked the moving figure, thereby causing an image to be "painted out" on the retina. Note that if the eyes move, the display becomes equivalent to one in which the slit is moved while the figure is fixed; thus the effect would not be a "new kind" of anorthoscopic effect at all. In support of this explanation, Helmholtz cited the fact that the figure is frequently seen as compressed in the direction of motion. This is exactly what would be expected if the eyes move more slowly than the target, for in these circumstances the retinal image would become compressed. It is plausible that tracking has a less than unity gain in these circumstances, because the only movement actually visible is that within the slit, which presents only a small fraction of the real target motion.

If Helmholtz's explanation is correct, the phenomenon resembles the one described by Mach (1872), in showing that there is imperfect compensation for changes in retinal location produced by smooth eye movements. The successive parts of the figure are presented in the same spatial location (inside the slit); but tracking will cause them to fall on different retinal points. If the result is that the figure is seen as spatially extended beyond the boundary of the slit, the conclusion that follows is that retinal extension due to eye movements is not distinguishable from retinal extension due to spatial extension in the outside world.

But is the "retinal painting" hypothesis an accurate account of Zöllner's anorthoscopic effect? Zöllner himself, and some later investigators, have asserted that the effect can be seen even if the eyes remain fixated on the slit. The literature has been well reviewed by Anstis and Atkinson (1967), who themselves supported the retinal painting hypothesis, thus I shall not attempt to describe it here. The most recent development is a paper by McCloskey and Watkins (1978), which claims that tracking eye movements are not necessary for the perception of shape. Thus this problem has not been resolved, despite more than 100 years of investigation. One reason for this may be that very little is known about the actual eye movements that occur when observers are attempting to recognize shapes moving behind a slit. If more data were available on this question, it might be easier to decide the theoretical issue. Another problem is that psychophysical data are lacking to demonstrate what kinds of shape recognition, if any, are possible when the observer is forced to make decisions between several alternatives. Nor are experiments available comparing the recognition of shapes moving behind slits with recognition of normally moving shapes of the same velocity. In the remainder of this chapter, experiments will be described that examine these issues.

In all the Experiments that follow, the appearance of shapes moving behind one or more slits was simulated on an oscilloscope screen under computer control. It is possible to do this by generating a moving shape on the screen using normal methods of $X-Y$ plotting and then to view the shape through a cardboard slit placed in front of the screen. In practice, the same result may be produced with greater convenience by intensifying the image of the moving shape only when it occurs within the boundaries of a notional slit on the screen. The difference between such a notional slit and a real one is that the notional slit is visible only when the shape is being plotted, whereas the real slit is visible all the time. As we shall see, there is no problem in observing Zöllner's effect through notional slits. But the possibility should be born in mind that some of the detailed results thus obtained might have been different if real slits had been used.

Since visual persistence is clearly crucial in these experiments, it is important that it should not be complicated by physical persistence of the signals. Therefore, a fast-decay P15 phosphor was used to ensure that the screen image disappeared within several microseconds of plotting. Further details of the display and computer-generated patterns will be found in a previous publication (Morgan, 1980).

Eye movements were recorded by locating the limbus with an infra-red reflection device (Findlay, 1974). The stem of a fibre-optic Y guide placed approximately 5mm from the front surface of the cornea acted both as the emitter of band-pass filtered infra-red light and as the collector of the reflected radiation, which was routed to a sensitive detector for conversion to an analog voltage signal. This signal was in turn sampled by the computer (Alpha LSI 20G) and stored on disc for further analysis. The subject's head movements were restrained by a bite bar and by a polystyrene vacuum head moulding. The recording system was sensitive to eye movements of approximately 2 min arc, but its accuracy was severely limited by DC shifts in the course of a recording session. In the following account I shall be concerned only with movements of the eye, and not with the absolute direction of the eye in space, the latter being difficult to precisely determine.

Experiment 1

The aim of the first experiment was to see if observers could in fact make pursuit eye movements to follow a target moving backwards and forwards behind a slit. Of particular interest were the following two questions: (1) How wide would the slit have to be before pursuit was possible? In other words, how much real as opposed to imagined motion is necessary for tracking eye movements? (2) Would the amplitude of tracking, if it occurred, be confined to the aperture of the slit, or

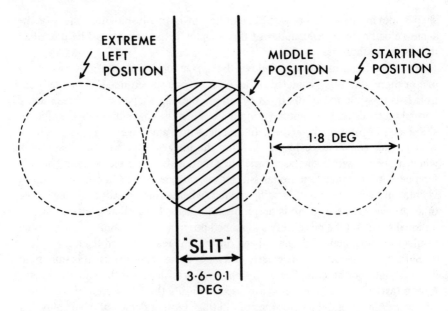

FIG. 2.   Representation of the stimulus for Experiment 1, in which an outline circle oscillated behind a slit. The circle was visible only within the confines of the slit.

would it to some extent follow the object outside the slit? This is important, because if the eye movements can occur only inside the slit, the image painted on the retina will be very compressed, while if tracking can follow the real target trajectory, the image will become more veridical.

The target in this experiment was an outline circle 1.8° in diameter moving behind a slit that varied in width between 0.1 and 3.6°. The circle oscillated in linear motion between left and right with a peak-to-peak amplitude of 3.6°. The velocity of movement was varied between 3.6 deg/sec^{-1} (0.5 Hz) and 18.0 deg/sec^{-1} (2.5 Hz). Figure 2 shows the display diagrammatically.

Phenomenal Impressions

There was a strong tendency to see an extended shape moving behind a slit on the screen. The boundaries of the slit appeared very clearly (like a "cognitive contour") even though they were defined entirely by the disappearance of the moving figure. The figure was rarely seen as exactly circular, but rather as an ellipse with the minor axis pointing in the direction of motion. Typically, the figure appeared to be wider than the slit. However, in the narrowest slit condition (0.1 deg) used, no extended shape was seen; the impression was rather of line segments moving up and down inside the slit.

Eye Movements

Typical eye movement records for an experienced subject under several different conditions are shown in Fig. 3. The separation between the horizontal lines to the left of each record represents the amplitude of an eye movement that would correspond to the slit width in that condition. This was determined by a calibration procedure before each condition, in the course of which the subject made repeated saccades between two points 3.6° apart. The eye movement amplitude corresponding to a given slit width was then determined by interpolation, after ascertaining that the record was linear over the 3.6° calibration range.

The records show a complicated pattern of pursuit and saccadic eye movements. Pursuit occurs even with slits as small as 0.22°, and was frequently of a peak-to-peak amplitude greater than the slit width. A particularly clear example of this is seen with subject AS in the condition where a 3.6 deg/sec^{-1} stimulus moved behind a 0.22° wide slit (see Fig. 3). Here the tracking movements tended to be more pronounced in one direction (left to right) than in the other. This was also clear with the 0.22° slit in the 6.0 deg/sec^{-1} and 9.0 deg/sec^{-1} velocity conditions.

To treat these data quantitatively a series of 5 trials at each slit-velocity combination was given to two subjects (the author and AS). Before each block of trials the eye movements were calibrated, and then on each trial 5 cycles of the stimulus were presented. Each trial was preceded by a 1-sec fixation point. Eye position was sampled every 10 msec and the records were stored on disc for later analysis. The analysis was aimed at determining, separately for each cycle of stimulus movement, the peak-to-peak amplitude of the longest period of unidirectional smooth pursuit, and the mean velocity of that same period of pursuit. Unidirectional smooth pursuit was considered to include those cases containing one or more saccades in the reverse direction to the pursuit, but not those cases where there was a saccade in the same direction. Velocity was calculated by taking a typical 100 msec period of the pursuit and multiplying its amplitude (deg) by 10 to obtain the velocity in sec^{-1}. Finally, the 25 separate samples (5 trials × 5 cycles) were used to calculate means and standard deviations of the amplitude and velocity measures.

Some representative results are shown in Fig. 4, with vertical bars representing standard deviation, to give an idea of the variability of the observations. In the top two panels the slit size is held constant while velocity is varied; in the bottom two panels the velocity is always 3.6 deg/sec^{-1} and the slit size is varied between 0.1 and 3.6°. Although the variability is quite large, it is clear that the amplitude of pursuit, except at the extreme slit widths of 3.6° and 0.1°, tends to be greater than that of the slit. With the smallest slit (0.1°) no pursuit occurred at all. Velocities seem to be quite well matched to actual target motion,

AS: 3·6 deg/sec

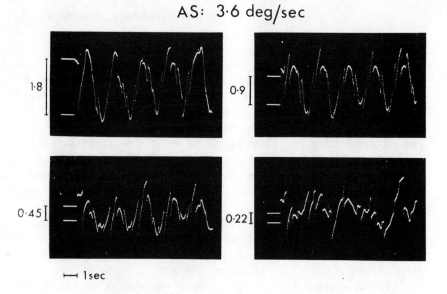

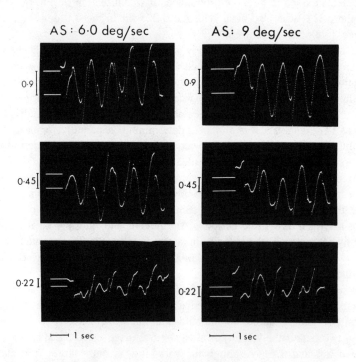

FIG. 3. Eye movement records from one subject (AS) tracking a circle moving behind a slit (see Fig. 2). The pair of horizontal lines to the left of each panel show the visual angle subtended by the slit. Representative records are shown for three different velocities: 3.6, 6.0 and 9.0 deg/sec^{-1}. Note that episodes of smooth pursuit often have an amplitude greater than the slit.

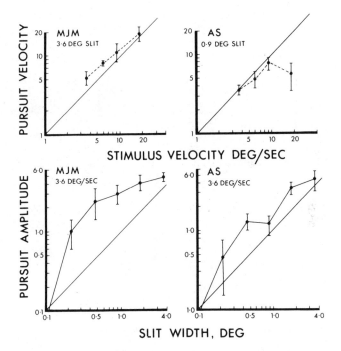

FIG. 4. Quantitative data derived from records such as those in Fig. 3. The top two panels show, for subjects AS and MJM respectively, the mean and standard deviation of the velocity of smooth pursuit episodes. The bottom two panels show corresponding data for pursuit amplitude. No tracking was observed in the 0.1° slit width condition. Points falling above the continuous diagonal line show a higher velocity or amplitude of the eye movement than that of the stimulus. Note that pursuit amplitude is typically greater than slit width. For further explanation of the method of analysis see text (Experiment 1).

except for a loss in gain at the highest velocity used (18 deg/sec^{-1}) for subject AS.

The results for all velocities and slit width for the two subjects are collected together in Fig. 5, which like Fig. 4 shows velocity as a variable in the upper panels and slit width as a variable in the lower panels. The figure shows that the effects just described hold over a wide range of conditions, except that with the highest velocity (18 deg/sec^{-1}) the pursuit amplitude is never greater than the slit width for AS, and is almost zero for both subjects with the 0.22° slit. In the slit-width range 0.22 – 1.8° and the velocity range 3.6 – 9.0 deg/sec^{-1}, the smooth pursuit typically goes outside the boundaries of the slit.

The main conclusion of this experiment is that an object can indeed be tracked with smooth pursuit eye movements as it moves behind the slit, and the movements can be greater than the angle of the slit itself. This could explain the classical observation that the object seen through the slit frequently appears wider

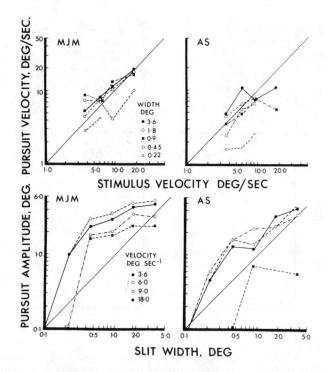

FIG. 5. The result from all combinations of slit width and stimulus velocity, plotted as in Fig. 4, but without standard deviation bars. Note that the amplitude of pursuit is typically greater than the slit width, except at the smallest slit widths and highest velocities. There was no pursuit when the slit width was 0.1°.

than the slit. It actually is producing by "retinal painting" a wider retinal image than would be expected if it were statically visible through the slit. Moreover, these observations show why the shape is compressed in the direction of motion: This could be predicted from the fact that the eye movement amplitude, while greater than the slit width, is not as great as the real stimulus movement. This must lead to a fore-shortening of the retinal image of the moving object, similar to that seen when taking a photograph of a fast-object with a relatively slowly moving focal plane slit-shutter. The undermatching of pursuit amplitude appears to be mainly due to slowing down at the ends of the cycle, rather than to undermatching of peak velocity, and this should lead to greater distortions at the end of the figure than in the middle. This was difficult to establish in the present experiment because the stimulus was a circle, but we did note that the stimulus typically appeared as an elliptical form, as predicted by "retinal painting."

Why is the stimulus pursued beyond the boundary of the slit? It is well known that tracking does not stop immediately as the pursued target disappears (Mitrani & Dimitrov, 1978) and this is an obvious explanation. Another possibility, however, is that tracking outside the slit boundary could be maintained by the extrafoveal movement of the object *inside* the slit. Winterson and Steinman (1978) showed that even inexperienced subjects could track a target located 6° below the line of sight. If the same can occur with a horizontally displaced target, this mechanism could account for tracking outside the boundary of the slit. There is no evidence available at present to decide between the two explanations.

Experiment 2

The previous experiment showed that a shape moving behind a slit could produce eye pursuit, provided that the slit is sufficiently wide. However, this does not decide the central question of whether such pursuit is necessary for perception of shape. To tackle this question we need to establish some method of preventing pursuit. A technique that has been used in other contexts (Westheimer & McKee, 1978) exploits the fact that smooth pursuit has a latency of about 150 msec; therefore stimulus presentations briefer than this are unlikely to elicit eye pursuit. If nevertheless a shape could be seen in these conditions, this would be a decisive demonstration that pursuit is not required. Of course, the converse is not necessarily true; if shape recognition were not possible, this might be for a variety of reasons, like the exposure being too brief to give rise to the perception of a moving oblect. Further controls would be necessary to investigate this and other possibilities. Unfortunately, when this method was attempted with a shape moving behind a single slit, severe problems were encountered. A single brief (150 msec) passage of the shape behind the slit was found to produce neither an impression of motion, nor one of shape. It appears that a single sweep of the stimulus behind the slit is not sufficient to produce Zöllner's effect; the to-and-fro oscillation is an intrinsic part of the proceedings. Equally, however, several fast oscillations within a 150 msec period failed to produce any impression of movement. One might wish to claim that this proves the importance of eye movements, but it could equally well be maintained that it is due to the absence of perceived motion in the display. Thus it was necessary to use a display in which even a brief exposure of the stimulus would still produce an impression of motion.

It turns out that this can be done quite readily by replacing the single slit with a series of slits, arranged along the direction of motion. Suppose, for example, that the shape is to be moved from right to left. The temporally-successive parts of the figure are first plotted all on top of one another in the leftmost slit, as described in Experiment 1. Then the plotting sequence is repeated in the next slit to the right, and so on. This provides a compelling impression of apparent motion from right to left, even for brief exposures. A further reason for examining such a display is that it has been suggested by Ross (1977) that it can produce an Anorthoscopic effect without eye movements. Ross has devised a display consisting of light-emitting diodes stacked in vertical strips spaced out on a long display panel. The diodes in each strip are turned on and off as if a picture were moving continuously along the display, causing each strip to light up in accordance with the column of the figure currently aligned with it. Although at any one instant of time the information presented on the display consists only of a number of vertically-aligned illuminated diodes, the display as a whole gives a very compelling impression of a shape in motion.

Such a display can be very readily simulated on an oscilloscope screen, using points of light instead of light-emitting diodes. In the following experiment this technique was used to simulate the appearance of an outline triangle moving behind slits. The sequence of events when the triangle passes by two such slits is shown in Fig. 6. Note that the abscissa of this figure is not space but time: the figure is plotted in vertical cross sections every 1 msec. Each of these vertical cross sections through the shape is plotted inside the same notional slit on the screen until the whole shape has been plotted: Then the whole sequence begins again in a slit displaced to the right, and so on. The top of the figure shows how

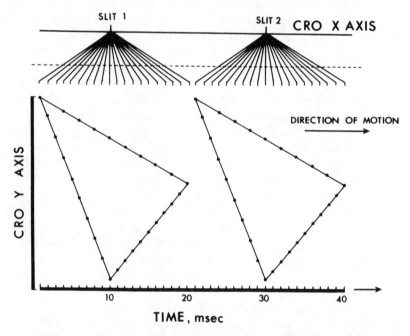

FIG. 6. The method of plotting shapes on a cathode ray oscilloscope (CRO) to simulate their appearance when moving behind narrow vertical slits. The shape, an outline triangle composed of dots, is plotted at one slit position in a number of successive 1 msec slices; and then is plotted in exactly the same way at the next slit position to the right. The converging lines at the top of the figure are meant to illustrate the mapping of time on to space. Thus the successive time-slices of the figure converge on to the same X position of the CRO and are plotted on top of each other. For further explanation see text.

the temporally-successive slices of the figure are gathered together at the same slit position. We shall refer to a shape plotted in this way as a zero-extended shape. Observers were required to carry out a shape recognition task in which the triangle was in one of 4 orientations (vertical and/or horizontal mirror images of Fig. 6.) The stimuli were designed so that time-averaged luminance at different heights in the slit was not a cue. Thus the triangle was never plotted as a spatially extended whole, and its temporally successive parts were plotted at the same spatial positions. Nevertheless, it was found that the display gave a compelling impression of a moving triangle, over a wide range of inter-slit widths and virtual velocities. The shape recognition task could be carried out with ease. It was also found that the display was producing pursuit eye movements in the direction of the apparent motion of the triangle. These movements would have painted the temporally successive slices of the figure on different retinal meridians, possibly accounting for the perception of the shape.

The next question was whether or not shape perception could occur in the absence of such eye movements. The moving triangle was therefore confined to a 5-slit sequence, and random direction of movement on different trials, for 100 msec. The interslit width was 18 min arc and the virtual velocity 12 deg/sec^{-1}. Three visually-psychophysically experienced (MJM, JMF, AJS) and two unpractised (DFE, CKK) observers attempted the shape recognition task in these circumstances. They were unable to perform above chance: The display simply appeared like a vertical bar in movement from slit to slit. Eye movement recording in these conditions confirmed that there was no pursuit.

The result might indicate that 100 msec is too brief for any kind of shape recognition. To examine this possibility, a real spatially-extended triangle was plotted in apparent motion with the same virtual velocity (12 deg/sec^{-1}) for 100 msec. The plotting sequence was exactly as in Fig. 6 except that now the temporally successive slices of the figure were plotted at different screen positions. (Consider, for example, the CRO X axis to correspond to the horizontal broken line at the top of the figure). In this way it was possible to vary the real width of the triangle on the screen between 0 (the original condition) and 18 min arc (the full inter-slit width). The results (Fig. 7) showed that accuracy of shape report rose markedly as the shape width increased. Recognition reached an asymptote at about 2 min arc in the experienced observers but increased more slowly in the two others.

Finally, we repeated a demonstration of Anstis and Atkinson (1967), showing that if eye tracking is induced in the opposite direction to the movement sequence of the shape, then the shape is perceived as its mirror image. A continuously moving spot on the same oscilloscope was used to induce tracking. When the tracking spot and the shape moved in opposite directions, the shape was indeed seen as its mirror-image around a vertical axis of symmetry. This meant that in the shape recognition task, the subjects' responses were the mirror image of those they produced when allowed to track the shape in the direction of apparent

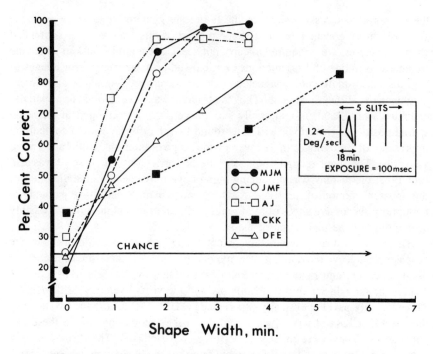

FIG. 7.   The ability of 5 observers to identify the orientation of a horizontally-moving triangle, plotted on a CRO as in Fig. 1. The differing shape widths (abscissa) were generated by varying the mapping of time on to space as in Fig. 1. For zero shape width, all the time-slices are plotted at the same X position; larger widths are obtained if the time-slices fall on different X positions, as would be the case with the dotted line in Fig. 1 corresponding to the CRO X axis.

motion. Such a result cannot be explained by supposing that the observers' deduced the hidden shape from its temporal fragments, because the sequence of fragments was the same under the two conditions, only the direction of eye pursuit differing. On the other hand, the effect is exactly predicted from the geometry of "retinal painting."

Supporters of "post-retinal storage" might argue that our simulation technique provided the observers with insufficient information about the moving shape to produce a true anorthoscopic effect. Rock and Sigman (1973) and Rock and Gilchrist (1975) have postulated that enough information must be present for the observer to form the correct perceptual hypothesis of a partly occluded shape. But our subjects were clearly informed of the purpose of the simulation, and none had any difficulty in perceiving the extended moving shape when allowed to track it with their eyes. We do not deny that shape recognition would have been facilitated if the virtual slit had been wider allowing more of the shape to be visible as oriented lines, as in Rock and Gilchrist's simulation. There is no doubt that even a shape as complicated as a letter can be deduced from the appearance of its parts behind a slit, if the slit is wide enough and if the observer is permitted to make a cognitive deduction. This point is unsurprising. But the more radical claim that a phenomenally extended shape can be seen from purely temporal information in the absence of retinal extension has no experimental support from this experiment, and the results show that, at the very least, orthodox shape perception from a retinally extended image is very much more rapid and accurate than any deductive process.

Experiment 3

The previous experiment is open to criticism because only a single, rather high, virtual velocity was used (12 deg/sec) and because only one kind of shape (triangles) was investigated. So the experiment was repeated using a lower virtual velocity (1.4 deg/sec), which implies also a smaller amplitude of movement and smaller inter-slit width. The height of each slit was 0.3°, and the exposure time was 125 msec. Eye movement was recorded and analyzed for directional asymmetries to see if these would correlate with differences in psychophysical performance in the two directions of motion. The experiment was carried out initially with the same triangles used in Experiment 2, the observer's task being to identify orientation. The triangles were either of zero real width or had a real width equal to the inter-slit distance, viz 2.7 min arc. Next the experiment was repeated using as a target a single oblique line, the orientation of which had to be discriminated by the observer.

1. Triangles. The stimuli were the same as in Experiment 3. They were presented either for an 11–slit sequence lasting 275 msec, which should have given sufficient time for eye movements to occur; or for only a 5-slit sequence lasting 125 msec, which was expected to be insufficient for eye tracking. Intermediate conditions of 7 and 8 slits were also investigated, although eye movement records were not taken in these sessions for all observers. There were also two different conditions of stimulus width, which were presented in random order within a single testing session. In the "zero width" condition all the temporally-successive slices of the triangle were plotted one on top of each other in the slit; whereas in the "real width" (2.7 min) condition the successive lines were spatially extended. The latter condition corresponds to a conventional apparent-motion stimulus, the former to a moving triangle visible only through a series of narrow slits.

The results of the shape discrimination task in Fig. 8 show that accuracy rose sharply with exposure duration. As in the previous experiment performance was not significantly above chance in the 5–slit (125 msec) exposure condition for the virtual (zero width) shape, but was above chance for the real shape. Analysis of

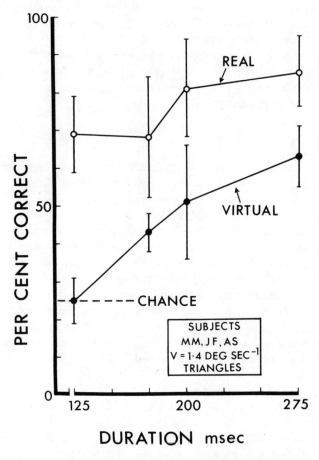

FIG. 8. The mean and standard deviations of the results in Experiment 3, in which 3 observers (MM, JF, and AS) attempted to identify the orientation of an apparently moving triangle. The triangle was presented successively in displaced positions with an ISI of 25 msec to give an impression of motion. At each position, the triangle was either plotted on the screen as a real shape of width 2.7 min arc, or as a "virtual" shape as shown in Fig. 6. The virtual shape condition simulates the appearance of a triangle in movement behind a series of narrow slits. The number of slits was varied in order to control the exposure duration of the stimulus (abscissa). Note that identification of the shape is chance with a duration of 125 msec (5 slits) but rises as exposure duration is increased. Results with the real shape are different; Performance is above chance even with the shortest duration.

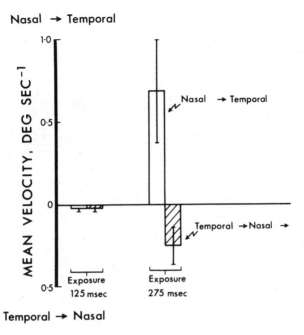

FIG. 9. The mean and standard deviation of pursuit velocity for three observers in Experiment 3, where a triangle had to be identified as it moved behind a series of narrow slits. Results are shown separately for the two directions of stimulus movement (shaded and unshaded bars) and for two different exposure durations: 125 msec (left hand pair of bars) and 275 msec (right hand pair). Velocity was calculated by dividing the amplitude of pursuit during the exposure by the total exposure duration. Note that the velocity in the 125 msec condition is very small and independent of stimulus direction, in contrast to the results with the longer exposure.

variance showed that the effect of exposure duration was significant $F (3,6) = 7.25$, $p < .02$ as was that of shape width $F (1,2) = 26.9$, $p < .05$. The interaction did not prove significant at the 0.05 level of confidence.

The virtual shape again could not be recognized in the condition designed to prevent eye movements, even though a real shape could be recognized in these conditions. To verify that no tracking eye movements were occurring in the 125 msec exposure, records were analyzed by comparing eye positions at the beginning and end of each exposure. The difference between these two positions was calculated, and the mean of these differences compared for the two directions of target motion. The results in Fig. 9 show that in the 125 msec exposure condition there was no difference in the direction of eye movement depending upon direction of target motion. In contrast, there was a very large difference in the 275 msec exposure condition, the eyes tending to move in the same direction as the target.

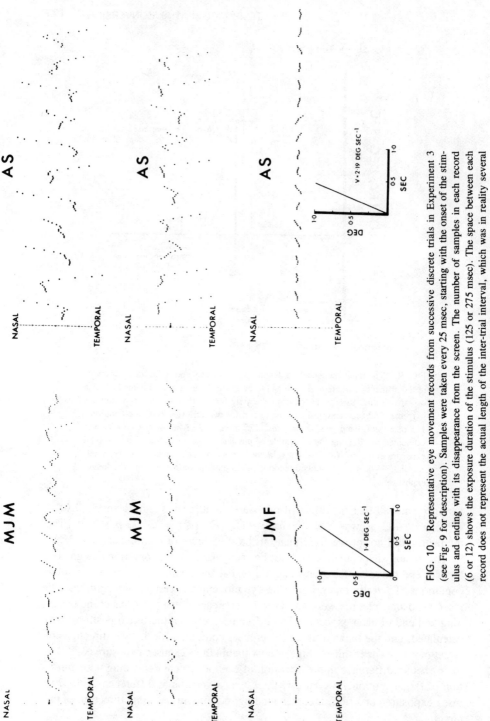

FIG. 10. Representative eye movement records from successive discrete trials in Experiment 3 (see Fig. 9 for description). Samples were taken every 25 msec, starting with the onset of the stimulus and ending with its disappearance from the screen. The number of samples in each record (6 or 12) shows the exposure duration of the stimulus (125 or 275 msec). The space between each record does not represent the actual length of the inter-trial interval, which was in reality several seconds. Left hand panels: subjects MJM and JF; Right hand panels: subject AS.

Examples of eye records from different conditions are shown in Fig. 10. These confirm that the latency of pursuit was not less than about 150 msec, and that there was negligible tracking in the 125 msec exposure. However, there were several interesting cases in which low velocity eye drifts occurred with zero latency. The direction of these tended strongly to be the same for a particular subject, irrespective of target movement direction. Could these have been anticipatory drifts similar to those recently reported by Kowler and Steinman (1979)? An attempt was made to see if they were due to head movements, by simultaneously recording the position of a black-white edge painted on to the subject's forehead. The results (e.g., Fig. 11) showed little correlation between the direction of eye and head movements. It can be tentatively concluded that these slow drifts were really due to eye movements, not to movements of the head. However, they do not appear to have aided shape recognition, since performance in the 125 msec exposure condition was not above chance.

The eye movement records in Fig. 10 also suggest that there were directional asymmetries in tracking even in the 275 msec condition. It is an intriguing question whether these correlate with psychophysical performance. A particularly clear example of such a correlation was found in subject JMF, who showed very little tracking of right to left (temporal) movement but quite clear tracking in

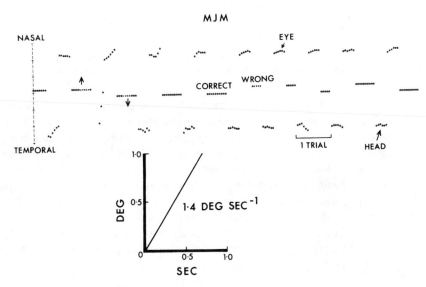

FIG. 11.   Representative records of eye and head movements for one subject (MJM) in Experiment 3. The record is plotted in a similar manner to Fig. 10, except that it shows separately eye movements (top) and head movements (bottom). The calibration refers to eye movements only. A marker has been added after each trial to show the direction of stimulus movement (arrows) and whether the subject was correct or wrong (length of marker).

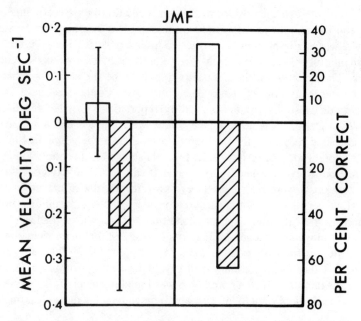

FIG. 12.   In Experiment 3, one of the subjects (JMF) pursued the apparently-moving triangle only when it moved in one of the two possible directions. He was also much more accurate at reporting the shape of the triangle when it moved in the preferred direction of tracking. This is seen in the figure, which shows the asymmetry of pursuit (left hand panels) and of shape recognition (right hand panels) between the two directions of stimulus movement (shaded and unshaded bars).

the opposite direction. He was also much less accurate at recognizing shape in the right-left movement condition. These asymmetries are shown in Fig. 12. To see if this correlation held over other subjects as well, each subject was given a velocity difference score, consisting of the mean difference of velocity between the preferred and nonpreferred direction, and a shape recognition difference score, consisting of the mean difference in percent correct between the preferred and nonpreferred directions of tracking. The results shown in Fig. 13 suggests that there was indeed a tendency for the direction of the aymmetry in psychophysical performance to correlate with the direction of tracking velocity asymmetry. This is strong evidence that the shape recognition task was being carried out with the aid of eye movements.

   2.   *Recognition of Oblique Line Orientation.*   The previous experiments strongly suggest that a moderately difficult virtual shape recognition task, discriminating between different orientations of a triangle, cannot be accomplished without pursuit eye movements. What about easier discriminations? Some data already exist to suggest that simple virtual shape discrimination is possible even

without tracking. I described an effect showing that a vernier offset between two moving bars was detectable through slits much narrower than the offset (Morgan, 1976). In fact the slit was no wider than the bars themselves, so that the real position of the bars were in exact alignment, with only a temporal difference between them. The vernier offset was detectable even with steady fixation, as measured by eye movement records. More recently, Burr (1979) has shown that the virtual vernier offset is detectable even in an apparent motion sequence of 150 msec, which was presumed to rule out the possibility of tracking. Thus it appears that some kinds of spatial analysis are possible even without eye movement. This was verified in the following experiment, which used a single tilted bar moving behind slits, the direction of tilt varying randomly between different trials.

The vertical bar was tilted 4.3° from the vertical, either clockwise or counterclockwise. This meant that the vertical/horizontal distance between the top of the line and the bottom as it passed the slit was 1.35 min of visual angle. As in previous experiments, a real shape condition equivalent to the vertical shape was also included. The observer's task was to report whether the line was

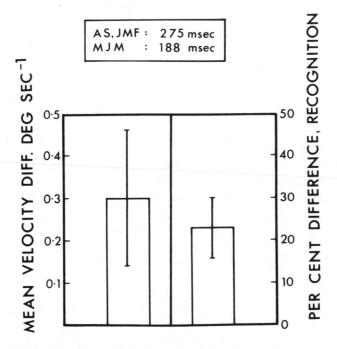

FIG. 13.   There was a tendency in Experiment 3 for observers to be more accurate at identifying the shape in their preferred direction of tracking (see Fig. 12 for subject JMF). The figure shows that the mean velocity difference between preferred and nonpreferred directions of tracking in the three subjects was about 0.3 deg/sec^{-1} (left hand panel). The mean difference in recognition performance between the preferred and nonpreferred directions is shown in the right hand panel.

tilted clockwise or counterclockwise, by pressing the appropriate one of two buttons.

The experiment was run with two subjects (MJM and AS) and the results were quite clear. In 50 trials with the real tilt both subjects were 100% correct; in 50 interspersed trials with the virtual tilt they were 78% correct (AS) and 72% correct (MJM). The mean velocity of tracking in the direction of target motion was 0.018 deg/sec (AS) and 0.022 deg/sec (MJM); thus it can be stated that essentially no target-motion specific tracking occurred.

The conclusion of this experiment is therefore that the orientation of a line from vertical can be discriminated under virtual shape condition, even when without tracking eye movements. The results are entirely different from those obtained in the more complex shape recognition task with virtual triangles.

Conclusions

I should like to draw two distinct conclusions from this rather complicated set of experimental findings. The first is that pursuit eye movements certainly *can* produce an "anorthoscopic effect." Tracking occurs both when the object is moving to-and-from behind a single slit, and when it is moving in one direction behind a series of slits. The evidence that such tracking is causally related to the perception of shape may be summarized: (1) In the single slit situation, the circle appeared wider than the slit but was compressed in the direction of motion— exactly as predicted from the eye movement records. Neither tracking nor perception of shape occurred when the slit was narrowed to 0.1 deg. (2) In the multiple slit situation, recognition of the orientation of a triangle was impossible if the exposure duration was inside the latency period of pursuit. The shape was recognized only in conditions where eye movement records showed pursuit. Individual asymmetries in left-right pursuit correlated with asymmetries in the detection of shape. When the direction of tracking was reversed, perception of the shape was mirror-imaged.

All these facts make it difficult to avoid the conclusion that pursuit eye movements are a sufficient cause of the "anorthoscopic" phenomenon, and also that in moderately complex kinds of shape recognition task, they are also necessary.

But this is not the whole story. We have also seen that at least one simple kind of shape perception, orientation of a single line, can definitely occur in the absence of smooth pursuit. We also know from other work that a vernier offset between two moving lines can be perceived even when they are visible only through a notional slit narrower than the offset (Morgan, 1976; Burr, 1979). Thus it appears that the resolution to the century-old argument about the perception of objects moving behind slits may be that both sides were partly correct. Perception of shape is severely restricted if the eyes do not pursue the target, but certain crude forms of analysis seem still to be possible. It remains to be discovered how far this simple ability extends. For example, could an "X" be discriminated from a single vertical line with the same time-averaged luminance?

ACKNOWLEDGMENTS

This work was supported by a grant from the Medical Research Council of Great Britain. I am very grateful to John Thompson, Malcom Rolling, and John Dobson for their help in constructing the apparatus; and to Chris McManus who collaborated in experiments (which will be reported elsewhere) on the effects of barbiturate drugs upon smooth pursuit and the anorthoscopic effect.

III PICTURES AND PICTORIAL PROCESSING

It is apparent that our understanding of how people view pictures is still very primitive. How is it that even though everyone looks at pictures differently, they are remembered equally well by all? Is is the presence of salient, critical features that are invariably absorbed by the viewer? Does the time course of viewing dictate changes in the ways that objects and scenes are viewed? Do certain items in a picture demand more or less gaze time to identify than others which are incongruent, and hence do not belong? What defines congruity? What are the dynamics of categorizing belongingness during brief glimpses?

Friedman and Liebelt describe the way that people look at objects that belong or that don't belong and hypothesize that the time course of viewing pictures is describable in terms of frame theory. Antes and Penland also examine congruency effects, both in pictures of scenes and of pictures of items in isolation. While their concern is predominately with understanding congruency, they conclude that portions of fixations are devoted to integrating information from previous fixations with the present. Findlay examines the compelling aspects of peripherally viewed stimuli and the dynamic aspects of saccades as they are executed in order that specific features of those stimuli can be identified. Intraub takes an interesting approach by mimicking fixation dynamics while presenting pictures in rapid sequences, providing only brief glimpses to the viewer, who must discriminate categories and identities of objects within these sequences.

Psychologists have traditionally felt that by partialing out pictorial information and making pictures simpler, a greater understanding of viewing pictures and scenes in the real world will come about. In keeping with that approach, we felt that these chapters examining congruency, contextual effects, fixation integration, peripheral and foveal viewing and dynamics within fixations will substantially aid our future understanding of picture perception.

On the Time Course of Viewing Pictures with a View Towards Remembering

III.1

Alinda Friedman
University of Alberta

Linda S. Liebelt
University of Colorado

Generally speaking, people process and recognize familiar surroundings on a continuous basis with little or no conscious effort and in many cases, with little or no awareness of what they have seen. This is perhaps because under most circumstances, the world offers little in the way of visual surprise. In contrast, witness the extremely conscious effort necessary to find your way around a new city, and how it is frequently the case that buildings that deviate a bit from the way city structures are supposed to be (e.g., the Sears Tower in Chicago, the World Trade Center in New York, anything at all designed by Antonio Gaudi) may readily function as landmarks. What are people doing when they look in order to remember? How does past experience, embodied in knowledge structures, interact with this process? Does the process change as a function of time, and if so, what is the relationship between past experience, recognition, and purposeful visual exploration?

In this chapter, we will infer several things about what people normally do when trying to remember their visual world from a situation in which they were trying to remember pictures. Although the objects in the pictures varied according to their contextual "belongingness," instructions to subjects emphasized learning as much as possible, about all of them, without regard to such things as context or a priori expectations. We will show that despite such injunctions, people consciously or otherwise sort their environment into things that ought or ought not be. We believe that sorting objects on the basis of belongingness is an automatic and natural byproduct of the visual recognition process. In addition, we believe that this automatic sorting occurs because it is the most sensible means of constructing a memory representation that allows people to distinguish among and therefore remember unique environments belonging to the same general class. We will further demonstrate that the functions describing the fixation durations accorded to belonging or nonbelonging objects do indeed change over the time course of viewing and are quantitatively and qualitatively different from each other.

Finally, we will argue that for pictures of coherent scenes, the measure of informativeness that is most useful for predicting both quantitative and qualitative differences in initial fixation durations, as well as differences in the pattern of durations over time, may be derived independently of the specific pictures used. In fact, the measure may be derived using a group of people who have never seen the pictures at all. This is because the type of informativeness that may influence fixations the most is informativeness defined with respect to the sort of world knowledge that is relatively invariant across specific contexts.

BACKGROUND

The approach taken here involves several underlying assumptions about the manner in which knowledge is represented, about how such representations influence both initial object recognition and the subsequent role played by a particular object in remembering the context in which it appears, and about the interaction between an object's relative informativeness with respect to a context and the manner in which visual exploration proceeds. Throughout the chapter, we will adhere to the view that knowledge about the world and the objects in it (e.g., the way things usually look, what they're called, where they belong, what they're for, etc.) is represented in an abstract memorial structure such as a frame (Minsky, 1975; see also Friedman, 1979; Norman & Rumelhart, 1975; Palmer, 1975a,b; Schank & Abelson, 1975). Two important features of frame representations are that they are organized into hierarchical systems and that the knowledge represented in such systems is stereotypical and relatively invariant. Thus, frames provide contexts, albeit internal ones; a global frame will represent the objects, actions, and events that are most usual and therefore most likely to actually occur within a particular type of real-world context.

Frames may exist at any of several levels of generality. For example, a professor's office, real or conceptual, is a likely context for a desk, which in turn is a likely context for a phone, ashtray, papers, pencils, books, and so on. The two levels of generality we will be primarily concerned with are the relatively global level of a place as contrasted to the less global level of a single object.

Under normal circumstances, that is, when people are in or *believe they are going to be in* a familiar environment, there are certain things that are expected (to be there; to happen) and others that are not. Thus, to be in or to expect to be in a particular environment will generally cause the frame (s) relevant to that environment to become activated, so that we become "ready to perceive" the objects represented therein. That is, since the frame for a global context consists of arguments for things that are supposed to occur there, and since these arguments can specify higher order visual "properties" of the objects they represent, such objects may be perceived relatively automatically and holistically. For example, in making the acquaintance of a new faculty member, one arrives at his or her office expecting to see some large, rather squarish-looking things that are readily identified: the thigh-high one is the desk, the chin-high ones are file cabinets, the tall ones are bookcases, and so on. These sorts of "features" are indeed global in comparison to the lines, angles, textures, corners, and other "pieces" that would need to be "put together" if recognition proceeded entirely from the bottom-up. Thus, when recognizing objects in a predominately top-down fashion by using an activated global frame, *ready to perceive* means ready to virtually automatically acknowledge the presence of objects that exist as arguments in that frame. This is how frame-driven or top-down perception facilitates visual recognition of expected things, thereby freeing resources for processing the unexpected.

Objects that are not included as arguments in the frame for a global context (1) cannot directly use that frame to aid their recognition and (2) are important for distinguishing among contexts that instantiate the same global frame. The implication that follows from (1) is that unexpected objects will take longer to initially recognize than objects represented in a frame because the frame-verification procedures necessary for recognition need to search at a less general level (i.e., a frame for a single object must be found), and thus cannot use higher order visual features. The implication that follows from (2) is that since unexpected objects provide a means of distinguishing among unique contexts that are otherwise generically identical (e.g., the offices of your various colleagues), the existence of unexpected objects is pragmatically important and hence they should generally be well-remembered. For example, you might chat with your new faculty acquaintance for a good hour or so, leave her office, and be unable to say whether she had a single or double pedestal desk, or two or three bookcases, yet quite clearly remember the Van Gogh print on the wall and the macrame plant hanger in the window for hours, days, or even months afterwards.

Thus, in general, when people perceive an event what they perceive most consciously (and hence, least automatically) are the differences between that specific event and their frame representation for others belonging to the same general class. The memory representation of a specific event resulting from its frame-directed perception will therefore be comprised of the global frame (and its contents) with an attached *difference structure* that's a kind of an inventory of things that occurred that were unexpected.

Both of the implications above (i.e., longer identification times and better memory for unexpected objects) have been experimentally validated in a situation in which location and duration of eye fixations was monitored as subjects viewed pictures of coherent scenes for 30 seconds each (Friedman, 1979). The subjects knew the topic (global frame) of each picture in advance of its presentation, and hence could be ready to perceive the objects expected to be there.

Logically, the first fixation made to an object should reflect the time necessary for its identification. Thus, if frames specifying higher order visual features are being used in this process, first fixations to expected objects should be shorter on the average than first fixations to unexpected objects. In fact, they were shorter by over 300 msec. In addition, subsequent recognition of changes made to expected objects, including changing their details and position, deleting them from the pictures altogether, and replacing them with other expected objects, was rather poor, while changes made to unexpected objects were generally well-noticed.

IMPLICATIONS FOR VISUAL EXPLORATION

Looking at the World

If frames can affect both initial recognition and subsequent memory, then they may also exert an influence upon visual exploration. Several aspects of exploration may be influenced, perhaps independently (e.g., what is looked at, when, and for how long). The particular aspect that will be affected probably depends upon both the purpose to be gained by looking and the characteristics of what is being looked at.

It should be clear that whether or not an object is represented in the frame for a global context will be at least one important factor in determining the relative informativeness of that object for remembering that context. If an object is represented as a frame-argument, then for most purposes it is generally uninformative when encountered in any specific real-world example of that frame. In general, an expected object would only be informative if, as an instance of its class, it violated the range of values given for the variables specified in its frame (e.g., an antique roll-top desk in a faculty member's office) or if it violated other, more general world knowledge (e.g., a floating desk). That expected objects are usually uninformative is especially true if your purpose is to remember a specific example of a global frame, but it is also true if you're just "having a look around." Therefore, upon initially assessing a new situation, expected objects should receive only meager amounts of attention.

It is possible, however, that after having briefly acknowledged the existence of expected objects during a first cursory look around, you might during later glances look more leisurely or more purposefully at them, in order to gather in more of their details. Even so, these later looks might not be especially effective for memory. For example, it has been shown that people are very inaccurate in reproducing the visual details of a building they either work or live in and that should consequently be very familiar (Norman & Rumelhart, 1975, pgs. 21–26). In addition, Nickerson and Adams (1979) demonstrated a remarkable inability to reproduce or recognize the details of an object encountered literally thousands of times during one's life (i.e., a Lincoln Head penny). Thus, while post-recognition glances at familiar, expected objects may be longer than initial glances, they may not necessarily result in a more detailed memory representation. For most pragmatic purposes, however, this is inconsequential. Further, the fact that the free variables in the arguments for expected objects might only become "bound" by specific details during a particular perceptual experience, and then return to their "unbound" or default state, preserves the invariance of the global frame to which the objects belong, and hence its usefulness for recognition across contexts.

In summary, then, although later fixations to expected objects might be longer than initial fixations, there are a number of reasons why unexpected objects might receive yet even longer fixations, both initially and over time. These include the desire to preserve the integrity of the global frame by unbinding the expected episodic and descriptive details of an event, while simultaneously creating a useful difference structure for those aspects of the event that are novel.

It should be noted that implicit in our assertions regarding the length of time people spend exploring expected objects over time are certain assumptions about motives. For example, although your own office might in most respects conform to those of your colleagues, in all likelihood you would know the exact or approximate location of a specific book, journal, paper, etc. This information is important and useful for you to know and you do know it, despite the fact that in a more general sense it is mundane. For that matter, the contents of your own home, office, kitchen, desk, broom closet, briefcase, etc., might have more weight in determining acceptable versus unusual objects for these contexts than would scores of other instantiations you may have experienced.

In a similar vein, during the second or third perusal of your new acquaintance's bookshelves, you might notice that she subscribes to *Neuropsychologia,* whereas during your first look that set of things might not have been consciously acknowledged at all, or might simply have been "checked off" in the argument for *journals.* However, even though these are expected objects, you might make a special mental note of their existence (e.g., by adding *Neuropsychologia* to the difference structure for that particular colleague's office) because the information could be of some future use.

In contrast to the relative uselessness of subsequent glances to expected objects, objects that are informative to begin with and that therefore capture an intially prolonged look as a requisite for their comprehension may remain informative over time. They may therefore continue to capture prolonged attention, especially in comparison to subsequent time spent looking at expected objects. This may be because first, if unexpected objects are represented in a difference structure, they will be the objects referenced in affirming that you have again encountered a specific instance of a particular global frame. Second, whatever attributes that made the objects informative to begin with (e.g., their absence from the global frame or any physical or perceptual anomalies they have) should generally continue to render those objects unusual (or interesting, or useful). For example, the World Trade Center is initially visually striking even for native New Yorkers, primarily because of its size relative to its surroundings, most of which are close to the "unusual" end of the size scale themselves. Over time, it remains an object of attention (i.e., if it is still visually striking), and in addition, one learns that it is a useful means of orienting around the Wall Street area which, unlike the rest of the city, is maze-like. Although this particular example describes an expected object whose unusualness is in part based upon exceeding the range of size values specified for *buildings* in a *city* frame, the example is meant to extend to objects that are unusual because they are not represented in the global frame at all.

Looking at Pictures

The discussion above referred primarily to what people might normally do with their visual world when they have relatively long opportunities for looking or when they have repeated experiences of the same visual environment. In the experimental world, the time period for looking has ranged from very brief exposures (e.g., on the order of milliseconds or a few seconds; Biederman, Rabinowitz, Glass, & Stacy, 1974; Loftus, 1972; Loftus & Mackworth, 1978) to durations long enough to approximate the amount of time you have to learn about a street corner while waiting for the stoplight to change (Antes, 1974; Mackworth & Morandi, 1967). It is the latter that are of primary interest here.

Both Mackworth and Morandi (1967) and Antes (1974) have explored the relationship between rated informativeness and fixation density, using independent groups of subjects to rate and view pictures. Fixation density is the proportion of total fixations made to a particular object divided by the proportion of area occupied by the object. The use of this measure therefore allows one to equate objects for size when comparing their ability to "capture" fixations.

Mackworth and Morandi's (1967) subjects viewed two pictures for 10 seconds each, their task being to determine which of the pictures was most preferred. These instructions should yield behavior that approximates what people do in a "free-looking" situation; that is, when they have no motives beyond the aesthetic. The measure of informativeness that was used was derived by having people rate each pictorial unit in terms of its "ease of recognition."

The pictures used by Mackworth and Morandi (1967) were relatively impoverished from the point of view of semantic complexity. One picture was an aerial photograph of a coastline and the other depicted the front of a person's head covered by a hood that occluded all facial features except the eyes. Moreover, each picture was divided into 64 equal-sized segments that were presented *individually* to the raters, who never saw the pictures as a whole. Thus, by dissecting the pictures into equal-sized pieces, the rater's task was similar to judging how easy it would be to recognize each piece of a jigsaw puzzle.

Considering the relative simplicity of the pictures, and the absence of a contextual whole, it is not surprising that approximately equal and high "recognizability" values were assigned to pieces that depicted some sort of visual contour (as contrasted to pieces that depicted simply texture), regardless of whether the contours were predictable or unpredictable in an information-theoretic sense. But since predictable and unpredictable only become meaningful concepts with respect to the pictures as a whole, the viewers made a further division of the pieces that had been rated as highly informative: They concentrated their gaze on the squares that had unpredictable contours, and they did so for the entire 10 second viewing period. Thus, fixation density was related to *contextual* informativeness and did not change over time.

Mackworth and Morandi (1967) concluded that

> a few outstanding areas within pictures received high concentrations of the gaze and these regions of the pictures were also judged to be highly recognizable. These dominant regions always contained unpredictable contours or unusual details. Simpler, predictable contours were estimated to be equally recognizable, but these outlines were seldom fixated [p. 551].

Although Mackworth and Morandi (1967) couched their discussion in terms of visual contour and texture, their data can be readily accommodated within the present view. When rating pieces of pictures for recognizability, contour is certainly more distinctive than texture. When placed in context, however, a contour may be more or less informative depending upon whether it is a contour of; that is, depending upon whether it is a contour of something that either is or is not in the currently active frame. Further, when pictures have very few details, (e.g., in the "eyes" picture only 12 of the 64 pieces had parts of the eyes, while the remainder were either hood or homogeneous background), it is not surprising that these details will capture the gaze throughout the time course of viewing.

Antes (1974) used more complex and meaningful pictures in his study (e.g., pictures from the Thematic Apperception Test), and rather than dividing them into equal-sized pieces, he divided them into units that for the most part could convey some meaning in and of themselves. His subjects viewed 10 pictures for 20 seconds each, and again, the task was to determine which picture was most preferred. The measure of informativeness he used was derived by having independent subjects rate each of the pieces according to the "informational contribution of that unit to the total information conveyed by the picture," and in this case, the pieces were rated in context.

Like Mackworth and Morandi (1967), Antes (1974) found a strong relationship between fixation density and rated informativeness, but unlike them, he found that both fixation density and duration changed over the time course of viewing. Relatively informative regions were fixated early but briefly, while less informative regions were fixated later but longer. Overall, fixation duration was a monotonically increasing function of viewing time. During the first tenth of the fixations made to the pictures, the average duration was 215 msec. This increased to 310 msec by the last tenth of the fixations. Antes concluded that subjects were "initially scanning the pictures as an orientation prior to close examination for detail (pg. 66)."

We do not believe, however, that Antes' (1974) data tell the whole story. First, to the extent that the pictures he used displayed relatively "normal" environments, subjects' ratings of informativeness had to be based upon the visual rather than semantic distinctiveness of picture segments comprised of objects or parts of objects that were all relatively uninformative. More importantly, recall that although both Mackworth and Morandi (1967) and Antes (1974) had their viewers look at the pictures from an aesthetic viewpoint, the rating instructions in the former experiment emphasized recognizability, while those in the latter did not. Therefore, the fact that Mackworth and Morandi's subjects did not differentially distribute their fixations over time while Antes' subjects did might be due to two different factors. The first, and less interesting, is the possibility that since Mackworth and Morandi's pictures were so informationally impoverished, their subjects effectively had nowhere to look except at the informative areas. The second possibility is that if our hypothesis about the relative usefulness of unexpected objects with respect to recognition and memory is correct, then it is possible that Antes' (1974) data reflect the time accorded to objects that are all more or less expected and usual, while Mackworth and Morandi's (1967) data reflect the time accorded to more unusual and informative objects.

It is difficult to tell which of these factors is more critical, however, because of the substantial differences between these experiments in both the materials used and the rating instructions. Furthermore, it is difficult to use the data from these experiments to test hypotheses about the influence of abstract knowledge on visual exploration because the informativeness ratings used were based upon subjects' having actually looked at the pictures or at segments of them. Thus, cues specific to the particular frame instantiations that were viewed may have played a large role in the ratings. Therefore, in order to determine the relationship between frame-like structures and visual exploration, we used pictures of coherent scenes in which the variable manipulated was the semantic informativeness of the depicted objects. In addition, rather than emphasizing either recognizability or informational content with respect to the pictures themselves, our rating instructions emphasized the question of whether or not particular objects belonged in particular places in a more generic sense of belonging.

The major purpose of these manipulations was to demonstrate that the time course of picture viewing, and by implication, the time accorded to different types of objects in the real world, is heavily influenced by abstract, invariant world knowledge. Further, we wanted to demonstrate that even when it is in their best interest to ignore differences between objects in terms of belongingness, subjects do not, and perhaps cannot, do so. To these ends, our raters did not rate pictures at all, but rather, they rated a written list of objects with respect to their contextual belongingness. Moreover, to ensure that differences in fixation durations to expected and unexpected objects would not be confounded with differences in the frequency with which they were fixated, our viewers were motivated to treat all objects equally by telling them they would have to later detect even small changes of detail to only one of the objects. These instructions made it likely that subjects would distribute their fixations evenly across all the objects without regard to their informativeness. Thus, we wanted to test our theoretical predictions regarding differences between expected and unexpected objects in the amount of attention they would capture over time in a "worst case" situation in which there was a good chance that the overall number of fixations to these objects would not differ. If ratings derived from written lists are reflected in the time course of picture viewing in this type of intentional learning situation, it would lend a great deal of credibility to the role played by frame representations in perception, subsequent visual exploration, and memory.

METHOD

Likelihood Norms

Since we have supposed that abstract structures such as frames will directly influence the length of time for initial fixations (i.e., recognition) as well as any changes in fixation durations over the course of the 30-sec viewing period, we deemed it most appropriate that our ratings of informativeness or belongingness be obtained independently of both the subjects who would be viewing the pictures, and more importantly, *independently of the pictures themselves.* To this end, a group of 15 subjects was asked to list as many things as they could think of that are *always, usually,* or *sometimes* found in each of 15 different settings.

Of the original 15 settings, the seven that yielded the greatest number of responses were chosen to be included in a rating study that used a new group of 51 subjects. These subjects received a packet in which the name of each place was typed at the top of a separate page, followed by an assortment of object names with the numbers 1 to 7 typed beside them. The objects listed for each place included all of the items generated by the previous group of subjects, as well as additional objects that were intuitively felt to be of medium to low likelihood.

The subjects were read instructions in which they were asked to rate the likelihood of seeing each of the objects in each particular place as a function of their experience (world knowledge) of such places. An example was given in which the objects mentioned were chosen on the basis of the frequency with which they were listed by the first group of subjects, and the context used was different from the seven that were to be rated:

> For example, suppose you were asked to list the things you would most often expect to find in the master bedroom of a nice house. You might almost always first mention a bed, and perhaps also a dresser and a closet. These are the sorts of things you should give a rating of 1. On the other hand, you would probably never mention an oak tree as something likely to be found in a bedroom, so that is the sort of thing you would give a rating of 7. Similarly, for bedrooms in general, things like TV sets and bookshelves fall somewhere in between *always* and *never*, and so for each of the places you'll be rating, you should use the numbers between 1 and 7 to reflect the range between highly probable and very uncommon things for that place.

It should be emphasized that according to our theory, the ratings given to the names of the objects would be entirely appropriate for their pictures, as long as the objects, when drawn, displayed neither physical nor pragmatic violations of frame knowledge (granting that this distinction is sometimes blurry). Therefore, in the pictures described in the following all of the objects were drawn as normal-looking as possible and were not displayed in physically impossible relationships. Further, each object was drawn with details that were sufficient to allow it to be recognized in the absence of any context.

Stimulus Pictures and Design

Complex and detailed line drawings of six different scenes (city, farm, kindergarten, kitchen, living room, and office) were used as the target stimuli. Each scene was drawn in correct perspective and was predominated by objects that had received relatively high or medium rated likelihoods. In addition, each picture contained a few objects whose likelihood of being seen in such a place was rated to be relatively low.

Each of 36 different subjects, 20 of whom participated to fulfill a course requirement and 16 of whom receive $2.00 for their participation, viewed all six target pictures. The picture presentation order was counterbalanced so that six subjects in each of six different groups saw every picture preceded and followed by every other picture exactly once.

For reasons discussed at length in a previous paper (Friedman, 1979), two of the six pictures (the city and the kindergarten) and seven of the objects in the remaining four pictures were not included in the discussion and analyses that follow. Briefly, our reasons involved the fact that across the six original pictures, there were 25 areas that depicted either an object with writing on it (e.g., a blackboard), or else a person or group of persons (e.g., the teacher and children in the kindergarten). Of these 25 areas, 18 were in the city and kindergarten. We found that subjects' initial fixations to people and objects with writing did not reflect their rated likelihood, whereas initial fixation durations to all the other objects reflected rated likelihood rather well. In addition, subsequent detection of changes made to either people or objects with writing was exceptionally good and similar to detection of changes made to unexpected objects, despite the fact that the people and objects with writing were for the most part highly expected. From the point of view of generalizing then, we do not feel that these areas are representative, and hence have excluded them from the analyses in this chapter. We will, however, report the means from these areas where appropriate.

The assignment of an object to a particular likelihood category was nonarbitrary and was determined as follows: The mean rating given to each object was obtained across the 51 raters, and then the standard deviations of these means were obtained within rather than across pictures, because some contexts (e.g., the living room) allow for a much wider range of "acceptable" objects than do others (e.g., the kitchen). The objects were then assigned a number from 1 to 4 according to whether their mean rated value fell within one of the following four categories: 1 = greater than zero but less than or equal to the value of one standard deviation, 2 = greater than one but less than or equal to the value of two standard deviations, 3 = greater than two but less than or equal to the value of three standard deviations, and 4 = greater than the value of three standard deviations. Thus, an object categorized as a "one" was highly expected with respect to its context and with respect to the range of objects originally rated for that context, whereas an object categorized as a "four" was highly unexpected.

Table 1 shows, for each of the four categories within and across pictures, the total number of objects in each category, the average proportion of area occupied by the objects, and both the fixation density and the average duration of the first fixation to an object in each category. Since the data for the first two categories (1 and 2) were strikingly similar across all of the variables investigated, these categories were combined for purposes of the discussion and analyses in this chapter. The objects belonging to categories 1 and 2 together, 3, and 4, will hereafter be referred to as high, medium, and low probability objects.

Procedure

Upon arriving, subjects were told they were participating in an experiment that would test their memory for pictures, that they would be seeing each picture for 30 seconds, that their eye movements would be recorded, and that they would have to later be able to distinguish between the original pictures and new pictures in which, for example, only a small detail on one object would be different. All the examples of possible changes to be detected were purposefully chosen to involve relatively high probability objects (e.g., subjects were told that if one of the pictures happened to be of a scene in the suburbs that originally had a boy's bicycle in it, the new picture could be exactly the same except that the boy's

TABLE 1
Average Area, Fixation Density, and First Fixation Durations to the Objects
as a Function of Picture and Rated Likelihood

Likelihood Category	Number of Objects	Proportion of Area	Fixation Density	First Fixation
Farm				
One	.2	.0332	5.11	271
Two	12	.0282	3.74	356
Three	6	.0103	4.25	374
Four	3	.0137	3.89	573
Kitchen				
One	13	.0179	2.57	295
Two	8	.0080	4.75	303
Three	7	.0131	2.70	328
Four	6	.0183	2.09	645
Living Room				
One	1	.0084	5.83	344
Two	9	.0210	2.92	238
Three	9	.0295	1.57	379
Four	5	.0092	4.80	559
Office				
One	1	.0060	6.83	285
Two	16	.0189	2.59	262
Three	10	.0135	3.69	344
Four	4	.0255	2.80	814
Across All Pictures				
One	17	.0183	3.31	294
Two	45	.0199	3.34	289
Three	32	.0173	2.98	356
Four	18	.0166	3.30	647

bicycle might be changed to a girl's bicycle. Most subjects groaned at this point in the instructions). Thus, the instructions emphasized that subjects should treat all objects equally, and attempt as best they could to remember as much about every object as possible.

After these instructions, the subject was seated in front of a rear projection screen and a Whittaker eye movement monitor, which determines the point of fixation by measuring the center of the pupil with respect to the center of the corneal reflection. The subject was asked to place his or her head in a chinrest, find a comfortable position, and remain still until the calibration procedure was finished and all of the pictures had been shown. After the eye movement monitor was calibrated, the experimenter repeated the instruction to look at each picture carefully and try to remember as much about every object as possible, and proceeded to show the pictures for 30 seconds each. The topic of each picture was announced in advance of the slide. The pictures subtended a horizontal visual angle of approximately 30°, and a vertical visual angle of approximately 20°.

RESULTS AND DISCUSSION

Every subject produced approximately three minutes of eye movement recordings, which consisted of a set of cross hairs superimposed on each target picture, representing the current point of fixation in real time. A "frame" of videotape was marked by the recorder every $\frac{1}{60}$ of a second. A tally was kept of the number of frames that occurred while the cross hairs were superimposed on a particular location, as well as the serial order in which each location was fixated. The number of frames per fixation was converted to milliseconds by dividing the total by 60, multiplying by 1,000, and truncating any remainder. The first fixation was defined as the location fixated at the end of the first saccade made by the subject after the onset of the slide.

The fixation density for each object was calculated by expressing the total number of times it was fixated across subjects as a proportion of the total number of fixations made to the entire picture and dividing this by the proportion of area occupied by that object relative to the entire picture. The fixation densities were then correlated with the mean rated likelihood of the objects, separately for each picture. The As expected, none of the correlations were reliable; they ranged from -0.02 for the farm to 0.15 for the living room. Thus, this preliminary analysis indicates that subjects were distributing their fixations evenly across all of the objects, regardless of informativeness.

To examine this issue in more detail, the total number of fixations made to each picture was determined for every subject, and was then divided into tenths that preserved their serial order, truncating the last few fixations when necessary. For example, if a subject made 74 fixations to one of the pictures, then there were seven fixations in each tenth, beginning with the first and disregarding the last four. For each subject, the percent of high (categories 1 and 2), medium (category 3), and low (category 4) probability objects that were fixated was determined across pictures for each of the ten segments of viewing. The denominators used for calculating the percents were the total number of fixations made across pictures during that particular segment by that subject. These data were subjected to a Likelihood (high, medium, or low) × Segment (1 to 10) repeated measures analysis of variance. The effect of rated likelihood was quite robust, $F (2, 70) = 576.19$, $MSe = 271$ and the interaction was also reliable, $F (18, 630) = 2.92$, $MSe = 202.19$. Figure 1 shows the data.

Overall, 56.7% of the fixations were made to high probability, belonging objects, 25.5% were made to medium probability objects, and 16.7% were made to low probability, unexpected objects. This distribution of fixations among the

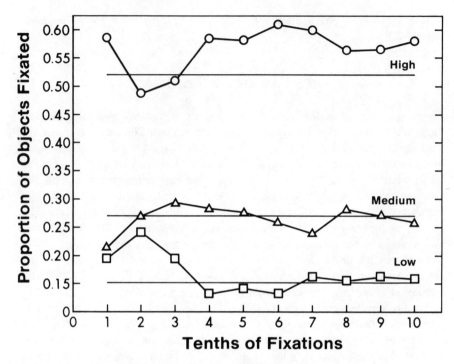

FIG. 1.   Proportion of total fixations per segment made to high, medium, and low
probability objects.

objects was basically identical to the distribution of high, medium, and low
probability objects that were actually in the pictures (i.e., 52.1%, 26.9%, and
15.1%, respectively, represented by the horizontal lines in Figure 1). For example, since there were more expected than unexpected objects in the pictures,
more of the total number of fixations were directed to them, but not proportionately more than there were expected objects to be looked at.

Polynomial regressions that included the first, second, and third-order components were performed separately on the data at each level of likelihood, and
none were reliable. Thus, subjects were indeed distributing their fixations
roughly evenly across all the objects in the pictures, regardless of their a prior
likelihood or the particular segment of viewing time. In view of the fact that they
were anticipating a difficult recognition test that could involve any of the objects,
this was a very reasonable strategy for them to use.

The absence of a positive relationship between informativeness and fixation
density renders the fixation duration data even more astonishing. If anything, the
fixation density data are opposite to what has been previously obtained, since of
the total number of fixations, there were always *more* made to the *less* informa-

tive objects across the entire time period of viewing. However, as Fig. 2 shows, there was no point during the viewing sequence that less informative, high probability objects received longer fixations than more informative, low probability objects, and it was only during the final segment of viewing that the fixation durations to high and medium probability objects became equal. The quantitative differences in fixation durations were tested in a Likelihood × Segment repeated measures analysis of variance. Both main effects were reliable, F (2, 70) = 104.37, MSe = 53490, for likelihood, and F (9, 315) = 2.97, MSe = 49501, for segment. The average fixation durations to high, medium, and low probability objects were 324, 379, and 562 msec. respectively. Across likelihoods, the average fixation to an object began at 349 msec during the first segment of viewing, increased to a peak of 474 msec during the sixth segment, and then decreased again to 445 msec during the final segment.

It can be seen from Fig. 2 that the durations for both the high and medium proprobability objects increased over the time course of viewing, while those for the low probability objects were noisier overall and did not show a steadily increasing or decreasing pattern. These qualitative differences in viewing time

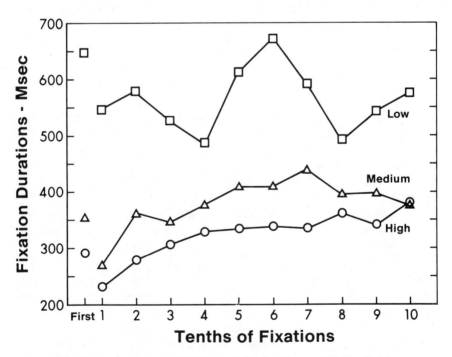

FIG. 2.   Fixation durations per segment as a function of the rated likelihood of the objects. The single points at the left of the figure indicate the average duration of the first fixation made to each of the high, medium, and low probability objects.

were examined by subjecting the average fixation duration per segment for high, medium, and low probability objects to separate polynomial regressions that included the linear, quadratic, and cubic components. Then, in accord with the recommendations of Cohen and Cohen (1975), the contributions of each component were investigated by determining whether the increment in proportion of variance accounted for by each was significant, rather than simply determining whether the cumulative proportion of variance accounted for as each component was added to the equation was significant.

These independent and conservative tests on each component showed that all three contributed significantly to the variance in fixation durations to high probability objects across segments. The linear effect was the strongest, accounting for 80.4% of the variance, $F (1, 8) = 32.74$, the quadratic component accounted for a further 9.7% of the variance, $F (1, 7) = 6.75$, and the cubic accounted for an additionally significant 6.8% of the variance, $F (1, 6) = 12.83$.

Recall that the fixation durations in Antes' (1974) experiment rose from 215 to 310 msec from the first to the last tenth of viewing. The durations for the high probability objects in the present experiment rose from 231 to 380 msec, which, considering the differences in materials and instructions, are roughly comparable to his. This suggests that our earlier contention that his data represent what happens to the time course of viewing when pictures contain objects that are all more or less expected is probably justified.

For the medium probability objects in the present study, only the first and second-order components accounted for a significant amount of the overall variance when these were examined independently. The linear component accounted for 41.8% of the variance in durations, $F (1, 8) = 5.74$, and the quadratic accounted for a further 43.8%, $F (1, 7) = 21.17$. Thus, while the linear component accounted for most of the variance in durations to highly expected objects, for medium probability objects, the linear and quadratic components accounted for roughly equal proportions of variance in fixation durations.

Finally, when the durations for the low probability, unexpected objects were subjected to the same analyses, it was found that none of the three components contributed reliably to the variance among fixation durations. Thus, the best estimate of fixation durations to unexpected objects for each segment of viewing time is the mean duration, or 562 msec. Fixations to these objects were uniformly longer than those made to high or medium probability objects and they did not change systematically across time. For purposes of comparison to the other types of objects, however, Table 2 shows the regression equations, standard errors of estimate, observed data, and predicted durations from the best-fitting equation for all three types of objects. In addition, the durations for the people and objects with writing are given, and it can be seen that these were roughly in between the

TABLE 2
Regression Equations and Predicted and Observed Fixation Durations
as a Function of Rated Likelihood

Regression Equations

I. Linear Effects
   High: $y' = 126x + 255$, s.e. = 20.096
   Med.: $y' = 100x + 324$, s.e. = 37.985
   Low: $y' = 12x + 555$, s.e. = 60.141
II. Quadratic Effects
   High: $y' = 317x - 174x^2 + 217$, s.e. = 15.311
   Med.: $y' = 546x - 405x^2 + 235$, s.e. = 20.243
   Low: $y' = 173x - 146x^2 + 523$, s.e. = 67.95
III. Cubic Effects
   High: $y' = 775x - 1166x^2 + 602x^3 + 165$, s.e. = 9.336
   Med.: $y' = 614x - 552x^2 + 89x^3 + 227$, s.e. = 21.772
   Low: $y' = 36x - 152x^2 + 181x^3 + 539$, s.e. = 67.947

Predicted and Observed Fixation Durations

	High		Medium		Low		Writing & People [a]	
Tenth	Y_{obs}	Y'_{cubic}	Y_{obs}	Y'_{quad}	Y_{obs}	$\bar{Y}$	Y_{obs}	$\bar{Y}$
1	231	231	269	286	547	562	409	465
2	279	278	366	328	579		443	
3	307	309	347	362	526		415	
4	329	327	378	389	484		464	
5	335	336	410	407	613		473	
6	339	340	409	417	673		505	
7	337	343	441	419	587		493	
8	363	347	398	413	490		479	
9	342	357	398	398	544		442	
10	380	376	378	376	576		526	

[a] These means are from the 25 areas across all 6 pictures, including the city and kindergarten, that depicted either people or objects with writing.

fixation durations to medium and low probability objects in terms of their distribution over segments of viewing.

CONCLUSION

The data from the present experiment may be summarized as follows. Subjects who viewed a small set of pictures for a relatively long time in an effort to remember them made fixations to expected objects that were relatively brief at first but that over the time course of viewing steadily increased in duration. In contrast, fixations made to unexpected objects were longer than those made to expected objects throughout the 30 second viewing period, and they did not show a systematically increasing or decreasing pattern. These data demonstrate that even when subjects are well-motivated to distribute their attention equally, and succeed to the extent of looking at everything about equally often, they nevertheless fixate longer on normal-looking objects that are contextually unusual. That they do so means it is possible to set up situations in which particular things capture a certain amount of attention no matter what people are trying to do. In addition, that subjects looked longer at unexpected objects in the type of experimental situation we contrived implies that at the very least, people would also look longer at unusual objects in a real-world environment they were trying to remember. Moreover, the fact that the pattern of fixation durations to high probability objects in the present experiment was similar to that obtained by Antes (1974), while the pattern of durations to low probability objects was similar to that obtained by Mackworth and Morandi (1967), both of whom instructed subjects to view and evaluate pictures aesthetically, implies that expected and unexpected objects may compel and receive different patterns of fixation durations even when people are just looking around.

It is important to emphasize that the contextual unusualness of the objects in the present study was determined prior to creating the particular stimulus materials used, and that in the absence of context, the objects were all normal-looking with respect to the class of things they were depicting. This lends a great deal of credibility to the existence of abstract knowledge structures such as frames, as well as to their influence on perception and visual exploration. The presence or absence of objects with respect to an activated global frame is clearly an important determinant of visual attention.

In a recent paper on divided attention and the deployment of resources, Navon and Gopher (1979) discuss the possibility that there may be certain types of stimuli that ''demand'' attention by their mere presence. The data from the present experiment suggest that because global frames are driving perception, we automatically deploy fewer resources to things represented in those frames, while at the same time, things that are unexpected or novel seem to demand a good deal of attention whether we like it or not.

The adaptive validity of an automatic division of resources between the expected and unexpected should be obvious. Under normal circumstances, we do not need to process those aspects of our environment that are expected, typical, commonplace, or mundane. On the other hand, things that are novel, unfamiliar, unusual, and unique may prove either dangerous or useful, but should compel our attention and interest in either case. We make use of such things to recognize specific instances of a class, to orient around familiar environments, to learn to navigate around new environments, and to appreciate the richness of visual experience that stands out against an ordinary and almost invisible background.

ACKNOWLEDGMENTS

Preparation of this chapter was supported by the Personnel and Training Research Program and the Engineering Psychology Program of the Office of Naval Research, and by the Air Force Office of Scientific Research, under Contract No. N00014-79-C-0679. We are grateful to Peter Holt, Mike Katzko, John Pullyblank, Dave Ross, and Lew Stelmach for their helpful comments on the manuscript, and to Jon Roberts for his advice on the data analysis.

III.2   Picture Context Effects on Eye Movement Patterns

James R. Antes and James G. Penland
University of North Dakota

The purpose of our research and much of our earlier work (e.g., Antes, 1974, 1977; Antes & Metzger, 1980) has been to investigate the factors influencing visual attention to complex scenes. This chapter deals specifically with the role of context as a characteristic of pictures in influencing attention, as measured by eye movement patterns. In general, our data support the following conclusions:

1. Contextual information in a picture provides rapid access to the picture theme that biases visual exploration in a manner consistent with that theme.
2. During the fixational pause semantic information of the object viewed and objects from the immediately preceding fixation are encoded and decisions, regarding the next object of fixation, are made on the basis of the semantic information of the surrounding objects.

CONTEXT EFFECTS

Recognition and identification of items are enhanced when those items are presented in context as opposed to an impoverished display. This has been shown for the recognition of speech (Bruce, 1956), letters in words (Wheeler, 1970), line segments in three dimensional-appearing arrays (Weisstein & Harris, 1974), and objects in pictures (Biederman, 1972; Palmer, 1975a). Although the existence of contextual effects using pictorial stimuli has been amply demonstrated, definitions of context have varied and attempts to determine precisely how context influences cognitive processing have only recently been made.

157

Most researchers do not explicitly discuss their definitions of context but seem to implicitly assume that context varies by degree from the mere presence of an item, adjacent to a target object, to a highly complex semantically coherent scene. Biederman (1980) has attempted to specify the characteristics of a contextually coherent "well-formed" scene that distinguish it from an array of unrelated objects in terms of relationships among objects. The well-formed scene is limited by two types of constraints on object relationships, syntactic and semantic. The syntactic constraints do not depend on referential meaning and include support (i.e., objects generally rest on surfaces) and interposition (i.e., most objects are not transparent). Semantic constraints include probability or the likelihood that an object appears in a scene; position, or the likelihood that an object appears in certain locations; and size, that objects in a scene have certain size relationships.

Two distinctions have been identified in the literature that have helped to advance thought regarding the nature of context effects. The global versus local information distinction is analogous to information apprehended as a whole and information apprehended in the parts comprising the whole. Researchers have suggested that processing of global information has priority over that of local information (Navon, 1977) at least when there are many elements in the display (Martin, 1979). Since the relations among objects contributing to context seem to fall into the category of global information, then processing of contextual information may precede processing of details of the scene. Consequently this early processing of contextual information may influence the course of later processing and provide the basis for certain context effects. Biederman (1980) supports this view by demonstrating that viewers have rapid access to semantic information in a picture, at least as rapid as their access to information that is not dependent on referential meaning.

The second distinction of data-driven (or bottom-up) processing or conceptually-driven (or top-down) processing, suggests that analysis of information may proceed through a series of stages determined by the current input information, or may be directed by expectations and organizational strategies. Ordinarily both types of processing occur simultaneously, but when the operation is conceptually-driven contextual information influences subsequent processing both through the precedence of global information and by expectations derived from previous inputs.

Friedman (1979) recently provided a theoretical framework characterizing the encoding of information in contextually rich pictures as a function of data-driven and conceptually-driven processing. According to Friedman, the latter form of processing is directed by a conceptual frame of the theme of the picture consisting of expectations about objects normally viewed in such scenes. In her research the theme was provided by oral information given prior to the exposure of the picture but the preceding analysis suggests that the contextually relevant global information in the picture itself may serve to "instantiate" a frame. Friedman contends that encoding of expected objects is automatic, dependent on feature *detection,* and thus memory for such objects is prototypical. Unexpected objects require feature *analysis* to be encoded, thus the interaction of data-driven and conceptually-driven processing. Consequently, unexpected objects are remembered in greater detail. Partial support for her position comes from her finding that first fixation durations on unexpected objects are twice as long as first fixations on expected objects, presumably representing the additional time required to fully analyze the unexpected objects via bottom-up processing.

Additional research, with manipulations of context, is needed to relate changes in context to eye movement patterns and perceptual processing. This was the goal of the present study. Subjects were required to view a series of line drawings that were either complex and contexually rich (high context) or consisted of an array of objects that retained only their spatial position from the high context counterpart (low context). The objects were either expected or unexpected with respect to the scene. Eye movements were examined for context effects and other factors that might influence the direction of gaze when viewing these scenes.

Method

The 23 pictures used in this experiment, taken from Antes and Metzger (1980), consisted of line drawings of varying themes, and contained a number of readily identifiable objects. They were modified by replacing two of the objects, one within 5° (at the viewing distance of 53 cm) of the center of the picture and one beyond that distance, with unexpected objects. Expectedness was determined by the experimenters and was later confirmed by subjective probability ratings (see the following). These pictures comprised the high context set. Six non-overlapping objects were selected from each picture and were reproduced at the same locations as they appeared in the high context set. All other objects and contours were eliminated. Four of the objects met the requirements of the two × two factorial combination of near (within 5° of the center of the picture)/far (beyond 5°) and expected/unexpected. These stimuli comprised the low context set and it was the fixations and saccades relative to these four objects in both sets that comprised the eye movement data in this experiment.

The pictures were prepared as achromatic slides and when projected onto the rear projection screen 53 cm in front of the subject, subtended approximately 18° vertically and horizontally. Figure 1 shows one of the pictures as it appeared in both context conditions.

The subjects were 21 undergraduates at the University of North Dakota who reported normal vision without eye glasses or contact lenses. Following three practice scenes, each subject viewed ten pictures in the high context condition and ten in the low context condition in a random order for four seconds each. Across subjects each picture was viewed in both context conditions equally

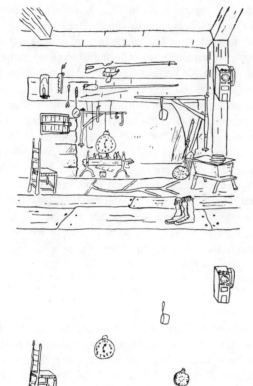

FIG. 1. Sample picture as it appeared in the high context and low context conditions. Unexpected objects are the pay telephone and clock.

often. The subjects were told to view the pictures in preparation for an object recognition test after each picture. For the recognition test an array of four objects was presented, one of which was from the picture while the three incorrect objects were not consistent with the picture context. The expected-near, expected-far, unexpected-near, and unexpected-far objects were probed as the correct object an equal number of times.

Eye movements were recorded by means of a Mackworth corneal reflection instrument from which a permanent data record was obtained on 16 mm film. A bite-board was prepared using a dental wax impression of the subject's teeth. Calibration adjustments were made and a film record of fixations on the center and the extremes of the screen was made prior to viewing the pictures. Between trials the adjustment was checked by having the subject fixate a spot at the center of the screen, which was to be fixated until the next picture appeared. The four-choice response matrix was also projected onto the screen, for about ten seconds, and subjects responded by pointing to a corresponding square of a facsimile matrix in the subject's view below and to the right of the screen.

The film records were hand scored using a film editor to determine fixation locations and durations and saccadic amplitude. The data were reduced to four major dependent variables: number of fixations; mean duration of fixation; gaze, the sum of the durations on a given object; and saccadic amplitude.

Expectations regarding the results were formulated under the guidance of the views of Friedman (1979), described above, and Hochberg (1970a), whose theory contends that attention is directed to confirm an evolving set of expectations and that perceptual processing involves the construction of a schematic representation of the scene. We anticipated that, in viewing the high context pictures, the global information relating to context would serve to instantiate a frame related to the perceived theme of the picture. Fixations would be directed to objects consistent with the frame and top-down processing would dominate. A representation of the picture, or schema, would rapidly evolve with each fixation. Thus the frame becomes the set of possible objects or events and their properties which are consistent with the schema. Peripheral vision locates potential fixation choices and the extent of processing of peripheral objects decreases rapidly with distance from fovea. Expected objects would be more completely processed at a given peripheral location than unexpected objects but eventually the latter would enter the "useful field of view" (Mackworth, 1976). This would result in a change in "visual momentum" (Hochberg & Brooks, 1978) and the unexpected object would be immediately fixated and a preponderance of data-driven processing would ensue. The schema would change as would the resultant expectations and viewing would progress in a manner consistent with the current schema.

We expected that the same process would be involved in viewing the low context scenes but the frame and corresponding expectations would be relatively impoverished. Processing would be dominated by data-driven analysis.

In terms of our data we expected, specifically:

1. Using Friedman's (1979) first fixation duration measure as an indication of time to encode an object, first fixations in the low context pictures should be longer than those in the high context scenes but only for the expected objects. Mostly data-driven processing should be involved for all objects in the low context scenes and unexpected objects in high context. Conceptually-driven processing of expected objects in high context should allow automatic encoding via feature detection and thus result in shorter first fixation durations.

2. For high context pictures saccades to expected objects should be longer than those to unexpected objects, reflecting a greater useful field of view for objects consistent with the frame. This pattern should not be present in the data from low context scenes.

3. An examination of cumulative fixation probabilities should show a preference for expected objects early in viewing and this preference should diminish with time. This pattern should not be evident for the low context scenes. It should be noted that this prediction contrasts with the results of Loftus and Mackworth (1978) who found unusual objects to be fixated more frequently throughout a

four second exposure. However, we believed that their results were due, in part, to the nature of their pictures, which did not appear to be as detailed as ours, a factor that would tend to make the unexpected objects more prominent.

Results and Discussion

In considering the following results it is important to view performance on the high context scenes relative to that on the low context scenes. In this way the low context pictures serve as a control and provide base level measures of the eye movement patterns (e.g., base encoding times as measured by first fixation durations) against which to evaluate the same measures on the high context scenes.

Means relevant to the first prediction are presented in Table 1. Per-subject means were computed and subjected to a Context × Expectedness × Location (near/far) analysis of variance, with all variables varying within subjects. The mean first fixation duration on any of the four target objects in the low context scenes was significantly greater than that in the high context scenes, as indicated by the significant main effect for context F (1, 20) = 4.69, $p < .05$, MSe = 52.75, and this effect in turn varied with Expectedness, as revealed by the significant Context × Expectedness interaction, F (1, 20) = 5.24, $p < .05$, MSe = 25.00. A Newman-Keuls analysis of the interaction showed the mean first fixation duration on expected objects to be significantly shorter in the high context condition than in the low context condition ($p < .01$). No other comparisons produced statistically reliable differences. The results support the prediction but the mean first duration on expected objects did not differ from that on

TABLE 1
Mean Duration of First Fixations
and Mean Saccadic Amplitude
for Expected and Unexpected
Objects in High and Low Context

| | Duration (msec) | |
Context	Expected	Unexpected
Low	352	332
High	305	325

| | Amplitude (deg) | |
Context	Expected	Unexpected
Low	6.95	7.02
High	6.17	5.61

unexpected objects in the high context condition as might be anticipated. However, viewing the first fixation durations during the low context exposures as a base level measure of encoding time, the expected objects in low context scenes required greater encoding time. With the added contextual information provided in the high context condition, mean first fixation values were reversed and were lower for the expected objects, in the predicted direction.

It was also predicted that mean saccadic amplitude to expected objects would be longer than that to unexpected objects and the means relevant to that prediction are also presented in Table 1. High context reduced amplitudes to unexpected objects more than to expected objects such that saccades to the latter were longer in the high context scenes. A comparison of amplitudes to expected and unexpected objects in the low context condition showed no differences, t (20) = 0.419, $p > .05$. In the high context condition saccades to expected objects were significantly longer, t (20) = 3.186, $p < .01$.

Figure 2 presents data relevant to the third prediction, cumulative probabilities of fixating expected and unexpected objects at both locations for each context condition. Several features should be noted. First, for near objects in high context, fixations on the unexpected items dominated throughout the exposure period. However, this was true even at fixation ''0,'' which represents where the eye was positioned when the picture appeared. Since subjects were instructed to fixate the center of the screen until the picture appeared, this result implies that the unexpected objects were closer to the center of the picture. An examination of the pictures revealed that in 13 scenes the unexpected object was closer to the center (by an average of 2.3°), in 5 the expected object was closer (by an average of 1.6°), and in 2 there was no difference. Obviously this situation could have affected subjects' schema formation and thus the course of subsequent scanning.

For far objects, after the first few fixations the expected items were fixated more frequently. In addition, for both near and far objects the pattern of fixation probabilities appears to be similar for high and low context. Given the earlier caution that the low context data should be viewed as a baseline against which to measure behavior during the high context exposures, Figure 3 was prepared, representing the cumulative fixation probability differences, where fixation probabilities for high context were subtracted from those for low context at each fixation number. Higher values in the figure thus represent *less* preference. The figure suggests that for near objects, after the second fixation, context depressed the number of fixations on expected objects relative to unexpected objects. The effect was reversed, although not so apparent, for far objects. Context reduced the probability of fixating an unexpected object in the periphery of the picture more than it affected viewing of similarly located expected objects. Thus the effect of content on fixation location depended on the position of the objects to be fixated. The probability of fixating unexpected objects near the center of the picture was relatively enhanced (less depressed than for expected objects),

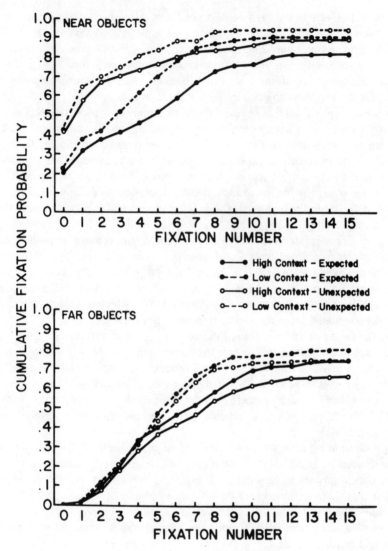

FIG. 2. Cumulative probability of fixating the near (above) and far (below) expected and unexpected objects in both context conditions.

perhaps due to the closer proximity of unexpected objects to the center of the pictures. The proability of fixating expected objects was slightly enhanced relative to unexpected objects when the objects were not near the center of the picture.

Thus, in general, the predictions were supported by the data. This lends support to the model generating the predictions, that of context contributing to

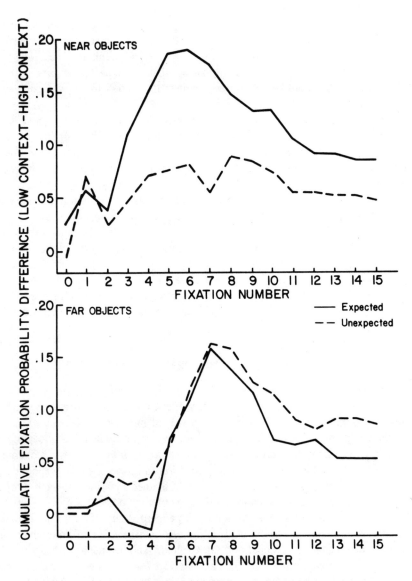

FIG. 3.   Low context versus high context differences in cumulative fixation probability on near (above) and far (below) expected and unexpected objects.

the rapid development of a schema that guides visual exploration with the aid of expectations consistent with the schema. Regarding the slight deviation in the latter prediction, it was suggested that unexpected objects near the center of the picture were located in such a position that they were immediately incorporated into the schema and thus received a consistently higher number of fixations than the near-expected objects. It is also possible that the expected objects near the center of the scene could be identified peripherally via top-down processing such that confirmation of expectations did not involve foveal attention.

Other models may explain these data. Indeed the view that attention is directed to confirm expectations seems superfluous in explaining the results. Rather, the view that attention is directed to unexpected, low probability objects appears to be more consistent with everyday experience. However, this approach cannot account for the result regarding useful field of view and we believe that attention to expected information better represents the situation in everyday viewing in which highly unusual objects are not normally encountered. In such situations, attention to information consistent with the general theme of the scene is an extremely efficient means of rapidly apprehending meaning. Notice that this does not imply avoidance of unexpected objects, merely that they are not noticed until such a time when they are brought close enough to the point of fixation that peripheral analysis can provide enough information to suggest that these objects might be of interest to the scene. At that point they would receive considerable attention.

OTHER VARIABLES INFLUENCING ATTENTION

Consistent with the general purpose guiding this research, additional analyses were performed in an attempt to identify variables that influence attention while viewing complex scenes. The analyses involved measuring as many variables within the pictures as could be identified and entering them as independent variables in a stepwise multiple regression routine along with eye movement measures. In addition to the variables of location and expectedness, we identified three other characteristics of the objects and obtained measures of them. Object *size* was simply the area in square millimeters of each object. Subjective *probability* ratings of the four objects by an independent group of subjects yielded a continuous probability variable and served as a confirmation of the dichtomous labeling of objects as expected and unexpected. Another measure, obtained by means of subjective ratings, was labeled *embeddedness,* and was an indication of the isolation of an object from surrounding objects and contours relative to the density of the rest of the picture. In addition to the eye movement measures described earlier of number of fixations, fixation duration, gaze, and saccadic amplitude, we also evaluated both duration and gaze of fixations immediately *before* and *after* a fixation on one of the four objects. In addition the eye movement amplitude *following* a fixation on one of the four objects was measured.

TABLE 2
Significant Predictors of Eye Movement Measures in Regressions
Performed on High Context Trials

Measure	Independent Variables				
	Location	Probability	Embeddedness	Size	R^2
Number of Fixations	2(−)		1(+)		.135
Duration Before					.004
Duration During		1(−)			.026
Duration After		1(−)			.019
Gaze Before	1(−)		2(+)		.048
Gaze During	3(−)	1(−)	2(+)		.093
Gaze After	1(−)	2(−)	3(+)		.081
Amplitude Before	2(+)	1(+)			.370
Amplitude After	1(+)		2(−)		.140

Note. The numbers indicate the rank of that independent variable according to variance accounted for among all significant ($p < .05$) predictors. The signs in parentheses indicate the sign of the b-value for that variable. Larger values of the independent variables are associated with far objects, higher probability, greater embeddedness, and larger size.

The regression routine computed the best one variable model, best two variable model, etc., in terms of maximizing R^2. Regressions were performed for the high context condition only, since ratings were performed using the high context pictures and they best represent normally encountered scenes. The discrete measure of expectedness was run in separate analyses from the probability ratings and since the results were virtually identical (the zero-order Pearson correlation between the two variables was 0.89), the following results are described for probability ratings only. Table 2 summarizes the results by presenting the significant predictors ($p < 0.05$) for each analysis. Results are presented for the models in which all possible variables were entered.

It is immediately evident that there was a considerable range in predictability of the measures from a low of about 3% of the variability in the duration measures to about 35% of the variability in amplitude of saccades preceding fixation on a particular object. The variables entered into the regressions consisted of measures both of the physical aspects of the objects (size, location, and embeddedness) and the semantic aspect of probability. It is apparent that size was not related to any of the dependent measures, neither class of variables predicted duration before, only probability predicted duration during and after, only physical variables predicted gaze before and amplitude after, and both types of variables predicted the other measures.

That size was not a factor in number of fixations and gaze, given much previous research to the contrary (e.g., Brandt, 1945) is somewhat surprising but explainable in that objects did not vary greatly in size. The mean size of all objects was 2.86° square and the standard deviation was 1.40° square.

Only probability of occurrence of an object predicted the duration of fixation on an object. It also predicted the duration of the *next* fixation, regardless of where that fixation was located, but did not predict the duration of the *preceding* fixation. If duration is taken as an index of time to encode an object then it would be expected, from the results previously described, that improbable objects would require greater time to be incorporated into the schema. The fact that object probability predicted the next fixation implies that encoding of an object continues into the next fixation. The failure of this relationship to hold for the preceding fixation suggests that no differential anticipatory processing was occurring. That is, whatever processing was occurring, it was not related to these variables. Thus the results involving fixation durations suggest that part of the fixational pause is devoted to processing the semantic information currently being fixated, that previously fixated, but not that about to be fixated. These findings thus lend support for Russo's (1978) "Anticipation of Location" model of the cognitive processes involved in the "eye movement cycle," which postulates a lag of processing into the next fixation. However they do not support his "Anticipation of Location and Stimulus $N + 1$" model, which postulates anticipatory processing of the object of the next fixation, at least to the extent that such processing is related to the variables in this study.

The predictors of amplitude after suggest that saccades after a fixation on an object in the periphery of the picture and one that is relatively isolated are relatively large. The fact that embeddedness was not related to amplitude before and negatively related to amplitude after in the high context scenes suggests a viewing strategy of moving the eye relatively large distances away from the more isolated areas but not selecting the distance to the object of the next fixation on the basis of the presence or absence of surrounding objects and contours. The finding that amplitude before was predicted by object probability and location suggests that decisions regarding the location of the next fixation involve the semantic as well as physical aspects of the surrounding objects. Since neither of these variables predicted *duration* before, it appears that the *time* required to make the fixation decision is not dependent on these variables. Thus although there is a tendency to fixate "informative" areas (Antes, 1974; Mackworth & Morandi, 1967), the decision to fixate those areas takes no longer than decisions to fixate other less informative areas.

It should be noted that it is difficult to interpret analyses like these and the explanations should be viewed as tentative and should serve only as hypotheses for study in future investigations.

CONCLUSIONS

The purpose of this research was to investigate the effects of picture context on eye movement patterns and, by inference, on cognitive processes underlying visual exploration. Predictions were guided by the view that attention is directed to confirm the changing set of expectations derived from an evolving schematic representation of the scene. It was suggested that contextual information promoted a rapid characterization of the picture theme, which contributed greatly to these expectations and helped guide the viewer via conceptually-driven processing. The results provided support for these predictions. First fixations on expected objects were shorter when they occurred in context. This was not the case for unexpected objects supporting the view that only expected objects receive the benefit of conceptually-driven processing. Context tended to reduce saccade length to expected objects less than to unexpected objects, supporting the idea of superior peripheral recognition of objects consistent with the frame. It was also predicted that expected objects in the high context scenes would be fixated more frequently early in viewing and unexpected objects would receive the higher concentration of fixations later. Instead it was found that throughout the viewing period increased contextual information resulted in fewer fixations on expected objects located near the center of the picture and more fixations on expected objects located in the periphery of the picture. This result may be confounded by the greater chance of having the eye fixated on the location of a central unexpected object when the pictures appeared, resulting in an earlier than anticipated schema modification. Or perhaps, because expected objects receive the benefit of top-down processing, they are more likely to be peripherally identified and do not need to be fixated to be incorporated in the schema.

The results also suggest that, in viewing a picture containing much contextual information, a portion of the fixational pause is devoted to integrating information from the preceding fixation to the object currently being viewed. Additionally, semantic and physical information contributing to the decision regarding the location of the next fixation is obtained but is not differentially processed. That is, decisions to fixate expected objects do not appear to take any more or less time than decisions to fixate unexpected objects.

The views of picture processing developed from the work of Friedman (1979) and Hochberg (1970a) from which the predictions were derived were supported in this study with one possible modification. Although attention may be directed to confirm expectations, some objects, which are highly probable within the scene, may be identified peripherally, then incorporated into the schema without the need to involve foveal attention.

This model has implications regarding the time course of object recognition. Brief exposures should result in superior recognition of expected objects if fine detail information is not required to make the judgment. When the task requires detail recognition, both kinds of objects should be recognized poorly, but for different reasons—expected objects because encoding did not involve detail and unexpected objects because they were not yet encoded. Longer exposures would lessen the difference in recognition of expected and unexpected objects when the task involves little detail information, and would result in superior recognition of unexpected objects when object detail was necessary to make the judgment. Friedman (1979) has demonstrated support for the latter implication in finding that unexpected objects from pictures exposed for 30 sec were remembered better than expected objects. We have some recent data (Antes, Penland, & Metzger, 1980) supporting the former, in which 100 msec exposures resulted in recognition performance for expected and unexpected objects attributable primarily to the global information provided by the context.

In this experiment we attempted to examine the effects of our manipulations on several different eye movement measures. The result was that the effects varied somewhat, depending on the particular measure of viewing behavior. We have viewed the results together believing that the pattern of findings would reveal more about the processes involved than would separate measures individually.

The extent to which these results may be generalized to other situations is unknown. The subjects were instructed to view the pictures in preparation for a recognition task and the results may not be comparable to a free viewing situation. Yarbus (1967) has clearly shown that instructions to subjects can dramatically alter the distribution of eye fixations. In the present study, comparability to free viewing was least probable for the low context scenes that presented the appearance of an array of unrelated objects. Subjects could conceivably have adopted a strategy of viewing the objects in, say, a clockwise order. We tried to reduce the possibility of this occurring by ensuring that the set of six objects in the low context scens represented widely differing locations across pictures and by randomly interspersing the high and low context scenes. Across subjects no particular viewing strategy on the low context pictures was evident but within subjects there appeared to be some such tendencies.

Finally, it should be emphasized that only a small fraction of the total variance for the various eye movement measures was accounted for in the regression analyses. It is possible that much additional variation could be attributable to subject differences and the pictures themselves. When entered as classification variables in a multiple regression equation, subjects and pictures accounted for, on the average, an additional 8% of the variance. Clearly much remains to be discovered regarding the factors influencing eye movement patterns.

ACKNOWLEDGMENTS

The authors wish to express their appreciation to Jim Clark, David Edwards, and Rich Metzger for their helpful comments in the preparation of this chapter.

III.3 Local and Global Influences on Saccadic Eye Movements

John M. Findlay
University of Durham, Durham, England

There is at present a recognizable gap between our understanding of the way in which saccades are generated to simple targets and our understanding of the way in which saccades occur in relation to complex pictorial material. In the former case one can point to a set of models of increasing refinement (Becker & Jürgens, 1979; Robinson, 1973; Young & Stark, 1963). The latter area has not, I believe, developed any similar theoretical coherence. The purpose of this chapter is to explore one key issue in this area. This concerns the way in which peripheral vision is used to select a saccade target and to direct the saccade.

It must first be noted that a variety of viewpoints exist concerning the importance of peripheral vision in saccadic behavior. At one extreme there is the position that makes no reference to peripheral vision but views the eye somewhat as a searchlight, capable of being directed to any desired position by means of internal processes. So, for example, Just and Carpenter (1976) in their interesting work on eye movements and mental rotation make the assumption that the visual picture can be treated as a set of symbols, spatially separated. Their analysis starts from the idea that "the eye fixates the referent of the symbol currently being processed." Likewise the detailed theory of Noton and Stark (1971c) ignores incoming visual information and assigns the direction of saccades, at least in the viewing of familiar material, to the internalized "feature ring." This is a type of perceptuo-motor memory that, having assimilated information at one fixation location, generates a precise saccade to the next required location. An account may, however, be given of scanpath phenomena, that assigns more importance to peripheral vision (Walker-Smith, Gale, & Findlay, 1977).

At the other extreme, Gibson (1966) says this about the process of saccade generation: "How are the exploratory shifts of fixation guided or controlled?

What causes the eye to move in one direction rather than another and to stop at one part of the array instead of another? The answer can only be that interesting structures in the array, and interesting bits of structure, particularly motions, *draw* the foveas towards them'' (p. 260). This seems close to the suggestion that events in peripheral vision essentially act as stimuli for saccades, an idea that Gibson has since explicitly denied (Gibson, 1979). Nevertheless it is well known, even outside psychology, that certain peripheral events can influence eye movements. We can quote Shakespeare who said, "Things in motion sooner catch the eye that what stirs not.'' It seems sooner reasonable to suggest that certain types of stimulation in peripheral vision might be particularly salient.

I have carried out a set of experiments (Findlay, 1980) to explore the possibility that there is a natural order of salience. The paradigm used, developed by Lévy-Schoen (1974), involved presenting two visual stimuli simultaneously on opposite sides of a fixation point. In this situation, the subject makes a saccade to either one or the other. It is then possible to vary the properties of the visual stimuli and determine their capacity to attract saccades. This does allow the development of a coherent psychophysics of saccade generation (Findlay, 1980), but it turns out that the important variables are the location on the retina (proximity to the fovea) and the amount of transient stimulation. Spatial detail, rather surprisingly, is ineffective. Thus a patch of black and white square wave grating when presented against a white background at an eccentricity at which the lines could be clearly resolved, was no more effective in eliciting eye movements than an equal sized, homogeneous, gray patch of the same space average luminance (c.f. Fig. 1).

I had started the experiment with the idea that the amount of contour in a region might be an "interesting bit of structure" in Gibson's terms and thus draw the fovea towards it. The results of many experiments on picture scanning can be encapsulated in the rather nebulous phrase that "the eye fixates on informative details.'' (Mackworth & Morandi, 1967). Frequently it may be expected that the areas that contain informative detail will also contain a lot of visual detail, leaving open the possibility that peripheral vision is involved in guiding the saccade. My results suggest, however, that amount of contour per se will not do this automatically.

The substitution of the word "informative" for Gibson's word "interesting" in what is otherwise a very similar idea makes one thing clear. What is informative will vary from one situation to another and so patterns of scanning might differ also. This is, of course, the case (c.f. the records presented by Yarbus (1967) of the effect of instruction on fixations when viewing the picture "An Unexpected Visitor"). Could the visual system be programmed to search for specific information in the periphery and then direct the eye to this location by means of a saccade? Hochberg (1970b) has used the term "peripheral search guidance" to describe this possibility. Although it would seem that any spatial detail that could be resolved in peripheral vision might be used in principle to

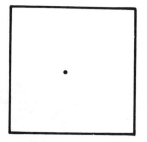

1. Fixation point offset from centre

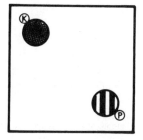

2. Targets and indicators 300 msec

FIG. 1.   Illustration of the type of stimulus used to study the effects of visual parameters on saccadic eye movements. The subject was presented with two stimuli simultaneously in peripheral vision and his task was to read off one of the indicator letters. A fixation point slightly offset from the central position was used to compensate for positional biases. It was found that a 4 cycles per degree grating patch was no more effective at eliciting a saccade than a gray patch of the same space average luminance when presented at 2.8° eccentricity, a region where the grating can be clearly resolved (From Findlay, 1980, with permission).

become the target of a saccadic eye movement, there appear to be quite severe limitations to the practical possibilities. Williams (1966) measured eye fixations in a task where a subject had to search a rather cluttered visual field containing objects of various sizes, shapes, and colors. He found that color information could be used effectively to guide the eye to targets, but that size and shape information were not effective.

However there are some situations in which shape information can be used effectively to guide the eye to targets. For example, Gould and Dill (1969), in a search task with an array of nine well spaced patterns, showed that a systematic increase in the probability of a pattern being fixated occurred as the shape of the pattern approximated more closely to the target shape. A possible reason for this discrepancy is that the direction of a saccade is normally influenced by stimulation present over quite a wide region of the visual field. This would mean that saccades can be accurately directed at a small target only if it stands in an isolated region of visual field. This possibility is supported by the following study (carried out while the author was a visitor to the laboratory of Ariane Lévy-Schoen in Paris).

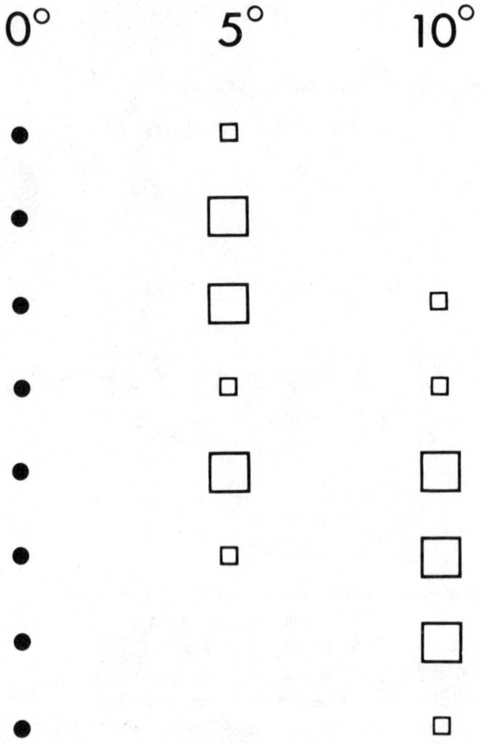

FIG. 2. Stimulus used in experiment to investigate the extent to which saccade amplitude is influenced by global stimulus properties. On each trial the subject was presented with one stimulus from the set of eight. These consisted of different combinations of large (0.42° side) and small (0.14° side) squares. On half the trials a small gap (4 min arc) was present in the side of one square.

Horizontal eye movements were recorded using a photoelectric method when subjects did the following. First, the subject initiated a trial by releasing a hand-held button. This caused the appearance of a visual stimulus, either on the right or on the left of the fixation point. The stimulus was one from the set illustrated in Fig. 2. Half of these consisted of a single square, either at 5 degrees in the periphery or at 10°, the other half comprised two squares one at each eccentricity. On half the trials, a very small gap was present in one side of one square. The object of the experiment was to discover, for the double squares, the extent to which the saccade control system would respond to them as a global configuration, as opposed to taking each target separately. Additionally, I was interested in the extent to which the processing was modifiable by instructions and consequently used two conditions. In the first, the task of the subject was to detect the gap and respond by pressing a second button if the gap was present. This task, termed "detection," was designed to demand accurate fixation on the individual targets. The second task, "comparison," used the same stimulus set but the subject had to respond only if the overall combination of square sizes was identical to that in the previous trial. Although the comparison task could be performed in peripheral vision, in practice a saccade was always made.

Four subjects were tested, the order of presentation of the conditions being counterbalanced. The amplitude of the resulting saccades are shown in Fig. 3. This shows a number of features of interest. For the double targets, the saccade is always directed to an intermediate position between the two targets, and this does not represent an averaging artefact—the variance of saccade amplitude is slightly greater than for single targets as explained in the following, but the mean position does represent the position where the saccades are most likely to fall. Thus the calculation of saccade amplitude is affected by the global properties of the target configuration. This once again suggests that local spatial detail is ignored by, and is possibly unavailable to, the saccade control system. This occurs identically in the left visual field and the right visual field. The saccade amplitude is also dependent systematically on the relative sizes of the two targets.

A most unexpected finding emerges when the results from the two tasks are compared. Paradoxically, the instructions that emphasize attention to target detail produce saccades for which the influence of the global target configuration

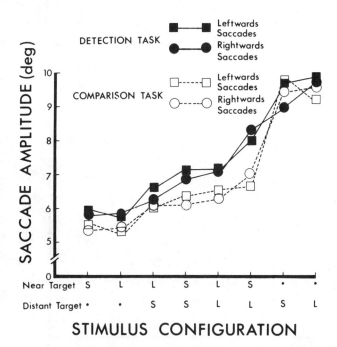

FIG. 3. Amplitude of saccades to the different stimuli shown in Fig. 2. Each point gives the mean of 32 trials and four subjects. The saccades to double square stimuli are directed to an intermediate position between the squares. The exact location depends systematically on the relative sizes of the squares. There is a significant interaction, F (7,21) = 5.32; p = 0.016, between the task performed by the subject and the stimulus configuration, but no significant differences to targets in the left visual field and those in the right visual field.

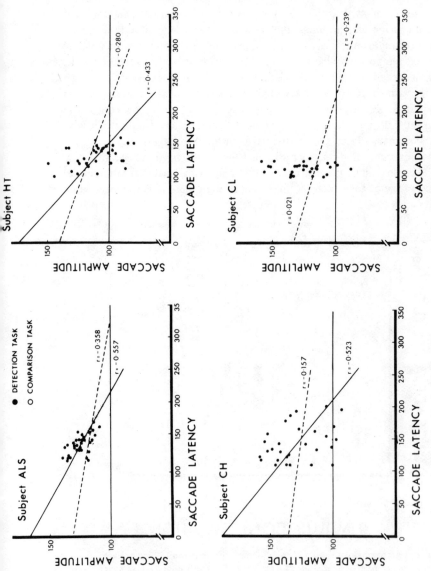

FIG. 4. Amplitudes of individual saccades made to two identical targets (either both large or both small), plotted against saccade latency for each subject. The saccade amplitudes are normalized relative to the mean amplitude for the block of saccades to single close targets (100). Regression lines are plotted for saccades in each task, showing that the more rapidly the saccade is generated, the more it is subject to control by the global aspect of the stimulus configuration. Filled circles and full lines show saccades from the detection task: Open circles and dashed lines show those from the comparison task.

176

appears greater. These saccades land further away from the individual targets than those in the comparision condition. For the target combination consisting of the small square at 5° and the large square at 10° the resultant saccades landed midway between the two targets and it was frequently found that the subjects needed two further saccades, one to each target, before responding. It seems that at one level of processing the eye was being directed to the individual targets, whereas at some other more basic level, the global visual properties of the stimulus were taking effect.

This doesn't explain why the eye should actually be worse at getting to the target position in the detection condition, the condition for which on-target saccades are required. Some light on this contrary behavior emerged from the observation that the average latency for the initial saccade in the detection condition was 133 msec whereas that found in the comparison condition was 165 msec. This suggested that there might be a general dependence of saccade amplitude on saccade latency. As illustrated in Fig. 4, such effects do occur for the double square stimuli, although there appears to be no such effect in the saccades to the single squares. Figure 4 illustrates individual saccades when the stimuli consist of two identical targets at 5° and 10°, plotted as a function of their latency from the trial initiation. For the results in each condition, least squares regression lines have been fitted to the data. Although the individual data show considerable variation (some of which may be ascribable to calibration inaccuracies), certain trends clearly emerge. It seems that in both conditions, the more rapidly a saccade is made, the more it is influenced by the global properties of the target configuration. In the detection task, a process appears to be operative in counteracting this tendency and directing the saccade to the nearest target. This process becomes increasingly effective as the trial proceeds. Three out of four subjects show this clearly, and in the case of the fourth it is possible that the range of saccade latencies is too small for the effect to become manifest. A similar process, although much weaker, is also present in the comparison task. One has the uncanny feeling here of seeing, in fine detail, the progression of a voluntary influence overriding a reflex tendency.

An even more direct approach to the question of the extent to which volitional influences can operate on saccades is shown in Fig. 5. In these trials, subjects were instructed explicitly to carry out the gap detection task but also to direct the gaze at one or other of the target locations whenever a target should appear there. Although this was not pursued systematically, the results do, nevertheless, show certain features of interest. As expected from the previous results, the occasion in which appropriate saccades were generated also showed long latencies. When instructions to fixate the closer target had been given, and a distant target only appeared, the first saccade was frequently hypometric. In this situation subject ALS frequently produced a flight of small saccades before reaching the target. It is possible, of course, that modifications in saccade behavior could occur with more practice (c.f. Festinger, White, & Allyn, 1968).

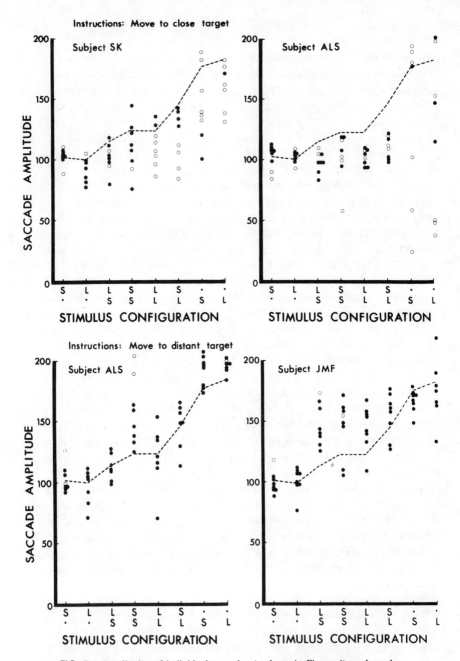

FIG. 5. Amplitudes of individual saccades (scale as in Figure 4) made under instructions to move to one or other target position. Open circles show saccades with latencies above 200 msec, filled circles those with latencies below 200 msec. Dotted line shows results from detection condition in Fig. 3. In general it does not appear to be possible for subjects to ignore completely the effects of the other target when present.

It is clear from the results presented that the triggering of a saccade is a complex process. Many workers in visual science in recent years have found it profitable to postulate that the visual signal is analyzed in several channels, more or less autonomously (e.g., Breitmeyer & Ganz, 1976). If this is accepted, the question of which channel or channels control eye movements becomes an empirical one. This was anticipated by Richards and Kaufman (1969) who said "It is not necessary that the feature detectors which mediate pattern perception also drive the oculomotor system." They introduce the term "center of gravity" to denote the position where the eye fixates in viewing simple geometric figures, and this term was also used by Coren and Hoenig (1972a) to explain results very similar to those presented here.

Two problems emerge with the use of the term "center of gravity," and I believe the term should be abandoned. Firstly, as shown here, the term suggests a single location at which saccades are directed, whereas it appears that the location varies as a function of saccade latency. Secondly, it has never been clear how the implied averaging process should be carried out. It might, for example, be argued that different regions of the visual field should be differentially weighted (Levy-Schoen, 1974; Findlay, 1980). Moreover, the term cannot encompass the important insights that have been obtained from analysis of the visual system in terms of spatial frequencies (Campbell & Robson, 1968; Sekuler, 1974). I believe that a more promising approach is to suggest that the reason why 'center of gravity' phenomena appear is that the oculomotor system is predominantly controlled by the low spatial frequency channels (c.f. Marr & Poggio, 1979).

These experiments have concerned stimuli that appear suddenly in the visual field and thus have a large transient component. Is it legitimate to argue from this situation to the case of scanning of static pictures? The answer is not obvious since it may be assumed that the processing of visual information for a saccade commences following a prior saccade, which will itself have moved the retina and produced a large quantity of transient activity. Situations can be found in which it seems clear that global factors affect the saccades when viewing static scenes. For example, when subjects are asked to estimate the lengths of lines in The Müller-lyer illusion, their fixations fall between the arrowheads. Yarbus (1967), in demonstrating this, refers to the "disobedience" of the eye. The arguments developed above might help to explain the eye's misbehavior.

III.4 Identification and Processing of Briefly Glimpsed Visual Scenes

Helene Intraub
Bucknell University

Remembering unrelated visual scenes that are presented for only a few seconds each is an easy task for the average observer. Hundreds and even thousands of pictures can be remembered with better than 90% accuracy when traditional recognition memory procedures are used (Nickerson, 1965; Shepard, 1967; Standing, Conezio, & Haber, 1970). If, however, the rate of presentation is increased to correspond to an average fixation frequency of 3 pictures/sec and faster (up to 8 pictures/sec), recognition memory suffers dramatically, approaching the level of chance (Potter & Levy, 1969). This observation that the ability to process pictorial information is severely limited when pictures are presented at the same rate that scenes are usually fixated is intriguing in that it provides an opportunity to study the nature of processes occurring at the level of a single fixation in normal viewing.

In this chapter I shall describe some recent work that has used brief pictorial presentations to simulate single fixations and sequences of briefly presented pictures to mimic the normal scanning rate. This research is concerned with two aspects of processing—identification and encoding. The first set of experiments is concerned with measuring the observer's ability to identify each briefly glimpsed scene in a sequence. The second set is concerned with the nature of encoding processes used to store briefly glimpsed pictures. This will include a discussion of the role of eye movements in encoding. The third will address the role of voluntary attentional strategies in pictorial encoding.

IDENTIFICATION OF SUCCESSIVELY
PRESENTED SCENES

One possible explanation of the poor picture memory following rapid rates of presentation is that the observer is not able to identify and understand most of the pictures that are presented. Although there is considerable evidence that the gist of an isolated briefly presented visual scene is rapidly grasped by the observer (e.g., Biederman, 1972; Biederman, Glass, & Stacy, 1973; Biederman, Rabinowitz, Glass, & Stacy, 1974), it does not necessarily follow that pictures shown in a rapid continuous sequence can be so readily understood. In these sequences, the presentation rate may be similar to the normal scanning rate, but the continuity and expectancy that are characteristic of normal viewing are eliminated through the use of unrelated scenes.

To determine if identification of individual scenes is the limiting factor for memory under these conditions, Potter (1975, 1976) compared detection of a cued picture in a sequence with recognition memory for pictures presented at the same rate. Sequences of 16 magazine photographs were presented at rates ranging from 113 to 333 msec/picture. Cueing was accomplished either by showing the target picture in advance or by describing it using a brief verbal title (e.g., "a road with cars"). The rationale was that to make the match with the verbal cue, the target would have to be analyzed at a conceptual level. The proportion of targets detected was, therefore, interpreted as reflecting the minimal proportion of pictures identified during presentation. Detection was measured as a key press response falling between 250 and 900 msec following target onset. A control group was shown the same sequences, each followed by a serial recognition test that included all the pictures from the sequence and an equal number of distractors.

The results showed a marked superiority of detection accuracy over recognition memory at all rates. On the basis of only the verbal description, at a rate of 333 msec/picture, approximately 80% of all targets were detected whereas the recognition memory subjects only remembered 40% of the pictures. At the rate of 113 msec/picture, much faster than the average fixation frequency, detection accuracy was extremely good, with more than 60% of the targets detected. Only 11% of the pictures were recognized by the memory group in this condition. This was interpreted as showing that despite the lack of visual continuity during rapid presentation, pictures are momentarily understood. Following identification many are then immediately forgotten.

An alternate explanation of these results, however, holds that detection superiority may actually have been the result of expectancy (Carr & Bacharach, 1976; Neisser, 1976). Even the verbal cue may have raised probabilistic anticipations about the visual attributes of the target, thereby facilitating perception. Rather than reflecting the number of pictures momentarily identified during presentation, detection superiority may simply reflect the fact that the cued picture was perceived more frequently than other pictures in the sequence. One way to test this possibility and determine the extent to which observers can identify unrelated pictures is to cue a picture in a sequence without providing any specific information about its visual characteristics or specific object identity. If pictures can be detected on the basis of such non-specific cues, this would indicate a striking ability of the observer to identify rapidly presented successive scenes even without the benefit of expectancy. One of the detection tasks used by Intraub (1979a) was intended for this purpose. It is described as a "negative detection" task, in which subjects are provided with a general category name prior to viewing a sequence and are instructed to detect and to describe the picture that does *not* belong to that category.

"NEGATIVE DETECTION"
OF RAPIDLY PRESENTED SCENES

Sequences containing a diverse set of 11 magazine photographs from a single general category, and 1 picture (the target) that was not a member of that category were presented at rates of 114, 172, and 258 msec/picture. General categories included: transportation, house furnishings and decorations, mechanical devices, food, body parts, people, animals, fruits and vegetables, and household appliances and utensils. Pictures were selected that were as visually dissimilar as possible. For example, pictures of "animals" included creatures as diverse as a frog, a dog, a giraffe, and a butterfly. The target picture did not differ distinctively in size or in overall coloration from the other pictures in the sequence. Prior to the start of each sequence, subjects were provided with the name of the general category and were instructed to find the picture that did *not* belong (e.g., "the picture that is *not* of an animal"). In this way, the target picture was cued without providing any specific information about its visual or conceptual characteristics. The subject responded by pressing a key upon detection (reaction times were recorded) and then was required to *describe* the target picture. By requiring a description of the target, the problem of screening out false detection responses was eliminated.

Once again, the relationship between identification and memory was studied by comparing detection accuracy with a control group's recognition memory. To allow a more direct comparison than the one made in Potter's experiments, detection accuracy was compared with recognition memory for the target itself, rather than being compared with overall recognition memory for all of the pictures in the sequence. The recognition test was made more sensitive to memory for the target by introducing the following two provisions. (1) Unlike Potter's recognition test in which *all* the pictures from a sequence were tested, in the present experiment only the target picture and one other picture from the sequence were tested. This eliminated the interference that a series of relatively long tests might provide. (2) The two distractors used in the brief 4-item test were neither visually nor conceptually similar to the target. Subjects in the recognition memory condition were instructed to pay attention to each picture as it appeared and to remember as many as possible. Subjects received the recognition test immediately following each sequence. No mention of categories or "odd" pictures was made. To determine if subjects had nonetheless spontaneously categorized the pictures they were asked at the end of the experiment to write a description of the sequences they had just seen.

The results showed that subjects could detect and describe targets specified by a negative cue at all three rates of presentation. At the rate of 258 msec/picture (a rate slightly faster than the average fixation frequency), 79% of all targets were detected. When the rate was increased to 172 and 114 msec per picture, 58% and 35% of the targets were detected, respectively. Memory for the same target picture, however, did not reach the level of detection accuracy. It ranged from 19% correct in the fastest condition to 49% and 58% correct in the slower conditions, respectively. Overall, more pictures were detected than were remembered, $F (1, 84) = 9.00$, $p < .001$. At the end of the experiment, all recognition memory subjects reported that the sequences seemed to contain pictures from a general category. In fact, 87% of those subjects specifically reported noting a "category plus odd picture" arrangement. Apparently subjects had seen enough to *spontaneously* categorize the pictures during presentation. In spite of this, immediate recognition memory for the targets was inferior to detection accuracy.

These results support the hypothesis that at rates of presentation that mimic the average fixation frequency of the eye, while retention of visual scenes may be poor, the ability to momentarily identify each glimpsed scene is remarkably good. The results show that expectancy alone cannot account for the superiority of detection ability over recognition memory that was reported by Potter. Using a conservative detection task (requiring description) and a highly sensitive immediate recognition test, more targets were "negatively detected" than were remembered. Of course the results do not imply that expectancy is not important in visual perception. What they do show is that under extremely adverse conditions, in which the continuity characteristic of vision is eliminated, conceptual information specific enough to allow relatively difficult decisions to be made is available at a very early stage of processing. Apparently, the poor recognition memory performance obtained under these conditions cannot be attributed solely to the observer's inability to identify the pictures. Instead, this poor performance reflects a limitation on encoding processes necessary for retention.

ENCODING BRIEFLY GLIMPSED PICTURES

Although the gist of a briefly glimpsed picture in a sequence is apparently available at an early stage of processing, recognition memory is poor immediately following presentation. One possible explanation is that for most pictures more than one fixation is necessary for storage of a memory representation detailed enough for the picture to be recognized later. It has been suggested that the eye fixation is a special "unit of encoding" (Loftus, 1972). According to this view, encoding takes place during the fixation, while the picture is physically present—perhaps specifically limited to the early part of the fixation (Loftus, 1976). The first fixation is seen as providing the observer only with general information about the picture; each additional fixation is thought to increase the probability that an informative detail will be encoded, thereby increasing the likelihood that a picture will be recognized later (Loftus & Kallman, 1979). The poor memory performance obtained following rapid presentation is attributed to the fact that only one simulated fixation is possible per picture.

There is a growing body of evidence, however, that disputes the notion that encoding is limited to the duration of the fixation. Rosenblood and Pulton (1975), for example, presented 400 pictures for as little as 80 msec each with a 5 sec blank interstimulus interval (ISI). Subjects recognized 74% of the pictures. This performance is far superior to that obtained when briefly presented pictures are shown in a continuous sequence. Intraub (1980) directly compared recognition memory for 150 magazine photographs presented for 6 sec each with no ISI, and the same pictures presented for only 110 msec each followed by a 5890 msec blank ISI. This drastic reduction in stimulus duration resulted in a surprisingly small decrease in recognition memory from 94% to 77% correct, even though the number of fixations probably dropped from about 18 to 1. When the same pictures were presented in a continuous sequence at a rate of 110 msec/picture, recognition memory dropped dramatically, with only 21% recognized. In another experiment, pictures were presented for 110 msec each, followed by blank ISIs of 1390, 620, 385, 165, or 0 (no ISI) msec. Recognition memory decreased from 92% to 83%, 74%, 57%, and 19% correct, respectively (Intraub, 1979b). This indicates that encoding is not limited to the duration of a fixation, although the nature of the encoding process is not readily apparent.

The decrease in memory obtained when the ISI between briefly presented pictures is reduced can be explained equally well by two general encoding hypotheses. (1) Encoding is an all or nothing phenomenon. For a given observer, a particular picture requires a fixed amount of time to be encoded in memory. If enough time is not allowed, the picture will be forgotten. As the time between pictures is diminished, although many pictures can be momentarily identified, fewer pictures can be encoded. (2) Encoding is a continuous process. Following identification, an increasing number of pictorial details will be stored. As the time between pictures is diminished, fewer pictures will be stored in enough detail to pass a recognition threshold at the time of the test. While both hypotheses predict a decrease in recognition memory when presentation rate is increased, they differ in their predictions regarding the stored representations of the pictures. According to the all or nothing interpretation, given equal stimulus duration, those pictures that are recognized following a rapid rate of presentation should be remembered in as much detail as pictures that are recognized following a slower rate of presentation. On the other hand, the continuous encoding hypothesis predicts that as the time between pictures is reduced, not only will fewer pictures be remembered but they will be remembered in less detail. A traditional recognition test that uses dissimilar distractors cannot distinguish between these two hypotheses because a minimal amount of information might be sufficient to elicit a recognition response. To avoid this problem, the following experiment was conducted.

RETENTION OF DETAIL
FOLLOWING BRIEF PICTORIAL EXPOSURES

To determine if less is remembered about each picture as the time between pictures is diminished, Intraub (1980) used a recognition test with two levels of difficulty. Subjects first were required to indicate whether or not they recognized a picture. Following that decision they then had to determine if the picture was in the same orientation as in the inspection sequence or if it was mirror reversed. According to the all or nothing hypothesis, with a constant stimulus duration if a picture is recognized, the ability to detect a reversal should remain the same regardless of the ISI. According to the continuous encoding hypothesis, the ability to determine that a recognized picture is reversed should decrease as the time between pictures is diminished.

Twenty magazine photographs were presented for 110 msec each with blank ISIs of 4890, 1390, 620, 385, or 0 (no ISI) msec, or for 5 sec each with no ISI. Ten subjects participated in each condition. They were instructed to pay attention to each picture as it appeared and to try to remember as many as possible. *No mention of mirror reversal was made at this time.*

Following presentation of the sequence, a serial recognition test was administered that contained 16 pictures from the inspection sequence (the initial and final pairs of pictures were not tested) and 16 dissimilar distractors (new pictures). Half of the 16 target pictures were mirror reversed for half the subjects in each condition. Subjects were informed that some of the pictures in the test would be mirror reversals of pictures they had seen in the inspection sequence. They were instructed to respond "yes" if they recognized a picture regardless of the picture's orientation, and "no" if not. Following a "yes" response they were told to respond "reversed" if they thought that the picture was mirror reversed and "normal" otherwise.

The proportion of pictures recognized ("yes" responses, corrected for guessing) dropped only from .96 to .84 when stimulus duration was reduced from 5 sec to 110 msec with a 4890 msec ISI. Recognition memory remained the same in the 1390 msec-ISI condition (.84), but decreased to .61, .48, and .20 as the ISI was further reduced (see Fig. 1). At all rates, however, recognition was better than chance. Reversing a picture did not affect the subject's ability to recognize it

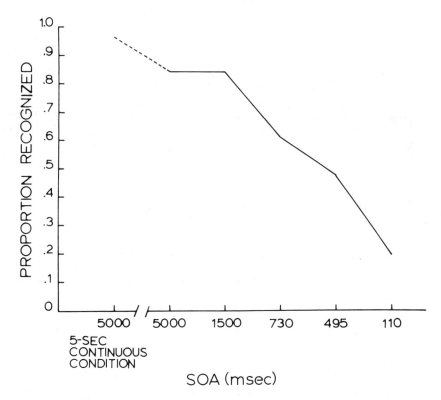

FIG. 1.   The proportion of 110 msec pictures recognized as a function of stimulus onset asynchrony (SOA) and the proportion of pictures recognized in the 5 sec/ picture control condition.

at any rate (an observation also reported by Standing, Conezio, & Haber, 1970, when pictures were presented for a few seconds each).

When a picture was recognized, subjects in the 5 sec continuous condition were able to detect a reversal 81% of the time. Reducing stimulus duration to 110 msec with a 4890 or 1390 msec ISI lowered but did not eliminate this ability (see Fig. 2). As the time between pictures diminished, the ability to detect reversal decreased sharply and was not significantly better than chance at the three fastest rates.

These results demonstrate that rather than being an all or nothing process confined to the initial part of a fixation, pictorial encoding is a continuous process. Although subjects could successfully recognize some pictures at each rate of presentation, the ability to determine that they were reversed was eliminated as the time between pictures was reduced, thus indicating reliance on a less detailed memory representation. This reduction in reversal detection occurred even though stimulus duration was held constant at 110 msec preventing the

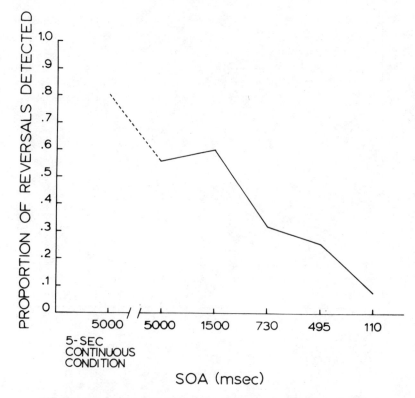

FIG. 2. The proportion of reversals detected as a function of stimulus onset asynchrony (SOA) with a 110 msec stimulus duration and the proportion detected in the 5 sec/picture control condition.

subject from making any additional eye fixations on the pictures during encoding. Since the pictures contained no alphanumeric characters, it is unlikely that left-right orientation of a picture was relevant to its meaning. Even so, after a brief glimpse, subjects were not merely limited to remembering the "gist" of a picture but frequently remembered the objects and scenes in enough detail to determine that they were mirror reversed provided that the time between pictures was long enough. To their own surprise, subjects reported that certain pictures simply *looked* backwards.

As would be expected, memory was somewhat better when pictures were presented for a full 5 sec each than when they were presented for only 110 msec followed by a blank 4890 msec ISI. In the former case the subject could continually scan the picture while encoding was taking place, perhaps storing additional details (e.g., Loftus & Kallman, 1979). The present results show that encoding of visual detail is not confined to the duration of the stimulus, nor is it necessarily dependent on the number of eye fixations made on a picture. Encoding of information necessary for reversal detection continued beyond the period of iconic persistence, and in fact beyond a 620 msec ISI. Under these conditions of presentation it appears that encoding of each picture is terminated when processing of the next picture begins. Does this mean that in normal vision, encoding of each "fixated" scene is terminated by the onset of the next fixation? Some recent work concerned with the role of attentional processes in encoding briefly glimpsed pictures suggests that this is not necessarily the case.

ATTENTIONAL STRATEGIES IN ENCODING BRIEFLY GLIMPSED PICTURES

Potter and Levy (1969) suggested that processing of each picture in a sequence is terminated by the appearance of the "next substantial visual event." Recent research, however, suggests that to some extent there may be voluntary control over whether processing will continue. Potter (1976) demonstrated that when briefly exposed pictures were interspersed with presentation of a colorful visual noise mask, recognition memory far surpassed that obtained when the same pictures were presented in a continuous sequence. Intraub (1980) presented pictures for 110 msec each followed by an ISI that either contained a blank field or a familiar picture that repeated throughout the sequence. Subjects were instructed to attend to the briefly presented pictures. Presentation of a repeating picture during the ISI interfered only minimally with recognition memory and did not affect the ability to detect reversal. Evidently, processing of a picture with a duration of at least 110 msec can continue despite the onset of a meaningless visual noise mask or a repeating picture.

In both cases, however, the ISI contained a familiar, expected visual event. During continuous presentation, each picture is followed by a new picture. To determine if observers can effectively ignore the onset of a new meaningful visual event, as they seem to be able to do with a familiar one, Intraub (1979c) presented pictures for 110 msec each with a 1.5 sec ISI that contained a blank field, a repeating picture, or a new picture each time. Again, subjects were instructed to attend to the briefly presented pictures. Recognition accuracy for the blank and repeating picture conditions was 89% and 80%, respectively. When a *new picture* was presented during the ISI each time, even though recognition memory for the briefly glimpsed pictures decreased significantly (dropping to 63% correct), it did not approach the low level of performance obtained following rapid continuous presentation. This level was reached when the subject was instructed to attend to the "long" pictures (the ISI pictures). As attention instructions were changed to place emphasis on "brief" pictures, all pictures, or "long" pictures, recognition memory for the brief pictures decreased dramatically from 63% to 12% correct. At the same time, memory for the long pictures (that had been presented for 1.5 seconds each) increased from 54% to 87%

correct. This indicates that not only can encoding continue in spite of the occurrence of a new visual event, but that to a large degree, the allocation of attention to sequentially presented visual information can be controlled voluntarily. In the case of rapid sequential presentation of unrelated pictures (no ISI), encoding of each picture may be disrupted when processing is initiated on the next pictures in the sequence (Intraub, 1980; Potter, 1976).

SUMMARY AND IMPLICATIONS

Without expectancy and continuity that characterize visual scanning, observers were able to conceptually identify unrelated, successively presented pictures at rates that mimic average fixation frequency. Identification did not necessarily result in retention. Detection accuracy (even with the use of a "negative" cue) was superior to immediate recognition memory for the same pictures. The ability to *momentarily* identify glimpsed scenes may function as a monitor in vision. For example, the ability to rapidly identify each fixated "scene" may play a role in controlling placement of subsequent fixations.

Apparently, following identification of a scene, the quality of the memory representation depends in large part on how soon encoding is disrupted. As the time between briefly glimpsed pictures was increased, the ability to remember a picture's left-right orientation increased. This superior memory was obtained without additional fixations having to be made on the picture. Although the factors that determine when encoding will be disrupted are not yet fully defined, it is clear that to a large degree the observer can voluntarily control the encoding process. When briefly glimpsed pictures are presented with an ISI that contains a redundant visual event, they are remembered nearly as well as when the ISI contains a blank field. Under conditions in which the ISI contains a new, unrelated picture each time, encoding of briefly presented pictures can extend beyond a single fixation if the observer is instructed to remember the briefly glimpsed pictures and ignore the intervening ISI-pictures. It seems likely that when scanning a coherent visual scene in which successive glimpses are related, encoding will not be limited to the duration of a fixation. The results suggest that the observer can rapidly assess the importance of each fixated "scene" during normal viewing and adjust the extent of encoding to be carried out. Perhaps these overlapping encoding processes play a role in the integration of successive fixations.

ACKNOWLEDGMENT

This research was supported in part by Advanced Research Projects Agency Contract MDA 903–76–C–0441 to Massachusetts Institute of Technology.

IV THEORY AND METHOD

With technological advances, software and hardware sophistication allows the researcher to challenge theory with method. Are the vector connected fixation sequences of scan-paths randomly generated within and between views and re-presentations of a scene? Are these patterns generated by stimulus features or cognitive processes? What are the nature and purpose of small, involuntary eye-movements? Do they have a place in the maintenance of vision? of fixation? Are these small movements real or artifacts of the recording device? Why does the programing of a new saccade take such a long time? Is there purpose to the "procrastination" of the oculomotor system? What refinements in technology are available that enable more precise "noise free" measurements and discrimination of eye movements and fixations?

In the first chapter of this section, Stark and Ellis continue, albeit more sophisticated, Stark and Noton's earlier inquiry into the nature of scan-patterns. Primarily, their focus is of the repeatability of these patterns with subsequent views. A model is presented that allows for both the stimulus and cognitive states to direct the gaze. Deterministic Markov matrices are used to construct simulated scan-patterns showing best fit to the model. Applicability of top-down and bottom-up notions of scan-pattern analyses are described for cognitive psychology, artificial intelligence and scene analysis.

Professor Ditchburn describes small involuntary eye-movements in Chapter IV. 2. He points out that our understanding of the mechanism by means of which the eye maintains its fixation is still not too well understood, but recent technological advances aid in more reliably measuring their activity. He uses knowledge about drifts and tremors to present problems still in need of solving. The ability of the eye to maintain fixation with peripherally unfocused targets is one of these. Deriving the mechanism whereby drifts and high-speed flicks continue to maintain fixation at a desired point is another. Ditchburn proposes that by examining the fine structure of these eye-movements the velocity spectrum will reveal internal processes and, perhaps, internal pathologies.

In Chapter IV. 3, Carpenter meticulously traces the time frame of stimulation to activity in the oculomotor system by neatly organizing a broad and eclectic data base. These latency data are then used to develop a new model of saccadic emissions which when applied to new data provides a quantum leap in our understanding of oculomotor system and new insight into the possibility that "procrastination" leads to efficiency.

Tole and Young describe a methodology using digital filters to detect saccades and fixations in Chapter IV. 4. The method allows for discrimination of saccades and nystagmus fast-phase movements by means of adaptive time domain template matching, rapidly and on-line in the presence of noise. In Chapter IV. 5, Sheena and Borah describe methodology for rapid, on-line identification of eye-point of regard with improved levels of preciseness and accuracy. Algorithms and mathematical analyses derived to compensate for noise and system non-linearities are presented in both chapters.

IV.1 Scanpaths Revisited: Cognitive Models Direct Active Looking

Lawrence Stark and Stephen R. Ellis*
*Departments of Physiological Optics,
Engineering Science and Neurology
University of California, Berkeley*

Our concerns are ''how we look'' and the role of eye movements in perception, visual memory and pattern recognition. Saccadic eye movements continually reposition the fovea (foveation) during active looking in the process of vision. These eye movements can at very least be considered as tags or experimentally accessible quantities that scientists can observe to understand underlying processes of congition. Stronger hypothesis is that eye movements play an essential role in vision; in particular that eye movements are controlled by cognitive models (either ideals or experientially generated) already present in the brain. These models are perceptual hypotheses to be tested against the complex world of sensory experience. In such checking phases of heirarchical pattern recognition processes, repetitious sequences of saccades are generated—''scanpaths.'' Noton and Stark (1971a,b,c) in originally putting forward the scanpath theory, postulated the feature ring, an ensemble or assembly of alternating sensory-motor-sensory-motor . . . . elements as shown schematically in Fig. 1. Sensory elements are semantic subfeatures of scenes or pictures being observed and motor elements are saccades that represent the syntactical structural or topological organization of the scene. Scanpaths, repetitive sequences of saccades, were observed to develop during first viewing of a picture and reoccurred early in a reviewing session with a recognition task.

*Presently with the National Aeronautics and Space Administration, Ames Research Laboratory Moffitt Field, California.

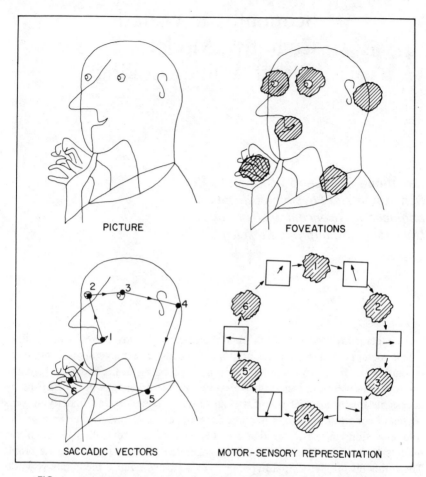

PICTURE

FOVEATIONS

SACCADIC VECTORS

MOTOR-SENSORY REPRESENTATION

FIG. 1. *Feature Ring.* Feature ring proposed by Noton & Stark as a format for
internal representation of a picture. Picture is identified by its principal subfeatures
and by successive saccades composing scanpath. Feature ring consists of sensory
memory traces of subfeatures and motor memory traces of saccades composing
scanpath. Scanpath is generated from this cognitive model by successively reading
out subfeatures and motor vectors in this checking phase of pattern recognition.

Although the scanpath story opened up a new experimental paradigm in
cognitive science (brief reviews of its interrelationship to artificial intelligence,
cognitive psychology, and epistimological philosophy will be put forward in the
discussion section in this chapter), there were important deficits in the original
Noton-Stark experiments. These included the requirement for a richer set of
pictures and scenes. Important also was the lack of a quantitative methodology to
evaluate the existence of a scanpath or to ascertain the degree of relationship of
one example of a scanpath to another—Noton and Stark unfortunately used their

own human recognition and biases for these crucial judgements. In the past ten years, however, a number of studies from independent laboratories, even with quite other interpretation of the role of scanpaths in recognition, have confirmed the experimental findings of Noton and Stark. Magnuski, Anliker, and Lai (1974, personal communication) and Lai (1975), used complex methodologies and computerized judgments with sliding thresholds for similarities between inter-fixational vectors and were so able to process the necessary large amounts of data; they provided impetus to our own computerized experiments to be described below. Locher and Nodine (1973) found scanpaths in their experiment requiring subjects to recollect complex and irregular polygons. Some subjects recognized well but had "poor" scanpaths, while other subjects produced "good" scanpaths but recognized poorly; they thus questioned an obligate relation of scanpaths to the recognition process. Further research however, by Fisher, Monty, and Perlmuter (1978), provided very strong evidence for the similarity between inspection and recognition patterns on simple and complex binary displays.

Parker (1978), from the cognitive science group of Norman, Mandler, and Rummelhardt in San Diego, used quite separated but detailed mulitcomponent scenes and asked subjects to detect changes in a scene on representation; his subjects showed the highest incidence of scanpath mode saccades. He chose to emphasize the ability of his subjects to use peripheral vision as a purported difference in interpretation from Noton and Stark. These new studies and other independent reports of like substance, (i.e., Luria & Strauss, 1978; Walker-Smith, Gale, & Findlay, 1977) taken together with experiments that preceeded the scanpath result and theory—Buswell (1935), Jeannerod, Gerin, & Pernier (1968), Llewellyn-Thomas (1963, 1968), Remond, Lesevre, & Gaversek (1957), Yarbus (1967)—established the experimental basis of scanpaths, raised new questions, and suggested new approaches to the problem of the role of scanpaths in cognition.

METHODS

The computer programs, illustrated in the flow-diagram of Fig. 2, were developed by Freksa, Ellis, & Stark (1980) and Stark, Ellis, Inoue, Freksa, & Zeevi (1979) and were embedded in an online laboratory operating system, On-Line-6, develped by John L. Semmlow, James Ferrigno, Robert V. Ken yon, and Frederick Hsu. It is convenient to delay discussion of these computer procedures until the actual results are illustrated. Our computer hardware system included two PDP-8 mini-computers with RKO8 and RF08 discs, A–D and D–A facilities, analog and digital tape recorders, a digital incremental plotter, several scopes for display of calibration and pictures to the subject, and also a hard-copy unit for display of results. The eye movement measurement used the inexpensive

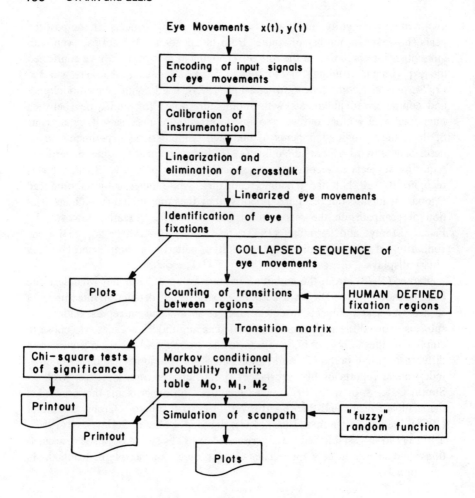

SYSTEM FLOW DIAGRAM

FIG. 2. *Flow Diagram.* Successive stages in program calibrate and linearize instruments, identify eye fixations, accept human-defined fixation regions, count transitions between regions to generate Markov matrix tables, perform chi-square tests of significance, and may simulate the scanpath.

scleral reflection technique (Stark, Vossius, & Young, 1962) sampled at 20 Hz by the computer. Although these require calibration, we feel they are probably more accurate, have a wider bandwidth, and are more precise than many other recording systems.

Choice of picture complexity, and of the task, as defined by instructions to subjects, were found to strongly influence results. We have, therefore, attempted to select a variety of pictures for presentation to reveal different aspects of the relationships between eye movements and perception. Similarily, the subject's degree of sophistication has been shown to influence scanning eye movements and therefore it was important in some experimental designs to use naive volunteers to study changes in cognition and recognition. For other purposes we could use more sophisticated and trained laboratory colleagues.

Linearization. When studying perceptual eye movements that cover an extensive vertical and horizontal range in angular degrees and include many oblique ones having both horizontal and vertical components, the problem of linearization and of independence of the horizontal and vertical components becomes an important one. Our calibration routine generates a sequence of 25 fiduciary marks that the subject is instructed to fixate successively. The values are transformed by the calibration routine so that subsequent recorded scanning eye movements over a picture can be accurately recorded. In Fig. 3, the upper left frame shows the recorded raw calibration data, while the lower left frame demonstrating the linearized and accurate results, shows the calibration algorithm operating. Note also elimination of noise exemplified by the extraneously vertical line in the raw data record in the upper left frame. The upper center frame shows the raw eye movement data recorded while the subject scans the social scene picture in the upper right frame. Note two blink artifacts appearing as hooked, almost vertical, double lines about the raw record in the upper center frame, but eliminated in the linearized and corrected record of the lower center frame. The lower center frame shows the same connected foveations after the linearization routine has corrected them with respect to the fiduciary points. Finally we show the "collapsed" foveations connected by their vectors superimposed on the picture in the lower right frame. The accuracy of the calibration algorithm can be seen by correspondence of the subject's fixation to points of interest in the picture. For example, the concentration of the fixations on the small objects of the table helps the subject understand the social situation that has brought this group of people together; the subjects task was to determine the time of day.

Fixation Identification. The next important part of the program is the identification of the automatic fixation sequence. The upper left frame, Fig. 4, shows three heads painted by a contemporary artist (Stefanie Stark, 1975). In the upper center frame, we show the fixation sequences after linearization by the calibration procedure described earlier. Fixation identification uses both duration of fixation and permissible extent of changes in eye position as criteria. As yet, we have not used a "fuzzy" algorithm, in the sense of Zadeh for fixation identification as described by Schwede and Kandel (1977). By changing the dimensions of the small boxes shown in the lower center frame, more or fewer fixations would be obtained. The algorithm starts by defining the center of a box (Fig. 4, center frame) at the first eye position and then continues to accept new eye positions

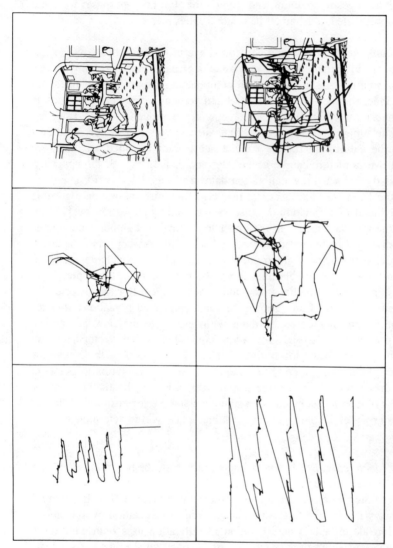

FIG. 3. *Linearization Procedure.* Left upper represents compressed readout from eye movement instrumentation of 25 successively presented and fixated fiduciary calibration points. Lower left shows calibrated fixations. Upper middle shows compressed eye movement recording, when subject views picture in upper right. Note two vertical loops representing eye blink artifacts. Lower middle represents eye movement data linearized by calibration and linearization procedures. Lower right shows (straightened) saccades and successive fixations superimposed on picture.

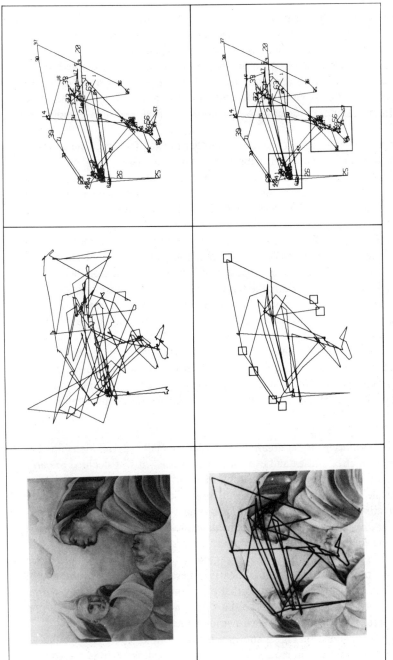

FIG. 4. *Fixation Sequences Identified*. Upper middle represents raw eye movement data after linearization. Lower middle represents fixation identification by computer; a half dozen fixation boxes have already been constructed. Upper right represents each of identified fixations numbered sequentially; physical size of identified number indicates duration of fixation. Lower right shows fixation regions identified by human experimenter. Lower left represents saccades (actually vectors between successive fixations) superimposed on picture shown in upper left.

within the box meanwhile averaging the coordinates. Finally, after the eye has moved out of the box, eye fixation is given as if it had only been at the center of gravity of the cluster of points within the box. This means that the center of the box and the final averaged eye position are not identical as can be noted in the examples presented in the lower center frame. This frame shows seven of the 60 or so identified fixations. The duration criteria is 150 msec or three consecutive samples; in averaging to determine position, the first and last sample are excluded.

The program next assigns a sequential number to each fixation. The physical size of each numeral is a function of the duration of time that the eye has spent in the fixation position. This sequence of numbers superimposed upon straight lines drawn between the fixation points is called the "collapsed sequence of eye movement," as shown in the upper right frame of the figure.

Fixation Regions.   The "collapsed eye movement" trace without the sequential numbers superimposed on the picture is shown in the lower left frame of Fig. 4. The fixations are not evenly distributed and tend to cluster on meaningful regions of the painting, especially the three faces. No specific task was given the subject; he was instructed simply to view the picture. This stage of the computer program involves a man-machine interaction. The experimenter locates "fixation regions," which are regions of clusters of fixations. Typical fixation regions are shown in the lower right frame of Fig. 4. Perhaps these fixation regions chosen for illustration are rather large, especially when compared with the idealized scanpaths described by Noton and Stark and supported by others; however, significant non-random structure, in terms of sequential dependencies can emerge.

Artificial Simulation of Scanpaths.   In order to study interrelationships between Markov matrix entries and eye movement traces, it was decided to carry out a series of simulation studies whereby matrices with sample sets of entries would generate artificial eye movements in an artificial scanpath pattern. Figure 5 shows details of such a simulation. For example, in the left frame is a deterministic Markov probability matrix with all values set to zero except for the supra-diagonal ones set equal to 1. Thus, if the eye is in fixation region 5, the probability of going to the sixth fixation region is 1. Thus, the eye would move from 5 to 6. This deterministic matrix clearly generates a directed, cyclic graph. A "fuzzy" operator has been used so that eye fixation occurs randomly within the fixation region. This contributes to the "fuzzyness" of the fixation position and to the spread of the superimposed eye movement traces.

The right hand frame of Fig. 5 shows a matrix with all coefficients equal to 0.1. If the eye is in fixation region 3, all the next fixation regions are equally probable. The resulting network of eye movements shows a rather disordered appearance. The center frame, labelled probabilistic, shows the Markov entries

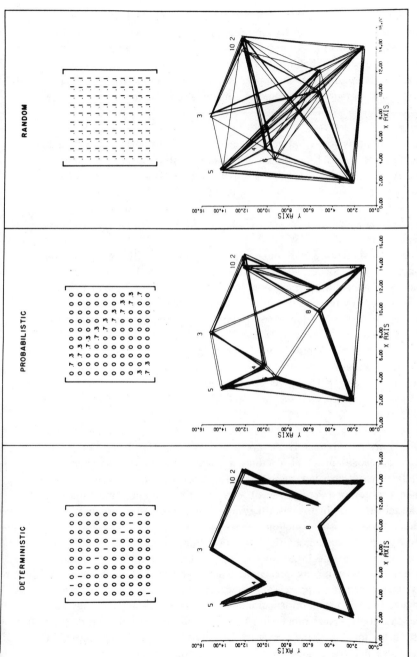

FIG. 5. *Simulation of Scanpaths From Matrix Coefficients.* Left matrix determines that in state n, simulated eye moves with probability 1 to state $n + 1$ yielding deterministic simulated scanpath below; some fuzzyness in fixation within fovea is introduced and presents line superimposition. Middle probabilistic matrix provides for transition probabilities as indicated and produces scanpath below showing some order and some randomness. Random matrix on right allows equi-probability of transitions from any state to any other state and results in completely disordered eye movement sequential pattern; note the $\mathbf{M}_{(0)}$ still provides structure.

in the superdiagonal line to be 0.7, in the next diagonal to be 0.3, and to be zero everywhere else. If the eye is in fixation region 8, there is a 0.7 probability of going to 9 and a 0.3 probability of going to 10. If the eye is at fixation region 8, it might have arrived with probability 0.7 from fixation 7 or a probability of 0.3 from fixation 6. This graph has an appearance intermediate between the deterministic and purely random forms and is somewhat similar to experiment eye scanpaths.

Fixational Eye Movements.   Eye movements occur during fixation although normal subjects are able to maintain the stability of their gaze within the 0.5° diameter of the "fixational fovea." The most prominent fixational eye movements are micro-saccades ranging in amplitude from 2 to 30 arc minutes; their velocities and other "main sequence" characteristics are appropriate to the motor definition of saccades in general (Bahill & Stark, 1979; Dodge & Cline, 1901; Zuber, Stark, & Cook, 1965).

Micro-drift movements are of three types. Conjugate drifts related to the smooth pursuit system occur with velocities of less than 0.25° per second. Slight head movements have been shown to be of significance (Steinman, Haddad, Skavinski, & Wyman, 1973) and some components of conjugate microdrifts may well be very low velocity vestibular ocular reflexes. Nachmias (1959) and St. Cyr & Fender (1969c) have described slow disjunctive or vergence drifts that may remain within Pannum's area, approximately 10 arc minutes at the fovea. Debate continues as to the relative importance of micro-saccades and micro-drifts in preventing fading or graying out of vision (i.e., as occurs in stopped image experiments (Ditchburn & Ginsborg, 1953; Ratliff & Riggs, 1950; and Yarbus, 1967).

Micro-tremors are seen only with very high resolution methods, since their amplitude is only approximately 10 arc sec with velocities less than 1°/sec and appear as quasi-sinusoidal oscillations with frequencies of about 70 Hz. Recently it has been suggested (Stark, Hoyt, Cuiffreda, Kenyon, & Hsu, 1980) that micro-tremor is composed of very small overlapping and truncated saccade-like movements. In any case, their amplitude makes them an unsatisfactory candidate for any visual function.

Most instrumentation methods used for recording the larger amplitude eye movements that play a role in active looking are too coarse to record micro-fixational movements with any precision. This becomes important when we consider visual information processing concepts like the necessity of a new saccade to take in more visual information. Thus a long duration pause may not, in fact, indicate more visual processing but less. Indeed, Intraub's work (this volume) suggests that the longer fixation durations as seen, for example, in reading saccades may be related to consolidation and utilization of cognitive models that have passed the checking phase. They can thus be protected by the longer inter-saccadic interval from a newly generated cognitive model with its sequence of saccadic and micro-saccadic eye movements. Abrams and Zuber (1972) have shown that the linguistic reading saccade has an approximate 250 msec fixational pause, whereas the "spatial" saccade has only a 180 msec fixation preceding its execution. These considerations suggest that high precision recordings be made to control experimental studies that show increased fixation durations. As an example, Ellis and Stark (1978) showed increasing fixation durations lasting about 400 msec that occur approximately 400 msec before organization of a new cognitive model in viewing the Necker Cube. Unfortunately, our recordings were not sufficiently precise to be able to rule out micro-fixational saccades occurring during this period, thus utilization of this data in formulating tighter relations between visual processing and saccadic eye movements is hindered (see also Kaufman & Richards, 1969; Richards & Kaufman, 1969).

EXPERIMENTAL RESULTS

Ambiguous Figures. In our recent attempts to collect evidence that a subject's cognitive model influences patterns of scanning, we have selected for study a variety of stimuli with alternative perceptual interpretations. Our general strategy has been to collect scanning eye movements while subjects view physically static but perceptually dynamic patterns and to identify changes in scanning contingent upon changes in perceptual organization.

Such a stimulus is the triply ambiguous figure shown in Fig. 6a (Ellis & Stark, 1979; Fisher, 1971). The overlaid scanning (Fig. 6b) shows the pattern of fixational eye movements collected over one subject's 25 sec period of viewing during which three alternate interpretations of the figures were seen. The subject's signal of which face he saw was recorded along with his eye position data and, with provision for his reaction time, allows the sequence of eye movements to be divided into sections corresponding to the alternative perceptual interpretations. Three scanning sequences corresponding to three signals of recognition of the old man's face, illustrate a somewhat repetitious scanning sequence beginning in the vicinity of the old man's eye, moving towards his nose, and doubling back (Fig. 6c). This pattern suggests a repetitive and stereotyped, spatial and temporal selectivity of fixation contingent upon the subject's current and cognitive hypothesis regarding the figure.

Necker Cubes. In a similar study, subjects' fixations were examined while they viewed a set of projections of Necker cubes (c.f. Fig. 7) in an attempt to identify the locii of fixation when the cube perceptually reverses (Ellis & Stark, 1978). A set of projections was chosen such that the "Y"-shaped features, which may be seen either as internal or external corners, systematically shift their relative positions (see also Brandt, 1940: Kaplan & Schoenfeld, 1966; McKel-

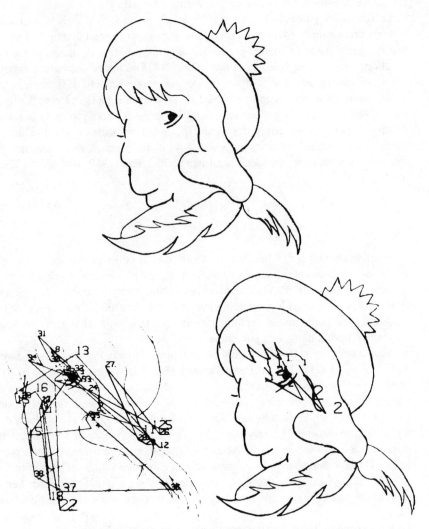

FIG. 6. *Triply Ambiguous Figure*. Upper picture shows old man with moustache, old woman with gnarled chin and nose, and young woman seen in profile with eyelash extending from silhouette (Fisher, 1971). Lower left figure shows eye movements and fixations during experimental run. Lower right figure shows eye movements during three successive occurrences with subject in that cognitive state wherein he saw old man.

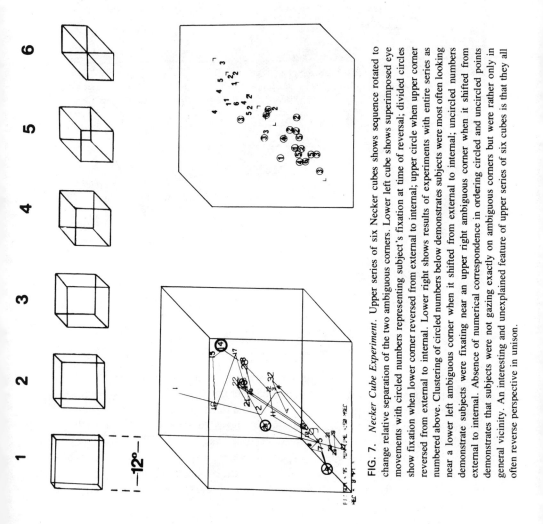

FIG. 7. *Necker Cube Experiment.* Upper series of six Necker cubes shows sequence rotated to change relative separation of the two ambiguous corners. Lower left cube shows superimposed eye movements with circled numbers representing subject's fixation at time of reversal; divided circles show fixation when lower corner reversed from external to internal; upper circle when upper corner reversed from external to internal. Lower right shows results of experiments with entire series as numbered above. Clustering of circled numbers below demonstrates subjects were most often looking near a lower left ambiguous corner when it shifted from external to internal; uncircled numbers demonstrate subjects were fixating near an upper right ambiguous corner when it shifted from external to internal. Absence of numerical correspondence in ordering circled and uncircled points demonstrates that subjects were not gazing exactly on ambiguous corners but were rather only in general vicinity. An interesting and unexplained feature of upper series of six cubes is that they all often reverse perspective in unison.

205

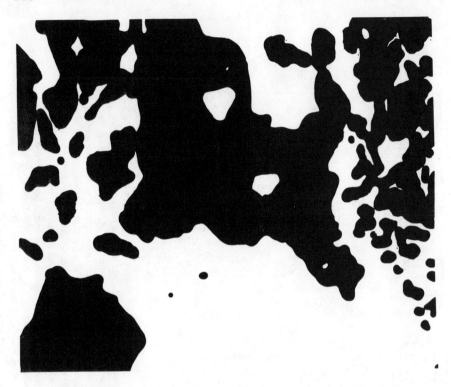

FIG. 8.   *Fragmented Figure*. A rather difficult hidden figure to recognize initially.

vie, 1973; and Shulman, Remington, & McLean, 1979). Subject's fixation positions were then associated with reported perceptual reversals, again allowing for
reaction times. In general our finding is that there was a rough association
between the fixation position during the two possible types of reversal and the
positions of the two "Y" intersections. The importance of the "Y"'s for reversal
also is shown by the distribution of fixations corresponding to reversals along the
axis of the change in the "Y" positions in the series of figures. These data
provide additional evidence that subject's three-dimensional cognitive hypotheses, in this case object hypotheses (Gregory, 1972), direct fixational eye
movements.

Fragmented Figures.   These fragmented figures varied a great deal in ease of
identification by our subjects. One of the most difficult (Porter, 1954), illustrated
in Fig. 8 and Fig. 9, upper left frame, is a heavily-shadowed lower face, inter-
mixed and surrounded by high contrast blotches so as to make the identification

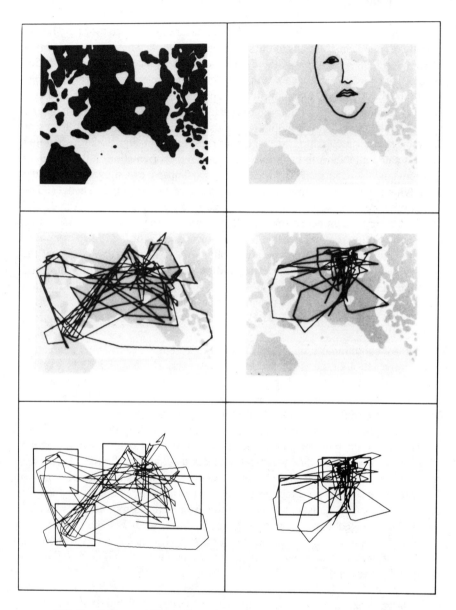

FIG. 9. *Fragmented Figure Experiment*. Upper left shows fragmented figure and upper right fragmented figure with outline drawing of face superimposed to help reader recognize hidden figure. Middle left represents eye movements during 75 seconds preceding identification; middle right represents eye movements during 75 seconds following identification. Lower left shows fixation regions before identification; lower right shows fixation regions following identification.

difficult. The upper right frame of Fig. 9 is an outline sketch that may help locate the hidden figure. Instructions to the subject were to look at the picture and signal when the sudden recognition of the figure had occurred (see also Mooney, 1956, 1958; Zavalishin, 1968; Zusne & Michels, 1964). In the center left frame of Fig. 9 are shown the "before recognition" collapsed eye movements (after linearization and fixation identification processes had been performed by the computer). An important experimental finding shows the collapsed eye movement traces of the subject, after recognition, in the center right frame of Fig. 9. Corresponding to the sudden alteration in cognitive state, marked reorientation in the scanning eye movements occurs. By considering the collapsed eye movements as the underlying, undirected graph, we can clearly see certain important changes. The extent of the eye movements greatly decreased once recognition occurred, and there are a greater number of small eye movements in the region of the identified face. Sub-fixation regions are drawn in the lower frames of Fig. 9 superimposed upon the two different before and after collapsed eye movements. Note that the fixation regions show changes corresponding to the alteration in the subject's cognitive state. The computer can now assign identifying numbers to the fixation regions and create a chain of "sequential transitions between fixation regions." This then is used to produce the Markov condition probability matrices as shown in Table 1.

Markov conditional probability matrices represent a quantitative abstraction of the information in the sequential eye movements. The $M_{(0)}$ matrix is a vector representing the unequal probabilities of the eye looking at a particular fixation region of the picture. An entry in the $M_{(1)}$ matrix represents the condtional probability of an eye movement between one fixation region and another. The values of the probability coefficeints in the $M_{(1)}$ matrix differ from those calculable from the $M_{(0)}$ matrix and represent part of the sequential structure of the eye movements. This is measured by the chi-square test. Analogously, an entry in the $M_{(2)}$ matrix represents the conditional probability of two eye movements representing two sequential transitions. An exact probability test is necessary here rather than the chi-square test. The statistical value quantitates our impression that the scanning pattern has changed after recognition. Note also the large 3-2-4 entry in the $M_{(2)}$ matrix again representing sequential structure. The $M_{(2)}$ matrix entries are here the numbers of occurrences of events rather than probabilities to enable ready understanding by the reader.

Spatial Schema.   In our search for more statistically reliable data with which to investigate the control of visual scanning due to cognitive models Ellis, has been collecting eye movement scanning data from a dynamic cockpit display (Fig. 10a) of air traffic information (CDTI) (Palmer, Baty, & O'Connor, 1978). The display was generated dynamically by a SEL840 computer programmed to depict a variety of encounters between a pilot's own ship (OS) located near the center of the display and a single intruder (I) represented by a circle. Both aircraft

TABLE 1
Experimental Markov Matrices Determined From Fragmented Figure
Experiment of Figure 6

Zero-order matrix M_0 represents percent time in each fixation region. First-order Markov matrix M_1 represents probability of transition from one of four fixation states to the other three states. Second-order Markov matrix M_2 represents the number of fixations occurring in transition from a state to any of other three states conditioned upon next but one preceeding state. Chi-squared and p values are shown for M_0 and M_1.

	Before Recognition	*After Recognition*
M(0)	(0.17 0.26 0.35 0.22)	(.07 .45 .24 .24)

	X^2	df	p.		X^2	df	p
	1.52	3	$\leqslant.68$		11.00	3	$\leqslant.018$

M(1):

$$\begin{bmatrix} — & .68 & .32 & 0 \\ .34 & — & .66 & 0 \\ .11 & .33 & — & .56 \\ .20 & .20 & .60 & — \end{bmatrix} \qquad \begin{bmatrix} — & 1.00 & 0 & 0 \\ 0.12 & — & .47 & .41 \\ 0 & .77 & — & .23 \\ .17 & .50 & .33 & — \end{bmatrix}$$

N=23 (Before) N=41 (After)

	X^2	df	p		X^2	df	p
	8.21	11	$\leqslant.69$		13.14	11	$\leqslant.28$

M(2):

$$\begin{bmatrix} — & — & — & — \\ 1 & — & 1 & 0 \\ 0 & 0 & — & 1 \\ 0 & 0 & 0 & — \end{bmatrix} \qquad \begin{bmatrix} — & — & — & — \\ 1 & — & 2 & 0 \\ 0 & 0 & — & 0 \\ 0 & 0 & 0 & — \end{bmatrix}$$

$$\begin{bmatrix} — & 0 & 0 & 0 \\ — & — & — & — \\ 0 & 1 & — & 3 \\ 1 & 0 & 1 & — \end{bmatrix} \qquad \begin{bmatrix} — & 3 & 0 & 0 \\ — & — & — & — \\ 0 & 5 & — & 3 \\ 1 & 2 & 1 & — \end{bmatrix}$$

$$\begin{bmatrix} — & 2 & 0 & 0 \\ 1 & — & 2 & 0 \\ — & — & — & — \\ 0 & 1 & 2 & — \end{bmatrix} \qquad \begin{bmatrix} — & 1 & 0 & 0 \\ 0 & — & 2 & 7 \\ — & — & — & — \\ 0 & 1 & 1 & — \end{bmatrix}$$

$$\begin{bmatrix} — & 0 & 1 & 0 \\ 0 & — & 1 & 0 \\ 1 & 1 & — & 0 \\ — & — & — & — \end{bmatrix} \qquad \begin{bmatrix} — & 1 & 0 & 0 \\ 0 & — & 3 & 0 \\ 0 & 4 & — & 0 \\ — & — & — & — \end{bmatrix}$$

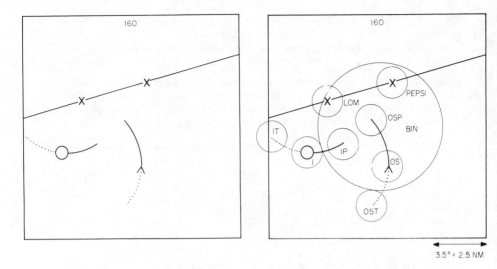

3.5° = 2.5 NM

FIG. 10. *Cockpit Display of Traffic Information.* (a) CDTI display showing a single intruder while both own ship and intruder are turning. Map shows a square region 10 miles on a side containing a jet route and two VOR navigation aids. Ownship's heading is shown at top center. (b) Circular fixation regions surrounding each of the points of interest on the display; fixations outside these areas were not analyzed. Entire display subtended 12 degrees and was presented to subject under mesopic luminance.

symbols were provided with predictors showing future position in 30 sec, as well as dotted trails showing previous position in 4 sec intervals.

The overall display was that of a track-up moving map with position of the intruder and of ground referenced symbols being up-dated every 4 sec. Turning of the OS, however, produced essentially continuous rotation of the entire display with respect to the OS and associated symbols. The subject's task while viewing the display was to determine whether the intruder would eventually pass in front or behind the OS. A variety of encounter geometries were used but all encounters were terminated before the intruder actually passed in front or behind. Thus, the subject had to estimate future positions in order to complete the task.

Direction of gaze data were collected with a pupilometer-type tracker during 24 different encounters that were each viewed for 28 sec. These data were processed to allow determination of the frequency of fixating each point-of-interest (POE) (Fig. 10b) on the display as well as the pattern of transitions among them (Fig. 11). Table 2a presents a summary of the overall frequency of viewing the various POE as well as the frequency of transitions between all pairs of points for one airline pilot subject. That fixations are not equally distributed across the POE is confirmed by a chi-square calculation made on the basis of a zero-order null hypothesis that frequency of viewing all POE should be in proportion to the area of the fixation region around each POE. Thus, the differential frequency of viewing the predictors and trails is statistically reliable and may reflect differential usefulness of the information they contain for the estimation of the intruders future position.

The actual distribution of fixation frequency across the POE can then become the basis of a first-order null hypothesis transitions among the points, equivalent to a stratified random sampling process (Senders, 1964). Elkind, Grignetti and Smallwood (1966) provided evidence for such a model but their original experimental situation may have biased their results by using statistically independent forcing functions to drive the displays the subjects viewed. This condition is somewhat unusual since displays on actual control panels are frequently intercorrelated. Nevertheless, Weir and Klein (1970; also see Spady, 1977, 1978), were able to use a similar model to describe scanning of aircraft cockpit instruments

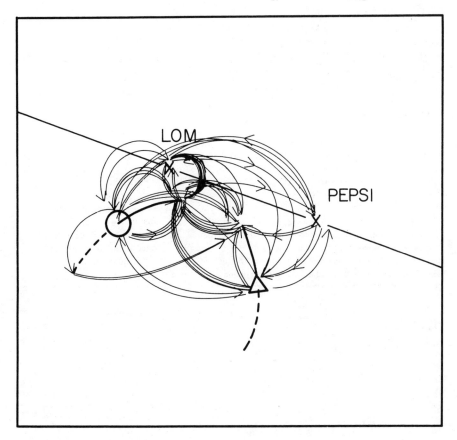

FIG. 11.   *Eye Movements Between Circular Fixation Regions*. Probability represented by number of lines in each arrow shift: < 10%, 10-20%, 30-40%, 40-50%. See also Table 2a.

during simulated instrument flight, a situation in which the instrument readings were clearly intercorrelated (see also Barnes, 1972, and Fitts, Jones, & Milton, 1950, p. 41).

For data collected while subjects scanned CDTI displays, the expected frequency of transitions between points on the basis of the first-order null hypothesis correlated well with our observed frequencies of transition (Table 2a; (Spearman rho $= 0.873$; $df = 70$: and Pearson $r = 0.932$; $df = 70$) and thus does not allow rejection of the null hypothesis. We have, however, pursued this question further by generalizing the model to examine second-order dependencies (Table 2b; comparison of expected and observed frequencies in this case *does* allow rejection of the null-hypothesis model).

Deviation between observed and expected frequencies primarily arises from pairs of transitions corresponding to movements first away from and then back to specific points of interest. Thus our preliminary analysis leads us to describe scanning as if the subject had a dynamically changing "home base" at the POE to which he frequently returns.

One might speculate, for example, that the shifting of this base back and forth between the OS and intruder might correspond to a shift of the subject in adopting the spatial point of view of either aircraft when attempting to judge future

TABLE 2a

Square matrix showing observed frequencies of transitions between all pairs of points of interest taken from one subject during one experimental run. Main diagonal is empty because transitions from a point to itself cannot be unambiguously observed and are excluded from our analysis. First column to left of matrix contains row labels for respective positions of interest (POE). First column to right of matrix contains sum of all transitions observed originating from each POE. Second column on right contains percentage of time subject spent looking at each point, clearly showing high percentage spent on ends of predictors. Chi-square in lower right calculated on null hypothesis that frequency of fixation should be in proportion to area corresponding to fixation region around each point. Chi-square below matrix was calculated model predicting frequency of transition between points from probability of fixation of points themselves. Small expected frequencies were collapsed together so that no more than 20% of remaining cells had expected frequencies less than five.

										Σ	%Time
OS	/	2	0	1	5	0	1	1	2	12	3.9
OSP	3	/	0	3	15	0	7	2	23	53	21.8
OST	0	1	/	0	0	0	0	0	0	1	0.05
I	2	8	0	/	13	2	3	0	8	36	11.6
IP	3	16	0	16	/	0	9	2	19	65	30.1
IT	0	1	0	2	0	/	0	0	3	6	2.4
LOM	0	4	0	3	14	0	/	0	9	30	10.6
PEP	0	2	0	3	3	0	1	/	2	11	1.7
BIN	5	17	2	5	14	3	11	2	/	59	17.9
			2							273	

$$X^2 = 33,8 \quad df = 31 \, p > .05 \qquad\qquad X = {}^2 169,2 \quad df = 8$$
$$p < .001$$

TABLE 2b

Five square matrices below show frequencies of successive transitions among triplets of POE for one run of one subject. Points receiving less than 5% of total transitions were excluded from analysis to reduce problems of small expected frequencies; remaining transitions amounted to 87% of original total. Each matrix shows transitions with first POE shown as matrix heading, second point in row labels to left, with third, and successive points in respective columns within matrix. All cells representing successive transitions from a point to itself are empty as in Table 2a. Small expected frequencies were collapsed as in Table 2a for chi-square, which tested for second-order dependencies.

	OSP						*I*						*IP*				
OSP	/	/	/	/	/		/	1	1	2	1		/	0	9	0	6
I	2	/	1	1	0		/	/	/	/	/		4	/	7	1	1
IP	2	4	/	1	3		5	4	/	0	2		/	/	/	/	/
LOM	2	0	3	/	0		1	1	1	/	2		0	2	4	/	1
BIN	7	0	5	1	/		1	1	0	3	/		5	2	4	4	/
Σ	13	4	9	3	3		7	7	2	5	5		9	4	24	5	8
		32						26						55			

	LOM						*BIN*			
/	1	0	2	1		/	2	3	1	9
1	/	1	3	0		1	/	1	0	3
3	3	/	2	2		3	0	/	3	6
/	/	/	/	/		0	1	3	/	6
1	1	2	2	/		/	/	/	/	/
5	5	3	9	3		4	3	7	4	24
	25						42			

$X^2 \geq 40.63\,df = 24$
$p < .03$

180

relative position. Such a shifting of point of view happens during the solution of problems like the missionary and cannibal puzzle (Levin & Hutchins, 1979). Clearly, this speculation requires further investigation, but for the moment we are satisfied to interpret the significant second-order transition probabilities experimentally found as further evidence that cognitive models control scanning behavior in a manner that lends insight into underlying cognitive processes.

DISCUSSION

Experimental Results

Our present computer-based experimental system objectively determines the collapsed sequence of eye movements as seen, for example, in the lower right frame of Fig. 3, the lower left and upper right frame of Fig. 4, and the middle left and right frames of Fig. 9. These represent adequate performance of the instrumentation, the calibration procedure, the linearization procedure, and the completely automatic fixation identification procedure. These sequential strings of eye movements from one fixation point to another represent the basic datum from which all other analyses depend.

The Markov conditional probability matrices represent an important aspect of our research. Given the fixation region identification process, we can now construct sequential strings of successive fixation regions and look to various statistical methods for investigating the underlying higher-level cognitive processes that control these eye movements. The first three Markov matrices, $M_{(0)}$, $M_{(1)}$, and $M_{(2)}$, succinctly summarize the stucture of the scanpath and other eye movements appearing while a subject looks at a picture. The $M_{(2)}$ matrix and high-order matrices represent the importance of past history of the eye movement sequence in governing the next movement. Simulation of these matrices is an interesting and helpful application of Monte Carlo methods for obtaining intuition about the non-randomness of sequences of eye movements serving visual perception, visual memory, pattern and cognitive recognition.

These new experimental results add considerably to the earlier Noton–Stark data. Rather than showing, as Noton and Stark did, that each subject has an idiosyncratic scanpath for each picture, we have rather studied the eye movements of the same subject looking at the same picture while his cognitive states change. In this way we use each subject as his own control, and we further control physiological processes of vision by using the same physical picture as the stimulus. Thus we can conclude that the only factor that has changed is the cognitive model in the subject's brain, "in the mind's eye". We have obtained clear evidence that eye movements change considerably with different cognitive states; this indicates that cognitive models direct scanpaths. The ambiguous figure experiment (Fig. 6) is most directly relevant to this point. Here the subject switches between three different cognitive states; the scanpath eye movements correlate well during successive occurrences of the same cognitive state, but are quite different when compared from one cognitive state to another. Lower level stimulus-controlled eye movements could not be the basis for this experimental difference. An earlier result of Noton–Stark indicated that a subject, under the influence of psylocibin, made much smaller scanpaths than physically appropriate for the visual angle of the viewed picture. The structure (angles and form) of the scanpath remained similar to the normal-sized scanpath obtained in sessions before and after the psylocibin session. This also indicated that the scanpath was not image-directed or controlled by lower-level processing, but rather was directed by a stored program or cognitive model.

It may help to think of a scanpath as a repetitive route of exploration for an explorer *with a map* who is proceeding from bench mark to bench mark, checking the accuracy of the map as a representation of the area being reexplored. This accounts for the idiosyncratic and repetitive nature of the scanpath sequence and serves as a metaphor for understanding the scanpath. Exploration without a map, and indeed without intent to make a map, would yield a much different journey. Although our data are not complete, we feel we can exclude this latter possibility as a viable model. Of interest in this regard are some preliminary studies in which we have attempted to utilize the travelling salesman problem (TSP) approach. On the one hand we are attempting to estimate the difficulty of generating algorithms whereby some type of economical scanpath could be constructed de novo with each repetition. (Such algorithms might be based on Karp's (1977) work obtaining approximating solutions of this non-polynomial (n-p) problem. Here one might divide the n fixation points to be visited into $\sqrt{n}$ regions; perform suboptimizations for each region; and then connect each region again in a suboptimal fashion). A further question has to do with the structural similarities that might ensue under these conditions (c.f. Barrow, Ambles, & Bersh, 1972). Finally, we have noted experimentally that while some scanpaths appear to be closed directed cyclic graphs as might be expected consequent to optimization of total path length, other scanpaths apparently do not conform to such minimizations.

Subjects can perceive and organize tachistoscopically presented pictures; that is, pictures presented as only brief flashes of light, thus not permitting time for successive eye movements. It is possible to postulate that such tachistoscopic pictures are stored first in short term memory; then shifts of attention, a cognitive computational process, substitute for the saccadic eye movements.

A further experiment by Noton and Stark (1971a,b,c) showed that for a particular subject each picture was scanned by a different scanpath. The fixations were generally on "informational relevant" subfeatures and the pattern of scanpath saccades provided an idiosyncratic and repetitive sequence. Even more interesting was the fact that for a particular picture each subject developed an indiosyncratic scanpath. This indicated to them that the scanpath was determined by higher level perceptual processes and not by such lower level mechanisms as the network "Lettvin feature detectors" discovered by Lettvin, Maturana, McCulloch, & Pitts (1966) to be characteristic of the frog's retina. This lower level procedure has been championed by Prokoski (1971) in an interesting modeling study of scanpaths, and by Didday and Arbib (1972).

In understanding our experimental results with fragmented figures (Figs. 8,9), we might consider that the human is able to "look without seeing" to "see without looking" and to "look and see." As the subject scans the fragmented figure before recognition, he is "looking without seeing." His eye movements are rather diffuse and may represent a number of different preliminary cognitive hypotheses for which our experimental techniques are unable to extract clearly recognizable scanpaths. Now all of a sudden, he "sees without looking." In less time than would be necessary for a second eye movement to occur, the subject has "clearly seen" the image (Mooney, 1956, 1958). Even contours far away from his fovea are "seen" clearly and without interruption by the fragmented components of the figure. To us it seems that he has "seen" his own cognitive model rather than any resultant from physiologically processing of image pixels.

Next the subject continues to "look and see." Now he makes a much more tightly organized sequence of eye movements that may be considered as a scanpath. This repetitive sequencing of saccades in the "look and see" scanpath phase apparently is part of a checking paradigm of the pattern recognition task. In many ways these experiments point the way for objective data support for both older and more recent cognitive science studies, both laboratory and theoretical (Brown & Owen, 1967; Egeth, 1966; Engel, 1976; Evans, 1965; Gould, 1967; Gould & Dill, 1969; Mackworth & Mackworth, 1958; McFarland, 1968; Schifferli, 1953; and also books by Monty and Senders, 1976; Senders, Fisher, & Monty, 1978).

Experimental Results in Light of Cognitive Science Developments

Cognitive Philosophy.[1]   Before approaching the relevant aspects of research in cognitive psychology it seems appropriate to point out the venerable history of different cognitive positions in philosophy.

Aristotle's point of view might be likened to a "bottom up" cluster analysis technique for formation of cognitive concepts. A "table" is an average or center-of-gravity in some feature space of all the tables we have visually experienced (or otherwise perceived). A new table will be so classified if it resembles the average table closely enough so as to fit easily into the cluster, "table." David Hume, the empiricist par excellence, thought that similarity and contiguity were at the base of not only perceptual or cognitive classification but even of concepts like cause and effect; and indeed were the only such base. John Locke's and his tabula rasa suggested that since we were born with no experience, we start with a "blank slate" on which such an Aristotelian process would then operate.

This is in stark contrast to the Platonic position. The immortality of the rational soul provides a complete preexisting catalogue of "ideals" for each of us. In so far as an object reviewed awakens or impels us to recollect an ideal that object can be so named or classified. In so far as a "table" resembles the ideal "table," it is so recognized. Socrates, when arguing with one of his disciples is trying to aid or to force him to recollect the same set of ideals that Socrates has in mind, at which time the disciple will clearly "see" Socrates' point of view.

In many ways the scanpath theory allies itself to the Platonic ideal. Visual experience is not enough to create a new cognitive model or ideal; indeed such new cognitive models like the different interpretations of the Necker cube (Fig. 12) are more likely to be formed propositionally—logically, formally, or by analogous reasoning from another realm of knowledge than that of sensory experience.

---

[1]One of us (SRE) holds his views on these matters in abeyance.

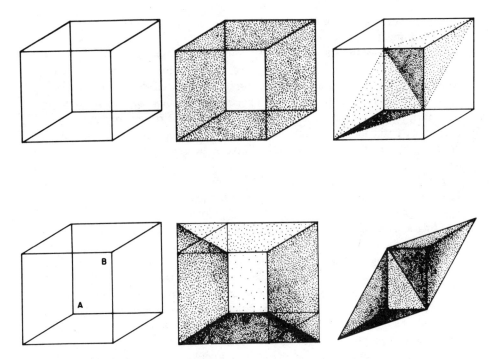

FIG. 12. *Propositional Construction of Necker Cube Cognitive Models*. Each of five models represents possible cognitive states for viewing Necker cube. Models A and B are the usual ones that are apparently most "natural" with either A or B as the external, forward projecting corner. Double pyramid and truncated pyramid are models that can be "seen" once verbal instructions concerning their description have been given; sketches below are exaggerations to help reader "see" these cognitive interpretations as models. Similarly "seeing" only a two-dimensional pattern of lines is a feasible interpretation after verbal instruction and can often be held between shifts from A to B. Double pyramid often has external sides more completely taking over entire sides of cube; shading used here would then only identify peaks of pyramids.

Kants' attempts to come to grips with this problem forced him to invent an a priori synthetic judgement; a priori indicating the concept was deductive and made before or without examination or factual study; and synthetic meaning to him that it arose from experience but *independent* of experience. Perhaps our cognitive model is such a concept, or even such a central nervous system phenomenon, generated to bring order into the pre-platonic chaos of sensory experience, but clearly not formed by or of that sensory inflow of information.

In some ways the scanpath theory is quite apart from Platonic thought. Clearly, biological evolution has shaped the central nervous system to be able with ease to form models of many aspects of the physical (and biological) world. Indeed, cognitive models may be present at birth—the mother's face and spatial frameworks, to name two. Evidence exists for the former from studies of infant development (Salapatek & Kessen, 1966); evidence for the latter is that the two most prominent models for the Necker cube are *three*-dimensional models for what is known by the subject to be a two-dimensional pattern of lines! Recall here also Kantian inherent notions of space. Also consider Herings (1868) clear demonstration of the inateness of the conjugacy of saccadic eye movements, disproving the Helmholtz theory of experiential learning of coordination for binocular vision. Nevertheless, like 'ideals,' cognitive models apparently pre-exist in the brain and are brought out in an hierarchical set of pattern recognition checking phases of which "scanpaths" give some evidence.

Historical.   Contemporary congitive approaches to the understanding of behavior may be traced from three styles of earlier research. The dept to the gestalt psychologists such as Koffka and Kohler is probably the clearest. Their understanding and research into the crucial role of behavioral structure and context established the basis for cognitive science.

A second major influence developed from the work of the American psychologists such as Lashley and Tolman who studied aspects of behavior illustrating the need for higher order explanatory constructs: grammars and cognitive maps. In particular Lashley (1951) recognized that nonlinguistic behavior, as well as language, had syntactic structure that was not parsimoniously modeled by Markov chains, a proposal implicit in many learning theories. And Tolman (1948) provided the evidence that even the lowly rat could more or less spontaneously construct an internal representation of its environment accessable for problem solving, eliminating the need for trial and error. The physiological bases for these representations remain speculative, but Hebb (1949) and more elaborate reports by McCulloch and Pitts (1943) have shown that this speculation can take concrete forms.

The third major development may be traced from Miller, Galanter, and Pribram (1960) who directed researchers towards a vocabulary and conceptual framework in which the theories of higher order behavioral phenomena could be expressed. A great number of contemporary investigators have been influenced by the search for processing algorhythms inspired by this book. For example, it foreshadowed research by Newell and Simon (1972) and Neisser (1967) and the application of formal models of linguistic structure (Chomsky, 1957; Fodor & Bever, 1965) to the study of languages.

The formation of a complex vocabulary for theoretical expression has required a corresponding increase in the complexity of behavioral data collected to test the theories. A certain amount of information regarding the underlying properties of our mental representations has been derived from relatively simple measures. Shepard and his colleagues (Shepard & Judd, 1976; Shepard & Metzler, 1971) and Kosslyn, Ball, and Reiser (1978) have, for example, attempted to deduce properties of our representation of spatial orientation from reaction time data. But while their reports have provided the interesting suggestion that the representation "preserves the metrical properties of space", the basis of this preservation is controversial (see Pylyshyn, 1973). Similarly, reaction times have been used to measure the processing complexity of sentences (Gough, 1966; Slobin, 1966), short and long term memory concepts (Sperling, 1960).

More intrisically structured information can be gathered from analyses of errors subjects make in a variety of situations. This approach has provided insight into the differential coding of information in short and long term memory. (Baddeley, 1966; Conrad, 1964; Wickelgren, 1966). Similarly, reaction time and error data have been useful in the identification of cognitive functions laterized in either of the cerebral hemispheres (Corballis & Beale, 1976). However, though analyses of behavior have passed far beyond simple Hullian concerns with response probability, many of the dependent measures available for study remain relatively unstructured.

More complex processing models, however, generate more elaborate expectations and require corresponding more elaborate predictions like behavioral protocols (Feigenbaum & Feldman, 1963; Norman & Rummelhart, 1975).

Underlying all of these types of theories is the assumption that abstract information processing structures interact with and structure the incoming information in complex ways.

Definition of Cognitive Model or Schemata.   Ever since the neurologist Head (1920) first used the term schema to refer to the context in which all behavior occurs, a variety of related terms have been proposed. Hochberg (1968, 1978) has stated one of the more useful definitions which we paraphrase: A schemata or cognitive model is the structure by which we encode, and can reconstruct, more information than we can retain from individual items or regions within our sensory world. This idea lies at the basis of many of the observations of the gestalt psychologists (Kohler, 1929), which pointed to the fact that the structuralist's alphabetic approach to perception was inadequate. The specific description of an individual's cognitive model in a particular situation has, until recently, remained elusive. The basic problem has been that the cognitive model is a mental construct that is accessible to neither observation nor introspection. Attempts, for example, to infer a model from unstructured data like reaction times or memory errors are indirect. Thus the analysis of scanning eye movements has proven useful with respect to this problem because it has provided a means to collect structured data externalizing aspects of the patterns of processing arising from the cognitive models. The following examples further illustrate how the scanning data provides this information.

Object Hypotheses.   If eye movements were under the control of the physical stimuli, then the spontaneous patterns of scanning would be generally determined by the physical properties of the stimuli. In accordance with this idea, Attneave (1954) proposed that irregular contours should attract disproportionately large numbers of fixations (see also Michels & Zusne, 1965). This type of proposal has been more elaborately made recently by Didday and Arbib (1972) who suggested that lower order aspects of the physical stimulus can generate cyclic patterns of eye movements. Although there is some evidence that lower order spatial properties like symmetry (Locher & Nodine, 1973) and density (Fisher, Monty, & Perlmuter, 1978) influence spontaneous eye movements, these influences are easily overridden by higher level processes associated with object recognition and scene interpretation. Yarbus (1967), for example, has shown that the pattern of eye movements while viewing a picture strongly depends upon the tasks or specific information the viewer is attempting to extract (also see Buswell, 1935). Indeed, the new experimental results we reported earlier in this chapter concerning viewing of physically static but perceptually changing stimuli confirms the important role of higher level processing. In general, the alternating patterns of eye movements while viewing scenes may reflect changes of the observer's "object hypotheses" (Gregory, 1972) on the manner in which the pictorial information is selectively processed. That there must be differential processing of the same physical stimuli is supported by experiments of Freedman and Haber (1974) and Weisman and Neisser (1974) which show that the recall of fragmented figures depends upon their recognition as nameable shapes.

Informativeness. The potential amount of information in a complex visual scene is exceedingly large and it is unlikely that all of it is continuously processed to an equal extent (Kahneman, 1973). Fortunately, the relevant information in a scene is not uniformly distributed. Viewers of scenes generally agree about the locations of these more "informative" regions. A variety of researchers (Buswell, 1935; Mackworth & Morandi, 1967; Yarbus, 1967) have shown that the regions of judged high "informativeness" disproportionately attract eye fixations. Since the informativeness of a part of a scene is related to the viewers expectations regarding it (Loftus & Mackworth, 1978), informativeness is best thought of as a relation between the viewer and the scene rather than as a property of the scene itself.

Mental Imagery. One of the more paradoxical cognitive effects on eye movements is a reported restriction of scanning associated with the generation of visual mental images (Marks, 1973; Singer, Greenberg, & Antrobus, 1971; Weiner & Ehrlichman, 1976). The effect seems most pronounced at the onset of the mental image and indeed, is not a dominating one since eye movements can be used to "measure" the angular size of mental images (Weber & Malstrom, 1979; also see Haber, 1969). Furthermore, eye movements while solving mental puzzles and during recall of spatially distributed stimuli appear related to the spatial positions of the stimuli recalled for solution of the problem (DeGroot, 1966; Gopher, 1973; Leask & Harber, 1969). The initial restriction of scanning may be explained from the increased information processing load during the initial creation of the image which restricts input, thus inhibiting eye movements.

Linguistic Influences.   The conventional placement of words in coherent text exerts substantial but potentially superficial influence on scanning during reading. The actual word ordering is apparently arbitrary and identical propositions can be presented by radically different lexigraphical conventions. However, careful analysis of eye movements during reading show numerous features pointing to higher level control. For example, Carpenter and Just (1976) found that after readers encountered pronouns with ambiguous referents, they frequently made regressive eye movements to the potential referents in a manner possibly indicating the time at which the pronoun's meaning was assigned. Linguistic influence is also evident in nonreading situations: Cooper (1974), for instance, showed that spontaneous eye movements towards textually relevant pictures are produced when subjects listen to recorded speech. The time course of these eye movements seemed related to the manner in which the speech was parsed and understood; thus providing a highly structured and detailed protocol against which models of speech processing could be tested.

Artificial Intelligence (AI) and Scene Analysis[2]

Historical.   Our eye movement studies of human visual perception and cognition led us to make distinctions between (1) serial and parallel processing, (2) BU (bottom up) and TD (top down) processing, (3) non-hierarchical, statistical recognition (cluster analysis) and syntactic and semantic organization of categories, and (4) 2D (two dimensional), 3D (three dimensional) and symbolic levels of operation (thanks to Prof. Irwin Sobel, Columbia University personal communication, 1978). These concepts are, of course, well known in the artificial intelligence (AI) and cybernetic community but may not be familiar to researchers in cognitive psychology or eye movements. It seems, therefore, worthwhile to point out and discuss the evolutions of AI since the early 60's (Minsky, 1961; Stark & Dickson, 1965 & 1966) that are pertinent to our present visual perception findings.

A brief list of the contents of Minsky (1961) indicates the scope of the field at that time: problems of search, especially hill climbing; problems of pattern recognition, including property lists, with generating and combining properties, descriptors and naming; learning systems with reinforcement, expectation and prediction; problem solving and planning, including logic theory, global and local heuristics, and planning with character-algebra methods; and finally induction and models, intelligence and models-of-oneself.

Stark & Dickson (1966) covered a wider variety of topics: von Neuman's contribution to the computer and the brain; AI including machine learning (checkers) and heuristic programming; psychological and behavioral metamathemati-

---

[2]Christian Freksa and one of us (Stark) are reviewing this subject (in preparation) and this section is abstracted from their work.

cal models; neuronal systems modeling with adaptive control; perceptrons; machine perception of 3D solids; physiology of neural operators; formal neuron theory; optomotor reactions; neural machinery; molecular architecture and molecular algorithms; mathematical versus computer modeling; problems of CNS redundancy, plasticity and spatio-temporal processing.

BU implies a well-defined algorithm that processes digitized image data, for example, and whose output is concisely structured information for the next level of the program. TD implies that a higher level structure superimposes control upon the lower level processing algorithms. We are here using TD and BU with respect to the perceptual and cognitive processes going on in human vision about which the scanpath eye movement sequence is giving us new research findings. By considering several different levels of processing in human or robot vision at once, TD and BU could become quite ambiguous. Also any BU algorithm must have been planned and pre-structured by a TD process to even be in place and working. Perhaps one should rather use "cognitively driven" for TD and "image driven" for BU.

BU—2D.   Selfridge and Neisser (1960) introduced feature extractors called demons and logical, as opposed to statistical, cluster analysis procedures (Okajima, Stark, Whipple, & Yasui, 1963; Stark, Okajima, & Whipple, 1962) for recognition of alphabetic characters (see also Duda & Hart, 1973; Nilsson, 1965). A different early approach was the Farley-Clark random neural network into which Rosenblatt (1958) introduced an important layered organization. This "perceptron" with its three levels—receptors, association neurons, and decision neurons really launched pattern recognition even though it has now been shown that simple linear perceptrons have important limitations (Minsky & Pappart, 1969). The neurophysiological work going on at this time by Lettvin, Maturana, McCulloch, and Pitts (1966) and Hubel and Wiesel (1962) lead Fukushima (1969, 1970) and Sutro and Lehrman (1973) to develop bionic models with even more structure than the perceptron. Blum (1973) developed a skeletonizing algorithm as a means of decomposing two dimensional contours; Binford and Tennenbaum (1973), Nevabia and Binford (1977), and Hollerbach (1975) have recent extensions of this method to three dimensions.

The segmentation operator (Horowitz, 1975; Pavlides & Horowitz, 1974) is an excellent example of the many low level two-dimensional image processing techniques that could be included here—region growing, normalization, pre-whitening, and chamfering (see also Muchnik, 1966). Another important technique is the "pyramid," which resolves problems of storage and data handling of the high number of image pixels (Tanimoto & Pavildes, 1975). Pavlides and Ali (1979), Pavlides (1977), Horowitz and Pavilides (1978) and Horowitz (1975) have developed seven symbols as a language for contour matching independent of resolution. Three structures have been developed for map features such as intersections that by putting semantically significant features into a syntactical relationship emphasizes the importance of a tile or strip structure for addressing portions of an image (Sobel, personal communication, 1978). Does saccadic foveation of the human eye act as a ''page turner'' to enable accession of high resolution portions of a hypothecated image?

3D—''Blocks World.''   A brilliant simplification of the visual scene to three-dimensional geometrical features—''the blocks world''—removed many extraneous semantic and syntactical problems. This then enabled Ai researchers to move out into the 3D world. Early computer programs by Shannon's pupils, Ernst (personal communication, 1962) and Roberts (1965), developed this blocks world; an important contributor was Guzman (1968) who used three-dimensional constraints to reduce complexity of a picture. Extensions quickly followed. Falk (1972) and Bullock, Dudani, Stafsudd, and Clark (1976) overcame absent information, like gaps in a line, by means of model matching techniques. Turner (1975) was able to handle curved objects and Ohlander (1975) natural landscapes, buildings, and city scenes. Bionic models were extended to work with polyhedra (Shirai, 1972). Sobel (1974) developed calibration procedures with projective geometric constratings. Davis (1976) mapped 2D images onto three dimensions by means of elegant BU relaxation algorithms. This latter work clearly related to our Necker Cube studies (Ellis & Stark, 1978) especially when one considers that human beings apparently continually generate 3D models for interpretation of two dimensional patterns of lines. Using two spatial dimensions and time, Jain and Nagel (1977) were able to construct three spatial dimensions, without time, again helped by constraints of physical processes.

Bu—Symbolic.   Symbolic methods provide names for structures. An important paper by Winston (1970) used a BU teaching method that provided a set of examples and counter-examples for an ''arch'' that eventually forced ''understanding,'' or at least characterization by the program of the arch structure. Barlow, Narasimhan, and Rosenfield (1972) review this and related methodologies. These AI studies provide precise examples helping to define various philosophical categories of visual information processes.

TD—Syntax.   By syntax we mean the utilization of relationships that, however, still fall short of scientific knowledge of the underlying mechanisms. The metaphor is clearly linguistic and suggests just as one can define a grammar, for a language without context or meaning of words in a sentence, so one can develop grammatical-like operations that proceed beyond simple non-hierarchical clustering techniques. Fu's (1974) book is an excellent introduction to this area. Mandelbrot (1977) deals with the mathematical theory of shapes but not with AI or pattern recognition. Freeman (1961) chose the resolution of the image representation and his program link the various parts of the picture together in a chain encoding system. Klinger and Dyer (1976) developed ''regular'',pyramids of relationships between segmented elements of a picture. Clearly these syntactical methods might be models for possible non-semantic brain mechanisms for generation of scanpaths. Parallel vs. serial processing schemes were contrasted by Noton and Stark (1971a,b,c) in formulating the scan-path hypotheses (see also Corcoran, 1967; Hanson & Riseman, 1974; Lindsay & Lindsay, 1966).

A further set of researchers relate to task-oriented knowledge about relationships in the 3D scene to be studied. Gravey's (1976) programs understood that a telephone might be looked for on a desk; Tenenbaum and Barrow (1975) used iterative relaxation of relational constraints that enabled their program to know that pictures frequently hang on wall; and Bolles (1975) similarly used his programs knowledge of relationships to guide performance of a robot inserting a ball into a hole. In general, Tenenbaum and Barrow (1975) suggested the importance of multisensory information such as language and disparity in judging distance; clearly a very close intuitive derivation from human performance. Finally, Minsky's (1975) concept of the "frame" provides an overview of syntactical structuring of organizational relationships—clearly an idea derivable from the scanpath feature ring by generalization.

TD—Semantic. As AI researchers proceeded to construct TD algorithms, they relied first on their intuitions about human performance, and then later developed techniques to expose how humans performed high level processes. Akin & Reddy (1977) used constrained human conversation for analyzing steps in image knowledge acquisition; Mackworth (1977, 1978) studied how people draw pictures to infer what the drawing really represents, and Firschein and Fischer (1972) utilized human naming of features to make such inferences. With respect to cognitive maps, Kuipers (1977) used verbal responses of people to infer how they performed, not necessarily consistent, procedures with only incomplete knowledge of the spatial relations in map-constructing and map-reading tasks, where Down and Stea (1977) took the geographer's point of view.

The difficult problem of how semantics or "knowledge" should be represented in a computer program has been approached in a number of recent studies—Bajcsy and Rosenthal (1975) have shown how TD knowledge informs BU procedures; Frender (1976) used TD knowledge about hammers in his programs to simplify BU operators in scene analysis; Fischler and Elschlager, (1975) and Ballard, (1978) discuss the importance of hierarchical representations; and Bajcsy and Tavakoli (1975) discuss how syntax relates to semantics (see also Barrow & Tenenbaum, 1975; Nagel, 1976; and Tenenbaum, 1973). Clearly studies like our early scanpath work have influenced AI concepts, like frames and chaining encoders; conversely, the scientific and philosophical world has been strongly influenced by the spectacle of robots carrying out visual processes that still seem mysterious when one only considers the psychology of human vision.

For the reader, we list a number of general references: (Barlow et al., 1972; Fu & Pavlides, 1979; Glezer, 1970; Riseman, 1978; Winston, 1975). Thus, AI by its very existence, engineers definitions in the form of working models of many formerly imprecise, vague and non-canonical concepts form cognitive philosophy and psychology.

To the above discussion of AI approaches to vision, several other contributions may be worthwhile to mention in connection with their relation to scanpaths. Graphic display techniques and image processing methodology are developing in a very rapid manner (Shantz & McCann, 1976). Vector graphic display for computer output, for man-machine interfaces like head's-up displays (HUD) for pilots, and in the map communication world, produces a cartoon-like output. This helps us realize that stimulation of appropriate cognitive models may be achieved with much less than full image detail presentation. Image processing is now employing much of the large computer resources in our society, although the theory of how to make a picture match the human eye has just begun to develop. Initially, lower-level processing, e.g., pseudostereopsis, has been found to be effective (Webber & Stark, 1971, 1972). It may be that we should now consider higher-level processes, like cognitive models, using scanpath eye movements and other information we have about TD human visual information processing. For example, a suggestion has been made that signal compression may be obtained for TV broadcasting by utilizing information similar to the scanpath mode of vision (L. Stark, personal communication to University of California re patent application proposal.) Supporting this are studies of human eye movements while viewing TW programm (Flagg, 1978) and related visual displays like montage (Hochberg, 1978) that apparently are made up of successive quasi-static scenes for which one may guess that "quasi-static scanpaths' may be an appropriate mode of active looking. Although scanpaths are idiosyncratic because of an enormous number of sequences of the order of n factorial connecting n fixation points whereas the locations of fixation points may be somewhat stereotyped. If most humans do share preferred fixation locations in the processes of checking out "important" and "relevant" subfeatures of a particular scene or picture, then it might be possible to utilize a signal compression scheme. The eye movements of a few subjects could be measured and a small set of high probability fixation locations determined in the TV station while broadcasting. Then broadcast transmission of especial high resolution of this small set of fixations could provide extra high resolution for apparently the entire video screen. Of course, the regular low resolution TV picture would be broadcast as well in an interwoven manner.

SUMMARY

Experimental evidence for the discovery of the scanpath by Noton and Stark is broadening with contributions from other independent laboratories. The exact role of the scanpath in pattern recognition, visual memory, and perception is still uncertain and subject to various critical issues.

New experimental evidence presented in this chapter makes clear that eye movement scanning patterns reflect changes in cognitive states. Thus we add support to the concept that cognitive models direct scanpath eye movements in active looking.

Brief reviews of recent work in cognitive psychology and in artificial intelligence make clear the burgeoning interest in cognitive models, active looking and both human and robotic higher-level visual information processing. Now with widespread availability of eye movement instrumentation and of online computers, we expect many research laboratories will be contributing new results to our understanding of the role of eye movements in vision.

ACKNOWLEDGMENT

We appreciate contributions from and discussions with our colleagues, Christian Freksa, Electrical Engineering and Computer Science, University of California, Berkeley and Hiromitsu Inoue, Nagoya, Japan.
The senior author wishes to acknowledge the stimulation he received from the MIT group: Manuel Cerrillo, Jerome Lettvin, Warren McDulloch, Oliver Selfridge, Claude Shannon and Norbert Wiener.

IV.2 Small Involuntary Eye-Movements: Solved and Unsolved Problems

R. W. Ditchburn

Engineering Department, University of Reading, Whiteknights, Reading, England

In this chapter I shall be concerned with the small eye-movements that remain during a fixation. Between 1930 and 1960, records that agree with the general picture shown in Figs. 1 and 2 were made by Adler and Fliegelman (1934), Barlow (1952), Ditchburn and Ginsborg (1953), and Riggs, Armington, and Ratliff (1954). Figure 1 shows two kinds of movements: (1) drifts at a velocity of about 5'/sec and mean magnitude about 2.5' and (2) sacadic movements whose duration is about 25 ms and whose average magnitude is about 5' so that the velocity of these movements is very high—about 200'/sec. Figure 2 (from Fender, 1956) shows (3) a high frequency irregular movement of small amplitude (30'' or less).

The eye-movements do not form a determinate signal in that knowledge of a piece of record does not enable us to calculate, in detail, the future course of the movements. They do, however, constitute a stochastic signal, i.e., there is a probability distribution for the direction of the visual axis at a given moment and a contingent probability dependent on the direction at a slightly earlier time. It is also generally agreed that the signal is stationary, i.e. these probability distributions do not change systematically with time. Provided these assumptions are correct, there exists a power spectrum, i.e., a function of temporal frequency that expresses the average properties of the signal.

SHOULD THE MOVEMENTS BE DIVIDED INTO THREE GROUPS OR ONLY INTO TWO?

It is not easy to make an analogue apparatus that produces a Fourier transform of records that contain many sharp movements as the eye-movement records do. Findlay (1971) devised an ingenious method of obtaining (1) a power-spectrum corresponding to the saccadic movements and (2) a power-spectrum correspond-

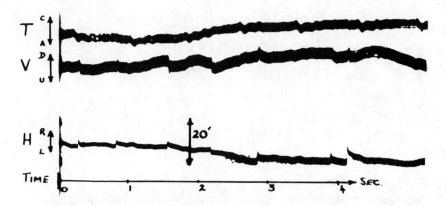

FIG. 1.   Horizontal (H), vertical (V) and torsional (T) components of eye-movements.

ing to the other movements. His results for one subject are shown in Fig. 3, which is an amplitude spectrum, i.e., the square root of the power per unit frequency interval is plotted against the frequency. Note that the unit for the ordinate is 1 second of arc per $Hz^{1/2}$ so that, except at low frequencies, the power per unit frequency interval is very small.

In order to obtain data in a reasonable time Findlay used a band width of 5 Hz. Thus, his measurements do not extend below 5 Hz and do not show whether there is a peak at about 1 Hz corresponding to the drift movement. A reasonable extrapolation of his curve to low frequencies would indicate a power of order 10 min arc^2 in the range 0.5–2.0 Hz, which is approximately the power for a movement of amplitude 2.5' and band width about 1 Hz. This reasonably corre-

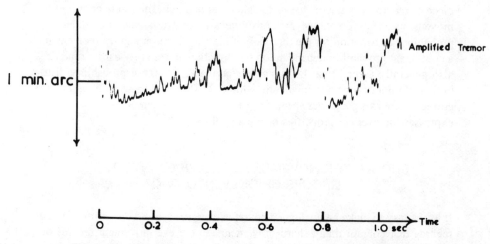

FIG. 2.   Tremor movement amplified (after Fender, 1956). Low frequencies are filtered out.

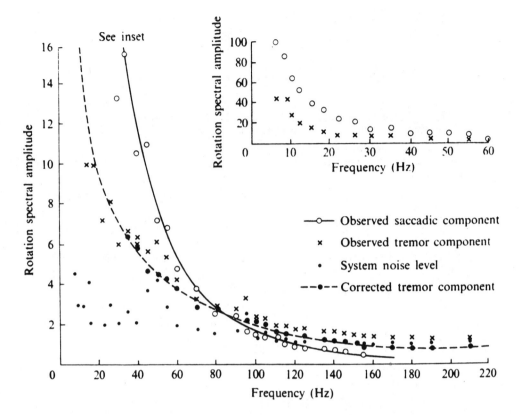

FIG. 3. Amplitude spectra for (a) saccades (b) other movements (from Findlay, 1971).

sponds to what we know about the drift movements. Thus Findlay's curve includes the drifts if we assume that the power spectrum has a maximum at about 1 Hz and falls to near zero at zero frequency. The existence of such a decline seems necessary on more general grounds because the drifts do not include a large overall displacement over a long time.

Most of the early workers on small eye-movements thought, from inspection of records, that there was a peak frequency for the tremor though this frequency was allotted different values from 30–80 Hz. Findlay's results do not support the existence of such a peak. It is unlikely that such a peak, if it exists, is very narrow (i.e., less than 5 Hz wide). Thus Findlay's results suggest that the drifts and the tremor constitute a single noise-like disturbance of the visual axis. He suggests that this irregular oscillation arises from random nerve impulses acting upon a system whose damping increases with frequency.

In passing, we may note that the low frequency part of this movement—up to about 10 Hz—operates to maintain vision while the high frequency part (about the CFF) effectively blurs the retinal image and impairs vision. Thus a damping system that nearly eliminates the high frequency components and has little effect on the low frequency components is advantageous to the visual system.

THE WORK OF THOMAS AND SHAKNOVICH

Thomas and co-workers (Bengi & Thomas, 1965, 1968; Davies & Plant, 1978; Thomas, 1958, 1967, 1969) have recorded the variation of velocity of eye-movements with time. They used tranducer systems that differ materially from those used by other workers and found a kind of tremor that has not been reported by others. It consists of short runs of a regular vibration at about 40 Hz interspersed between irregular movements (Fig. 4). They give a velocity spectrum that peaks at 40 Hz. They have also measured the response of the eyeball system when driven by sinusoidal forces and find a reasonance at 37 Hz with a bandwidth of 40 Hz in the velocity response.

Shaknovich (1977) found that this tremor is markedly different in patients suffering from certain kinds of brain tumors. For example, in the case shown in Fig. 4, the bursts of regular vibration are absent. He further states that there are obvious changes in the movements when brain function is beginning to fail, in some cases, a change in the eye-tremor was the first sign that terminal failure of brain function had commenced.

Davies (1976), who has analyzed some of the records suggests that, even in normal subjects, the character of eye-tremor (e.g., the length and frequency of bursts) changes from time to time so that the assumption that the eye-movement signal is stationary (in the sense defined earlier) is not valid. This, if true, is of considerable importance in relation to theories of eye-movements and to their analysis.

The work of Thomas, Shaknovich and co-workers provokes a number of questions. Why are the bursts of tremor of one frequency not observed in any of

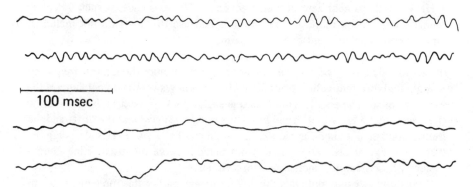

FIG. 4.   Velocity spectrum of tremor (after Shaknovich, 1977).

the records of *displacement* made by various other workers and why is there not any corresponding maximum in the amplitude spectra of Findlay (1971) and Fender and Nye (1961)? Four answers appear possible. The first is that, for any one frequency the mean velocity is f times the amplitude (where f is the frequency). It is possible that the amplitude corresponding to the effect found by Thomas is so small that it is less than the experimental errors of the amplitude spectrum. Thomas does not give—as far as I can see—any absolute value for his velocities so this idea cannot be tested now. The second answer is that the results of Thomas are an artefact of his method. Boyce (1965) investigated the response of contact lens systems and found that, in certain circumstances, subharmonics of the resonant frequency could appear as artefacts. The third possibility is that Thomas has recorded a sideways translation of the eyeball in its orbit and not a rotation. The fourth possibility is that by instilling an anaesthetic into the eye he has reduced the damping of the eyeball and allowed a resonance that is normally strongly damped to build up.

On the whole, I believe that Thomas has found something important, but until his work is repeated by other workers using different techniques the possibility that his results are artefacts of his apparatus must remain. It is very important that independent experiments be made. If his results are genuine they are of considerable importance both for military and for medical applications.

ACCURACY OF FIXATION FOR VARIOUS SIZES OF TARGETS

There are a whole series of unsolved problems connected with the high accuracy of fixation and its variation—or, in most cases its lack of variation—with various experimental conditions. I will briefly mention some of the more important.

1. How Is Fixation Maintained as Accurately as It Is?   I have listed twenty-two determinations of the root-mean-square of the difference between two directions of the visual axis (taken two seconds or more apart) when the subject is fixating (Ditchburn, 1973). The lowest is 1.4' and the highest is 4.7' with an average of 2.5'. The direction of the eye-ball is controlled by three pairs of muscles that are both capable of moving it very fast when that is required and of holding it steady to 2.5' for periods of 60 seconds or more. Start considering how you would build a servo-system using six rubber bands and a ball-bearing to perform both of these functions. This is not an easy problem. How is it done so well?

2. Why Is Fixation So Good?   One could understand that it might be advantageous to hold the retinal image of a point of interest within the fovea—or even within the central fovea of 15'—but what is the advantage, what is the survival

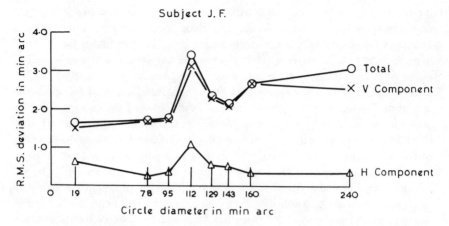

FIG. 5.   Variation of r.m.s. deviation of direction of visual axis, when subject fixates centre of a circular target, vs. diameter of target. (Reproduced from Optica Acta by kind permission).

value of a control that holds the point of interest within a very small central area that is only 1% of the area of the fovea? Why has such an accurate control been evolved?

I can suggest only one clue. One subject who had the most accurate fixations of all the subjects tested was also a very high scorer on other visual tests. This suggests the possibility that accurate fixation is a by-product of a system en- volved to meet some other need—and not an end in itself. If you ask "what other need?"—I can't make any suggestions.

3. Variation of Accuracy of Fixation With Size and Type of Target.   Stein- man (1965) measured the variation of accuracy of fixation when the diameter of a circular target was altered in the range 2' to 87'. Rattle (1969), whose results are shown in Fig. 5, made similar measurements over a range from 4' to 240'. The r.m.s. deviations of the horizontal component and the vertical component are each about 50% larger at 240' than at 4'. There is also a maximum in the r.m.s. deviation at 95' for one subject and 120' for another.

Disregarding the maximum for the moment, it is very difficult to explain why the r.m.s. deviation does not increase more rapidly with size of target—at least in proportion to the size of target—by a factor of 60 instead of a factor of 1.5.

At one time, I proposed the following explanation. As the size of the target increases the length of the circular boundary increases and this tends to increase the available information. On the other hand, the information obtained at the boundary has to be interpolated over a larger distance when the target is large. Hence there are two opposing tendencies, one tending to increase accuracy and the other to decrease it and the result is a small decrease of accuracy.

If this theory were correct, the r.m.s. deviation when the subject is asked to fixate the central point between two dots should (1) always be much greater than for a circular target whose diameter is equal to the separation of the dots and (2) should increase very much when the separation of the dots is increased. Rattle measured r.m.s. deviation when the subject fixated the center of two dots and his results are shown in Fig. 6. Neither of the predictions is fullfilled. The r.m.s. for the two dot target is only about twice the r.m.s. for the circular target and the variation with separation of dots is much the same as the variation with diameter of the circular target. The above explanation of the results obtained with circular targets cannot be correct and I have no alternative theory to suggest.

Thus, there are two unsolved problems: (1) the variation with size of target and (2) the maximum value of the r.m.s. deviation when the target points fall on the edge of the fovea.

There is a considerable field for further work: (1) to repeat the Steinman-Rattle tests with more subjects and (2) to use different kinds of targets. Rattle made a few (unpublished) measurements on the r.m.s. when subjects fixated either (1) the center of an equilateral triangle and (2) the center of a gap in a line. In both cases the r.m.s. deviation was much higher than that obtained with two dots.

4. *Variation With Luminance and With Color.* It has been found (Boyce, 1967a, 1967b; Gliem, 1967; Steinman, 1965; and Steinman & Cunitz, 1968) that accuracy of fixation varies by less than a factor of two when the luminance is varied over the main part of the photopic range—3000cd/m^2 to 1 cd/m^2. The

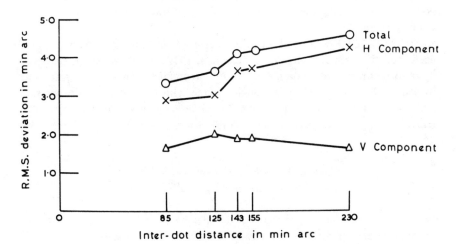

FIG. 6.   Variation of r.m.s. deviation of direction of visual axis, when subject fixates centre of two dots, vs. separation of dots. (Reproduced from Optica Acta by kind permission).

pattern of eye-movements is also little affected when the luminance is varied within the photopic range. Of course, it changes completely when the luminance is so low that the target cannot be seen with the fovea (Gliem, 1964, 1967; and Steinman & Cunitz, 1968).

Steinman (1965) and Boyce (1967a) found that the accuracy of fixation and the pattern of eye-movements were much the same (for equal luminance) when white, red, or blue illumination is used. When we consider the many experiments that tend to indicate blue-blindness of the fovea, this result is astonishing. The question why fixation does not fail with blue light is important and I have no answer. I can only suggest that the blue used in these experiments may not have been pure enough. It is desirable that tests be made on fixation with monochromatic sources (using interference filters).

5. *Effect of Blurring the Target and of Low Contrast.* There are no experiments, as far as I know, on the accuracy of fixation and pattern of eye-movements when the target has blurred outlines. However, Gliem (1964) Gliem and Gunther (1967) measured saccades for subjects with defective vision and found no difference when the acuity varied from 1.0 normal to 0.25 normal. Campbell (personal communication) claims that accuracy of rifle shooting is little affected when lenses are used to put the target outside the marksman's range of focus.

It is almost certain that subjects can fixate the center of a moderately blurred circle almost as well as that of a sharply outlined circle. If this is so, how it is done is another unsolved problem. I think systematic work on accuracy of fixation and pattern of eye-movements with blurred targets is very desirable. Also, I do not know of any systematic work on targets of low contrast and I think such work is required.

Steinman and Kowler (1979) have suggested that micro-saccades have no useful function (see also Kowler & Steinman, 1977). While accepting the validity of their experiments, I do not agree with their conclusion and have responded by letter (Ditchburn, 1980), although I agree with them that we do not fully understand the function of saccades and there are certainly some unsolved problems.

HOW DO SMALL EYE-MOVEMENTS
MAINTAIN GOOD VISION?

We know from the experiments with stabilized retinal images that eye-movements are essential to maintain vision. We also know something about the size of imposed movements needed to maintain vision. (Ditchburn & Drysdale, 1977a & b; Ditchburn, Fender, & Mayne, 1959; Gerrits & Vendrik, 1970, 1974; King-Smith & Riggs, 1978). So far we are in an area of solved problems. The information required for vision must come from boundaries.

We do not know what kind of signals are generated by the eye-movements at boundaries. If dI is the difference of luminance across a boundary, is the signal that reaches the cortex proportional to dI or to log dI or to dI/I? For a sloping as opposed to a sharp boundary is it proportional to dI/dx or to ldI/Idx or to d^2I/dx^2 as has been suggested to explain the Mach bands?

There is still a very large area of unsolved problems here—the answers can only be obtained by a combination of experiments on electrophysiology with electrodes implanted in animals and psychophysical tests on humans.

It is particularly important to understand how the eye-movements generate information about color. I hope shortly to publish two papers on this topic (Ditchburn & Foley-Fisher in preparation, a & b), but they still leave a number of unsolved problems.

To sum up, I suggest that we have one area of solved problems and three areas of unsolved problems, as follows:

1. Area (A) of Solved Problems

We understand fairly well how the drifts and saccades combine to maintain the direction of the visual axis within a small range of angles. The work of St. Cyr and Fender (1969a & b) adds a great deal to our understanding, particularly with binocular fixation.

2. Area (B) of Unsolved Problems

These concern the high accuracy of fixation and the fact that accurate fixation is maintained under conditions that we should expect to be adverse. Why do the signals that maintain fixation depend so little on luminance, hue, sharpness of target, etc.?

Further work is needed on various aspects of these problems as I have indicated earlier. We need to remember that while instrument designers can easily produce sharp symmetrical fixation targets, nature offers us targets that are asymmetrical, blurred, colored, low contrast, etc. and we are far from understanding how fixation on such targets is maintained.

3. Area (C) of Unsolved Problems

The work of Thomas and of Shaknovich on the velocity spectrum of high frequency oscillations raises a series of unsolved problems. Their results may be artefacts, but if they are not, then they are of great importance, especially to clinical medicine. It is very important that their experiments be repeated with different methods of eye-movement recording.

4. Area (D) of Unsolved Problems

The understanding of what and how signals are generated at boundaries.

IV.3 Oculomotor Procrastination

R. H. S. Carpenter
University of Cambridge, England

"The secret of science," Sir Henry Tizard once remarked, "is to ask the right question" (as quoted by Snow, 1962). For those who are actively engaged in research, this may hardly seem a problem: There is no shortage of questions, and frequently we find that to dispose of one reveals two more growing in its place. But, just as in everyday life, there is a tendency to tackle urgent tasks in preference to those that are merely important. My brief for this chapter was to try to stand back a little from the more pressing and immediate questions that arise naturally enough from the discoveries of recent research, and, with a more distant view of the oculomotor system, attempt to identify some area of *real* ignorance, of the kind that might be more obvious to an outsider than to those too involved in the field.

With this in mind I asked one of my second-year students what *he* thought was the most puzzling thing about the oculomotor system. The reply was unhesitating: Why do saccades take such an extraordinarily long time? His question, on reflection, seemed a rather pertinent one. On the one hand, the saccade itself is a masterpiece of control engineering, in which the eye—a distinctly sluggish member that, left to its own devices, likes to take up to a second to settle down in a new position—is smartly accelerated and decelerated to bring the fovea to rest on its goal with a time-course that frequently lasts little more than 20 msec; yet typically it doesn't *start* doing all this until some 200 msec have elapsed since the first appearance of the target. An analogy may serve to emphasize just how odd this situation is, for those who have come to accept it through familarity. A fire station receives an urgent summons by telephone. But for nearly an hour absolutely nothing appears to happen; then all of a sudden the firemen leap into action: The doors are flung open and the fire-engines rush off at

237

break-neck speed with their bells ringing, arriving at the fire in less than five minutes.

Now, of course, it is true that neural communications are very slow by computer standards, having to rely on propagated action potentials rather than ordinary electrical currents; yet 200 msec would allow conduction by an ordinary central nerve fiber over a distance equivalent to some fifty brain-diameters. Even if we allow for synaptic delays as well, to account for the 200 msec we have to imagine something like a hundred neurons in series, each on average conducting over a few centimeters. But such a scheme could not account for this great *variability* in latency that is characteristic of saccades (one frequently finds 20% of responses lying outside a central range of 100 msec or so), and in any case is an order of magnitude too big in relation to what we know of oculomotor anatomy. On the input side, as few as five neurons connect the retina with the visual cortex or superior colliculus, and only a very few more connect with the very highest levels of visual integration. As far as the output is concerned, commonly-accepted schemes of connections amongst neurons in the brain-stem (e.g., Buttner, Hepp, & Henn, 1977) suggest that only three or four intervene between the trigger stimulus for a saccade and the eye muscles themselves. Neurophysiological studies in various parts of the brain confirm the shortness of latencies both between visual stimuli and the first electrical responses in different visual areas, and also between electrical stimulation in the oculomotor system and actual saccadic movement (Fig. 1). So what on earth is going on in-between?

In the first place, it does not seem to be true that this time is simply needed in order to make frantic computations of what to do to get the right size of saccade. Under special circumstances one may observe visually-evoked saccades with very much shorter latencies (Barmack, 1970), and as Becker and Jürgens have recently shown (1979), there is no tendency for short-latency saccades to be any more inaccurate than those that occur later. The bulk of the saccadic latency seems to be simply some kind of oculomotor *procrastination*. Teleologically, of course, procrastination is not necessarily a bad thing: "don't do today what you can put off until tomorrow" can be sound advice if by that means we avoid unnecessary and self-defeating overactivity. There are good reasons for this to be particularly true of saccade generation. A typical saccade of 10° lasts about 50 msec, during which the high rate of visual slip, amongst other factors, renders the visual system all but blind. Thus, paradoxically, the more frequently the oculomotor system tries to improve things by getting the fovea exactly on target, the less time remains actually to *see*: so that a suitable balance must be struck between not seeing quite what we want, and not seeing at all. The saccadic system cannot in fact be permitted to fiddle about making adjustments at its own speed: Some restraint must be imposed from above that forces it to wait a little before proceeding to action; and if meanwhile some change in the visual stimulus has rendered the proposed saccade inappropriate, it may be cancelled (Becker & Jürgens, 1979). Furthermore, the oculomotor system alone is not the best judge

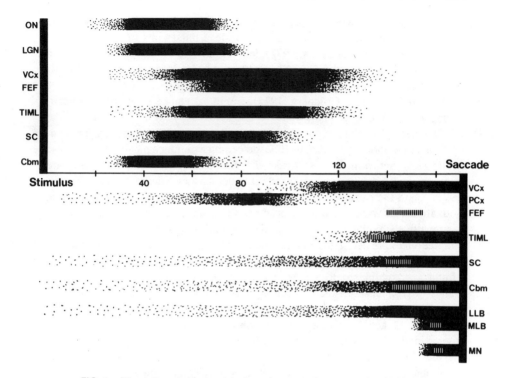

FIG. 1. The timing of neural activity in various central areas associated with the generation of visually-evoked saccades. Above, activity related to the onset of a visual stimulus; below, activity related to the occurrence of the saccade itself, here taken to have an overall latency of 180 msec. The horizontal bars and stippling are intended to represent the approximate spread of observations by various authors and in different units, though in the case of parietal cortex, superior colliculus, cerebellum, and long-lead reticular burst units the stippling also indicates the period of build-up of excitation. The vertically stripped areas represent the spread of latencies of evoked saccades obtained by electrical stimulation in the indicated regions.

ON, optic nerve; LGN, lateral geniculate nucleus; VCx, visual cortex; PCx, parietal cortex; FEF, frontal eye fields; SC, superior colliculus; TIML, thalamic internal medullary lamina; Cbm, cerebellum; LLB and MLB, long- and medium-lead burst units of the pontine reticular formation; MN, oculomotor neurons. The sources of the data used are given in the footnote.

of what is *worth* looking at; again, I would expect to find some over-riding mechanism of directed attention, able to delay or prevent saccades when they are not thought to be important, as well as deciding between conflicting alternative targets.

How might such attention-dependent procrastination be achieved? Figure 1 perhaps illustrates an answer. In several of what might be termed ''higher'' regions of the oculomotor system we find units that show an irregular increase in firing rate during the whole or part of this saccadic dead time. These include the "ragged prelude" of discharge seen in long-lead burst units of the brain-stem (Keller, 1974; Luschei & Fuchs, 1972), and the slow and steady increase in mean firing rate seen both in the cerebellum (Llinas, 1974; Noda, Asoh, & Shibaki, 1977), units in the superior colliculus (Schiller & Koerner, 1971; Schiller & Stryker, 1972; Wurtz & Goldberg, 1972), and in parietal cerebral cortex (Lynch, Mountcastle, Talbot, & Yin, 1977). (The latter may well be related to the steadily-rising "readiness potentials" described by Kornhuber and Deecke, 1965, as a component of human EEG preceding voluntary movements.) These responses are much more closely related to the subsequent saccade than they are to the original stimulus evoking it, and it is perhaps significant that Lynch et al. (1977) found the parietal responses to be most marked when there was a strong motivational drive to make the saccade, rather than in circumstances of casual fixation. In the colliculus, similarly, the responsiveness of such units to visual stimulation is greater if the corresponding part of the visual field is about to become a saccadic target, a phenomemon likened by Schiller and Stryker (1972) to turning a searchlight onto a potential target before shooting at it. Wurtz and Mohler (1976a) describe the colliculus in this context as "an agent of a readiness and selection process" rather than as an initiator of saccades. Could it be that this steady rise of activity might also provide the timing mechanism for saccadic procrastination? For example, the rate of increase of such a response—initially triggered by the appearance of a potential target—might be determined by some attentional or motivational factor: When this activity subsequently reaches some threshold level, a trigger signal could be sent to the brain-stem to initiate the saccade itself (Fig. 2). Such a mechanism would also allow selection between conflicting alternative targets in the visual field, essentially by running a race between the build-up of excitation in the corresponding areas, in a manner reminiscent of Robinson's (1973) model of saccadic selection, recently amplified by Becker and Jürgens (1979). The greater the attention directed to a particular part of the field, or perhaps in some sense the greater its significance, the faster the associated rate of increase of activity would be, and the sooner the threshold for triggering a saccade would be reached.

Perhaps I can be more specific. Let us suppose that in some cell or group of cells in the brain, the degree of excitation rises steadily in response to the appearance of a target stimulus, at a rate r, until at a time t it reaches some threshold value θ, at which point a saccade is triggered. The latency t in these circumstances will therefore (neglecting simple conduction delays) be given by θ/r. The variability that is a puzzlingly characteristic of saccadic latencies must then be due to variation in r, or θ, or possibly both. Now one of the obvious properties of the actual variability of saccadic latencies, that any model ought to be able to explain, is the fact that the distribution of latencies is not Gaussian, but has a distinctly elongated tail on the far side of the median.

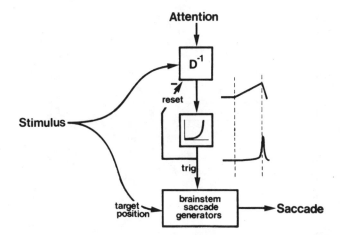

FIG. 2. A possible model of saccadic procrastination. A saccadic stimulus in-
itiates a steady rise of excitation, at a rate dependent on such factors as attention, in
a central neuron or group of neurons corresponding to that part of the visual field.
When this excitation reaches some threshold level, it triggers the execution of a
saccade of appropriate size. For further details, see text.

This skewness can be seen clearly in the circles of fig. 3, which show the
cumulative distribution of 1400 20° saccades from one subject, plotted on a linear
time-axis on probability paper, so that a Gaussian distribution would result in a
straight line. Now if the observed variation in t were simply the result of random
variation in θ on different trials, I would be no nearer explaining the skewness of
saccadic latencies, since θ, being proportional to t, would have to be distributed
in the same asymmetrical way. Of course, there is no reason why it should not
be; but such an *ad hoc* assumption does not explain the origin of the skewness. It
would be rather more satisfactory if the asymmetry could be predicted from the
model on the basis of the more economical hypothesis of Gaussian variation in
some other parameter: A priori one must postulate Gaussian distribution of a
random variable unless one has a specific reason to expect some other law. What
would happen, for example, if it were r rather than θ that was subject to random
fluctuations on different occasions? Let us suppose in particular that r is distributed normally about a mean μ and with variance σ^2. Then the distribution of the
excitation at a time t will also be normal, with mean μt and variance $(\sigma t)^2$; thus
the probability $P(t,\theta)$ that at time t the excitation exceeds θ—i.e. that the trigger
for the saccade has already occurred—will be

$$P(t,\theta) = \frac{1}{2}\left[1 + \mathrm{ERF}\left(\frac{\mu t - \theta}{\sigma t \sqrt{2}}\right)\right], \text{ where ERF}(x) \text{ is defined as } \frac{2}{\sqrt{\pi}}\int_0^n e^{-\mu^2}\,du$$

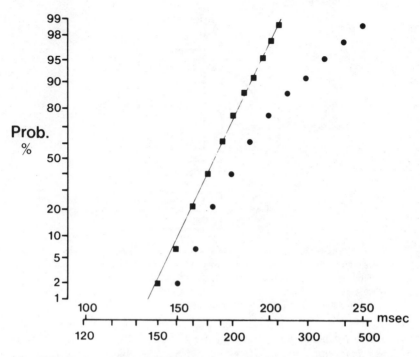

FIG. 3. Cumulative distributions of saccadic latencies: 1400 trials with
amplitude 20°, in a single subject. The ordinate is a cumulative Gaussian probability scale. •, plotted on a linear time-axis (upper scale); ■, the same data, but plotted
as a function of the reciprocal of the latency (lower scale).

If we take θ to be fixed, we can write the cumulative distribution of saccadic
latencies as

$$P(t) = \frac{1}{2} [1 + \text{ERF}(m - k/t)], \text{ where } m = \frac{\mu}{\sigma\sqrt{2}}, \text{ and } k = \frac{\theta}{\sigma\sqrt{2}}$$

We can clarify this a little by defining a new variable s as $-(1/t)$, so that

$$P(s) = \frac{1}{2} [1 + \text{ERF}(m + ks)]$$

In other words, if I plotted the cumulative saccadic latencies on probability
paper, not as a linear function of t, but rather on a reciprocal time-scale in s, I
would expect to obtain a straight line of slope k and intercept (at $s = 0$,
corresponding to infinite latency) of m. The filled squares of fig. 3 show exactly
the same set of data as the circles, but plotted now in this reciprocal fashion, and
it can be seen that they lie quite satisfactorily on a straight line. Figure 4 shows

some cumulative plots of saccadic latencies under various conditions from previously-published data, plotted on a reciprocal time-axis as in fig. 3, and again it can be seen that most of the points are reasonably co-linear, although both the median latencies and the slopes of the lines are noticeably different under different circumstances. In fig. 5 a similar reciprocal plot has been made of some of Fuchs' data (1967b) on saccadic latency in the monkey—to illustrate there is nothing peculiar about humans!—and again (allowing for the fact that the number of observations is here rather small, and the scatter correspondingly greater) the points fall convincingly on straight lines.

Now it is well-known that saccadic latencies may alter for a given subject under different stimulus conditions like amplitude or luminance. Is it possible to identify which of the various parameters in the model may be changed in such cases? Alterations in μ, the mean rate of increase of excitation as a result of the stimulus, will change m, the intercept of the reciprocal plot, but not the slope k; alterations in θ, the threshold, will alter the slope but not the intercept; while alterations in σ, the degree of variability of r, will cause changes in both slope and intercept. Causal inspection of the data already presented reveals that stimulus conditions certainly affect k. In the particular case of changes in target

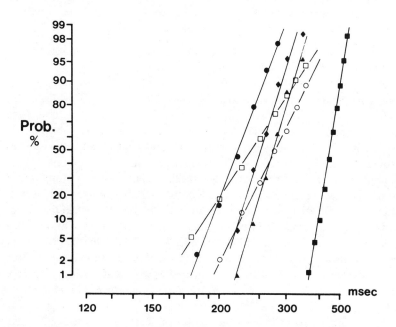

FIG. 4.   Cumulative saccadic latencies, on a reciprocal time-axis, under different conditions. Filled symbols, data from Wheeless et al. (1967) at various target luminances: •, +2; ◆, +1; ▲, 0; and ■, −1 (log units relative to foveal threshold). Open symbols, data from White, Eason, & Bartlett (1962): □, 20°, and ○, 40° saccades.

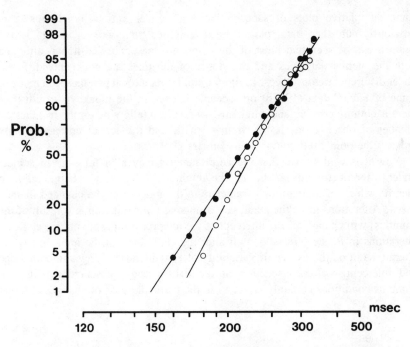

FIG. 5. Cumulative simian saccadic latencies, on a reciprocal time-axis: data from Fuchs (1966). Amplitude 5–10°: •, nasal; ○, temporal.

luminance, for which Wheeless, Cohen, & Boynton (1967) have published latency histograms (fig. 6), extrapolation of straight lines through the cumulative distributions appear to intersect at a single point (with the exception of the data relating to stimuli 1.5 log units below foveal threshold, which more than probably involve a somewhat different visual mechanism). Since this point lies on the origin, implying a constant value of m across all the data, in terms of my model this means that the effect of such changes in luminance is to alter the level of excitation at which the triggering of a saccade takes place, rather than the rate of build-up of excitation, and it is perhaps not implausible to imagine that this trigger-level might depend on the level of background noise that is present. m simply represents the probability of not making a saccade at all; in this particular case, its actual value is of the order of one in 10^{24}, a probability so low as to have little empirical meaning. But it is easy to imagine circumstances in which there might be a significant and measurable probability of no saccade at all taking place—for example, when the target is nearly masked by artificial visual noise—and it would be interesting to know whether under these circumstances saccadic reaction times follow the relationship that would be expected from prior knowledge of the proportion of trials on which no response is made.

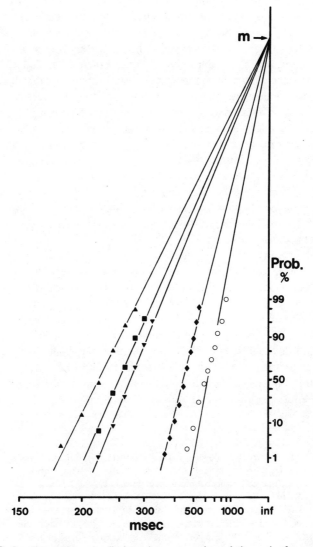

FIG. 6. Cumulative saccadic latencies, on a reciprocal time-axis, for various target luminances (data from Wheeless et al., 1967): ▲, +2; ■, +1; ▼, 0; ◆, −1; and ○, −1.5 (log units relative to foveal threshold).

One fundamental conceptual problem with the model as presented here has to do with the supposed random fluctuations in r. For Gaussian variation in the rate of increase of excitation to result in the observed skewed latency distributions, it is necessary to propose that r, though different in different trials, should not vary *during* the latent period in any one trial. If this were not so, the resultant distribution of $P(t)$ would not be skewed at all, but merely Gaussian. Thus r must not be allowed to vary much during the 200 msec or so of saccadic latency, yet may do so between one trial and the next. To find out whether this is in fact true, we would need to measure the autocorrelation function of latencies for different intervals of time between trials; while this kind of data has been published for the special case of double-step targets less than some 200 msec or so apart, it seems likely that more specialized mechanisms may influence the timing of the second saccade under such conditions. If we suppose that it is fluctuation in the level of attention given to different regions of the visual field that gives rise to the variation in r, then it seems likely that the first of a pair of target steps would influence the level of attention associated with the second. Thus it may in principle be impossible actually to estimate in any informative way the time-dependent statistical properties of r.

While the data that have been presented here are at least compatible with the proposed model of oculomotor procrastination, they are equally clearly insufficient to support it very strongly, and unfortunately a technical disaster involving our PDP-11 at Cambridge prevents me from being able to present more complete and original data on such matters as the effect of stimulus parameters on the form of saccadic latency-distributions. But from the purely empirical point of view, and leaving aside the possible merits or demerits of the model itself, I hope that the notion of plotting cumulative distributions of latencies on reciprocal time-axes may in future at least help to simplify the description of such data-sets by reducing them to a simple pair of variables, m and k.

The data in Fig. 1 is from the following: Bartlett & Doty (1974); Buttner, Hepp, & Henn (1977); Cohen, Goto, Shanzer, & Weis (1965); Cohen & Komatsuzaki (1972); Donaldson & Hawthorne (1979); Dow (1974); Evinger, Kaneko, Johanson, & Fuchs (1977); Goldberg & Robinson (1977); Guitton & Mandl (1974); Guitton & Mandl (1977); Keller (1974); Keller (1977); Llinas (1974); Luschei & Fuchs (1972); Lynch, Mountcastle, Talbot, & Yin (1977); Mohler, Goldberg, & Wurtz (1973); Moors & Vendrick (1979a); Moors & Vendrick (1979b); Mountcastle, Lynch, Georgopoulos, Sakata, & Acuna (1975); Noda, Asoh, & Shibaki (1977); Robinson (1970); Robinson (1972); Robinson & Fuchs (1969); Robinson & Goldberg (1977); Ron & Robinson (1973); Schiller & Koerner (1971); Schiller & Stryker (1972); Schlag, Lehtinen, & Schlag-Rey (1974); Schlag & Schlag-Rey (1977); Snow (1962); Sparks, Holland, & Guthrie (1976); Strashill & Schick (1974); Wolfe (1971); Wurtz & Goldberg (1972); Wurtz & Mohler (1974); Wurtz & Mohler (1976b).

IV.4 Digital Filters for Saccade and Fixation Detection

J. R. Tole and L. R. Young
Biomedical Engineering Center for Clinical Instrumentation and Department of Aeronautics and Astronautics M.I.T.

Rapid detection of saccadic eye movements using a digital filtering scheme has been applied to the on-line processing of vestibular nystagmus. Although saccadic eye movements made during changes in direction of gaze/fixation involve different mechanisms than those of the fast phases of nystagmus, the temporal characteristics of the two events are sufficiently similar that computer processing methods for one type of eye movement may be equally suitable for the other.

SACCADE CHARACTERISTICS

Before discussing our detection scheme, it is worthwhile reviewing some of the relevant temporal and spatial characteristics of saccadic and nystagmus eye movements that are of importance in the detection process. The latency to a single step change in target position is typically from 120 to 300 msec. If the initial saccade misses the target, however, subsequent corrective saccades may occur with much shorter latency. Normally voluntary saccades are separated by a minimum psychological refractory period of about 200 msec.

The amplitude of saccades may vary from microsaccades of a few arc seconds (which may be used to recenter the image on the fovea) up to greater than 90°. Saccades up to 15° to 20° are most common for changes in fixation (Bahill, 1975), while peak eye velocities during these movements may exceed 600 deg/sec. The velocity is influenced by the amplitude of the saccade with peak velocity occurring approximately at the midpoint of the movement and the duration of the peak velocity segment increases with amplitude. Acceleration and deceleration of the eyes may be quite large at the beginning and end of saccades, approaching 80,000 deg/sec². This value depends on the magnitude of the saccade but it is usually smaller for smaller movements. The deceleration appears to be typically somewhat lower than the acceleration, as if the eye is braking at the end of the movement, but is more ballistic at the onset. The duration of a saccade is related to its amplitude and velocity, increasing roughly in proportion to both of these parameters (Robinson, 1964). Families of time course of saccadic position and first and second derivatives as a function of saccade amplitude may be found in the literature (e.g. Clark & Stark, 1974).

PREVIOUS WORK ON IDENTIFICATION

A number of workers have investigated the automatic detection of saccades and/or fast phases of nystagmus, and several hardware methods have been reported (Voots, 1969; Engelken & Wolfe, 1977; Michaels & Tole, 1977). These methods generally employ analog and/or digital circuits that detect saccadic events on the basis of their velocity or acceleration exceeding a threshold. Software methods generally employ min/max searches for saccadic end points (Gentles, 1974; Sills, Honrubia, & Kumley, 1975) or require that velocity exceed some threshold for longer than a prespecified duration (Baloh, Kumley, & Honrubia, 1976; Allum, Tole, & Weiss 1975). At least one algorithm (Evans & Gutmann, 1978) is used to classify fixations as well as saccades in an off-line fashion using techniques similar to ones used in the present work. Most of the reported algorithms appear to depend on fixed thresholds for the detectors. One method (Gentles, 1974) employs several adaptive methods for establishing thresholds and rejecting artifacts. A least mean squares fit to slow phase segments is used to calculate slow phase velocity. The variance in this fit over a number of segments is used as an estimate of the noise level and segments are rejected as artifacts if this level becomes too high. Although these programs may be adjusted to yield good performance on a particular record, performance may be much poorer on a new record. Some algorithms may also include provision for manual editing of program output for further elimination of artifacts. These features suggest that a certain level of user knowledge of both eye movements and of computers is required for successful operation of the programs. This limitation may prove a considerable problem if large quantities of data are to be processed as might occur in a clinical testing situation.

PROBLEMS IN AUTOMATIC RECOGNITION OF SACCADES AND FIXATIONS

In studies in which a subject is asked to fixate a target that may move either periodically or aperiodically, the analysis of the data is somewhat simplified by the knowledge that a stereotyped response to the stimulus is likely to occur within certain known time intervals. This type of experiment is reasonably amenable to automation (e.g., Jernigan, 1979).

When subjects scan instruments, have fixation disorders, or make nystagmus, the problem is usually one of identifying actual events versus artifacts even though the temporal characteristics of an event (saccade or fast phase) are reasonably stereotyped. This problem is challenging since the sequence of events may or may not be stationary in a statistical sense, or synchronized to the stimulus, and the magnitude of the noise may be difficult to predict in advance. Furthermore, nonsaccadic eye movements like smooth pursuit or slow phases may cause false triggering of certain event detectors unless precautions are taken.

One of our goals in recent years has been to develop algorithms that will work well without user interaction, that can handle a variety of records that can occur in use, and that operate in near on-line fashion. The requirement for near on-line operation is not absolutely necessary but we have retained this as a desirable feature because much of our work is devoted to clinical vestibular function testing. Having results readily available at the end of a test procedure allows immediate repeat of the test if necessary.

The fundamental approach of our algorithms is the on-line, beat to beat detection of saccades or fast phases of vestibular nystagmus based on current estimates of signal to noise ratio on the incoming data signal. Although the work described here is only for a single channel of eye position, we are currently working on applying some of these techniques to simultaneous recording of horizontal and vertical eye position.

The general form of a system for processing of eye movement data in near on-line fashion is shown in Fig. 1. The eye position sensor output is amplified and band limited according to the sampling frequency to be used. The data is sampled by an A/D converter and read into a circular buffer, BUF1, on an interrupt basis. A main program loop operates in parallel with the sampling process. This loop processes the raw data to extract features necessary for event classification and/or desired output. These features include time derivatives of the input data as well as certain timing characteristics of the raw waveform. When one second of processed data has accumulated in circular buffer BUF2, the event classifier is allowed to look for events in the waveform. These events may include saccades, fixations, slow or fast phases of nystagmus, or artifacts.

AN EVENT CLASSIFIER FOR SACCADES/FAST PHASES

The event classifier used in our current program employs a template matching approach. The optimal filter or detector for an event is a filter that "looks" like, i.e., has the same time domain characteristics, as the event one wishes to detect. If one convolves an incoming data signal with such a filter, the largest response should occur when the matched event occurs in the data. In order to develop a template for saccades or fast phases of nystagmus, one needs to consider their

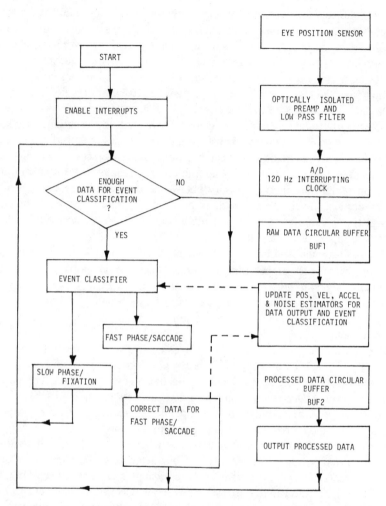

FIG. 1.   General form of eye movement classification algorithm.

characteristics as reviewed above. An idealized example of a saccade and its first and second derivatives is shown in Fig. 2A. As seen in the figure, a velocity pulse and an acceleration impulse pair are associated with the saccade.

Actual saccades do not start or stop quite as abruptly as in the ideal case. They are better represented by the example in Fig. 2B. The velocity and acceleration responses are similar to the ideal case, but reflect the non-instantaneous nature of the real movements. It is also interesting to note that the deceleration at the end of a saccade tends to be smaller than the acceleration at the onset of the movement for larger saccades (Hyde, 1959). Ideal and actual waveforms for a single isolated nystagmus beat are given in Fig. 2C and 2D, respectively. The velocity and acceleration are very similar to that for the saccade, however the velocity baseline is non-zero, reflecting the slow phases preceding and following the fast phase.

Figure 3A shows a finite impulse response filter that is sensitive to acceleration and is used in our event classifier. This particular filter was chosen for several reasons. It has all integer weights, thus allowing the use of fixed point arithmetic. It is of short duration (9 samples), thus filter delay is minimized to avoid aliasing associated with vestibular nystagmus of high frequency (up to 10 beats/sec). These were important considerations since the filter was to be implemented on an 8080 microprocessor in our vestibular test instrument.

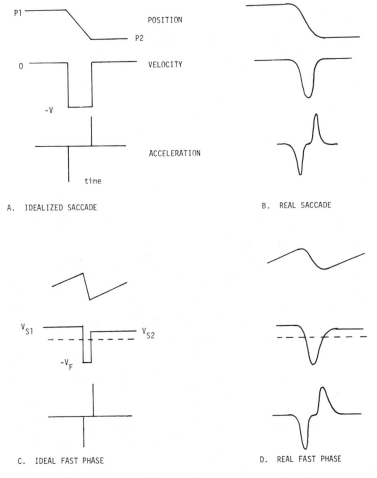

FIG. 2.   Ideal and actual saccades and fast phases of nystagmus. (Axes labels for A are typical.)

The incoming data are convolved with the acceleration filter of Fig. 3A requiring 9/120 or 75 msec delay. Eye velocity is also calculated using the FIR filter of Fig. 3B. One half second of raw and processed data is maintained in circular buffers. Whenever the event classifier is entered, the output of the acceleration filter is compared with the current value of a threshold (the criteria for which are discussed in the following). If the acceleration exceeds this threshold, the acceleration buffer is scanned forward to check for a second peak in acceleration of opposite sign to that at A and greater in magnitude than

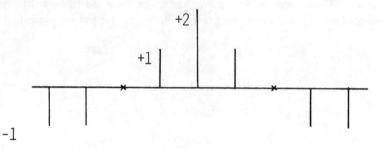

ACCELERATION

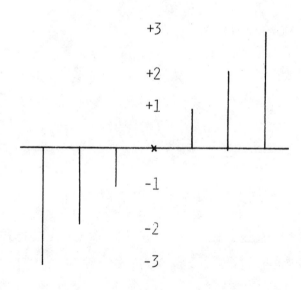

VELOCITY

FIG. 3. Integer weight finite impulse response filters used for saccadic event detection.

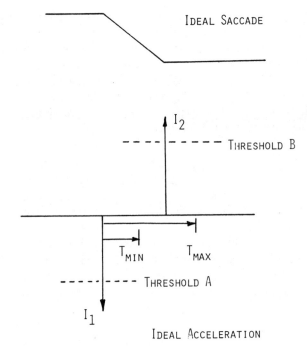

1. $\left| I_1 \right| > A$

2. $\left| I_2 \right| > B$

3. $\text{SGN } I_2 \neq \text{SGN } I_1$

4. $T_{MIN} < I_2 - I_1 < T_{MAX}$

FIG. 4. Basic criterion for saccade/fast phase event classification.

threshold B. Minimum and maximum durations for this search, based on theoretical limits discussed earlier, are applied. If all these conditions are met a saccade is said to be present in the record. The conditions for fast phase/saccade classification are summarized in Fig. 4.

ADAPTIVE METHODS FOR SETTING THRESHOLDS

The above scheme appears to work quite well on low noise data where velocity of non-saccadic eye movements is low. Unfortunately, the general eye movement recording scheme is neither noise free nor solely concerned with fixations. Thus noise may cause false event detection as may non-saccadic eye movements of high velocity/acceleration (e.g., smooth pursuit or slow phase of nystagmus). These difficulties point out that the methods by which thresholds for event detectors are set are at least as important as the actual detection method chosen.

Several schemes are employed in our algorithm to estimate noise levels and set thresholds for the template filter. The first technique estimates the peak to peak amplitude of fluctuations on the input signal when the average eye velocity over the last two sec is less than 4 deg/sec. It can be easily shown that, to first order, the noise in acceleration may be estimated as

$$\text{accel/DC noise} = 2|\Delta p|/\Delta t^2$$

where Δt is the sampling interval and Δp is the current peak to peak estimate of noise in position. This noise could be estimated once during eye position calibration if the signal to noise ratio could be expected to remain constant over a test session. In the more general case, noise may vary dynamically due to changes in ambient illumination, extraneous muscle noise pickup if EOG is used and so forth, hence the need to estimate the noise level whenever eye velocity is low.

The second estimator of noise operates on the output of the acceleration filter. The notion here is that the acceleration signal of interest is a series of impulse pairs and that all other output from the filter is "noise." Note that this output will include estimates of eye acceleration at all times, not just during saccades, but that the impulses related to beginning and end of saccades will typically be the events of largest magnitude in the filter output. The impulse pairs are further assumed to make little contribution to the total RMS power of the acceleration, allowing one to argue that the current RMS of acceleration reflects the current "noise" level on the signal being processed. If the thresholds A and B in Fig. 4 are also made functions of this RMS estimate, they become adaptive to recent acceleration history of the input signal resulting in better performance of the event detector. This adaptive process becomes especially important in vestibular nystagmus resulting from high frequency periodic stimuli where the acceleration of slow phase segments may be quite high.

The practical implementation of the estimate of the RMS level of acceleration requires several further assumptions. First, it is assumed that the acceleration can be assumed to be a zero mean signal for time windows greater than 4 sec. Second, in order to avoid taking square roots and to use more simple calculation methods, the following approximation is made:

$$\text{Accel}_{\text{RMS}} = \sqrt{\frac{1}{T} \int_0^T (\text{Accel}^2(T) - \overline{\text{Accel}^2})\, dT}$$

In discrete form:

$$= \sqrt{\frac{1}{T} \sum_{i=1}^{T} (\text{Accel}^2(i) - \overline{\text{Accel}^2})}$$

For nystagmus and fixation data, $\overline{\text{Accel}} \to 0$ as $T > 4$ seconds. Then:

$$\text{Accel}_{\text{RMS}} \simeq \sqrt{\frac{1}{T}\ \Sigma\ \text{Accel}^2(i)}$$

since $\sqrt{\Sigma\ \text{Accel}^2} \leq \Sigma|\text{Accel}|$, one obtains

$$\text{Accel}_{\text{RMS}} \leq \frac{1}{T}\ \sum_{i=0}^{T}\ |\text{Accel}(i)|,\ T > 4 \text{ seconds}$$

Since there will usually be some residual noise that will not be estimated by the above methods, a constant term is also added to each of the thresholds to make each of them have an absolute lower bound. The thresholds are thus given by:

Threshold A = 4000 deg/sec^2 + Accel/RMS + Accel/DC noise

Threshold B = 4000 deg/sec^2 + Accel/RMS

EXAMPLES OF OPERATION OF THE ALGORITHM

Figure 5 shows the saccade detector in operation on horizontal eye movements recorded with EOG during reading. The lower recording is the horizontal eye position recorded with D.C. coupled EOG. The upper tracing is the corresponding acceleration record. The detection of saccades by the event classifier is shown in the Saccade Indicator channel. Figure 6 shows the response of the adaptive threshold A to an increase in the noise level of the EOG signal when the subject is asked to grit his teeth. Note that the threshold (which is shown increas-

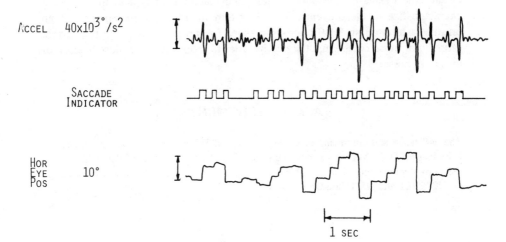

ACCEL   40x10^3°/s^2

SACCADE
INDICATOR

HOR
EYE   10°
POS

1 SEC

FIG. 5.   Identification of saccades during reading.

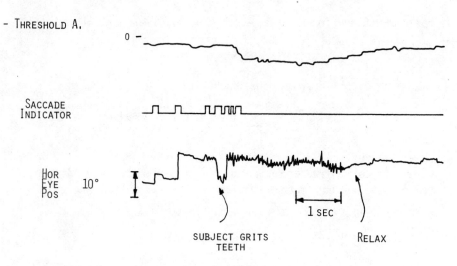

FIG. 6.   Response of threshold A to peak to peak noise changes.

ing in the negative direction) rapidly adapts to the increased noise level and that no events are detected on the basis of this increased noise. When the subject relaxes, the threshold decreases to a lower level once more.

SUMMARY

We have developed a practical means for the automatic recognition of fast phase or saccadic events on the basis of template matching of typical time domain characteristics of these events. The algorithm for this purpose operates in an on-line fashion on an 8080 microprocessor. The program adapts to the current estimate of noise on the input signal in order to minimize false identification of events in noise.

ACKNOWLEDGMENTS

The assistance and comments of C. M. Oman and W. A. Morrison are gratefully acknowledged. D. L. Michaels performed some of the work on matched filters which led to the current processing scheme. This work was supported by NIH Grants NIH-1-P01-GM22392-01 and NS 15862-01.

IV.5 Compensation for Some Second Order Effects to Improve Eye Position Measurements

David Sheena and Joshua Borah
Gulf + Western, Applied Science Laboratories

THE GOAL OF EYE POSITION MEASUREMENT INSTRUMENTATION

It has always been the goal of eye position measurement technology to maximize instrumentation performance by:

1. allowing subjects the maximum possible psychological and physical freedom;
2. extracting a large amount of information with the highest possible accuracy;
3. enabling successful eye position measurement of the greatest possible subject population (different eye pigmentation, different eyelid shapes and positions, glasses, contact lenses, etc.).

These goals may mutually conflict because it is possible to approach one at the expense of another. For example, the greatest accuracy can be obtained by the use of very restrictive contact lenses or bite boards at the cost of reduced subject freedom. With a contact lens system, eye movement measurement precision and accuracy may be fractions of a minute of arc; whereas, the precision possible with a free-head, remote, television-type system is generally about half a degree with an accuracy of one degree (Young & Sheena, 1975).

Note that there is a difference between precision and accuracy of eye movement measurement. Accuracy indicates how closely the measurement corresponds to the true eye position, while precision is a measure of the reproducibility of the measurement. In some applications, like reading, accuracy is important, while in others, like the study of eyeball dynamics, only precision is important.

257

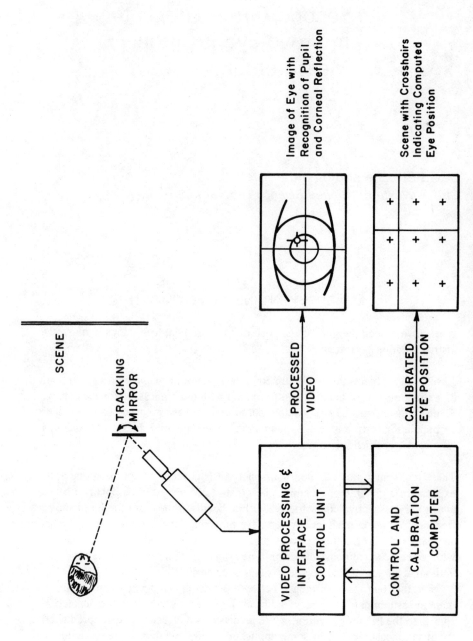

SCENE

TRACKING MIRROR

VIDEO PROCESSING & INTERFACE CONTROL UNIT

CONTROL AND CALIBRATION COMPUTER

PROCESSED VIDEO

CALIBRATED EYE POSITION

Image of Eye with Recognition of Pupil and Corneal Reflection

Scene with Crosshairs Indicating Computed Eye Position

FIG. 1. Representative bright pupil eye position measurement system.

The state of the art, as it stands, is barely sufficient for many experiments in which the subject must be relatively unencumbered. It is difficult, for example, to distinguish small fixations from noise or to discern small saccades with this class of instrument. In reading studies, the stimulus must frequently be enlarged to enable unequivical determination of the line and word being viewed.

Since the experimental situation precludes us from restricting the subject in order to improve accuracy, we attempt to solve the problem by keeping things "fixed" mathematically. We attempt to find and measure as many parameters as possible that seem to cause variations in the measured eye position, and then compensate for these variations. The resulting computations yield only second order improvements and with diminishing returns; but since the instrumentation is at the borderline of suitability for some applications, small improvements in performance are very worthy of pursuit. Finally, it is extremely important that these performance gains be achieved in a practical fashion.

REPRESENTATIVE EYE MOVEMENT SYSTEM

Computers have become a boon to eye movement instrumentation. They can handle complicated computations and perform convoluted calibrations and mapping of what are essentially very non-linear phenomena. Most importantly, they make practical some second order accuracy improvements that would be prohibitive or impossible without them.

The general approach and techniques described here are not peculiar to any one eye movement measurement method or instrumentation. A particular system will be described, however, as a representative one and is the system to which the various computational improvements discussed in this chapter have actually been applied. It is a member of an important class of devices that operate by determining the positions of two elements of the eye; in particular, the center of the pupil and the center of the corneal reflection. In other cases, the center of the corneal reflection and the fourth Purkinje image are used; the concept, however, is the same.

The system employed is shown schematically in Fig. 1. The sensor, a television camera, views the eye of a subject through a head tracking mirror, and the video signal is processed to extract the features of interest, i.e., the pupil and the corneal reflection. The coordinates of all the boundary points are fed to a computer that, in turn, determines the centroids of the two elements. The vectorial difference between the two centroids is the "raw" computed eye position, which varies monotonically with true eye position, and, to first order, independently of head motion as shown in Fig. 2.

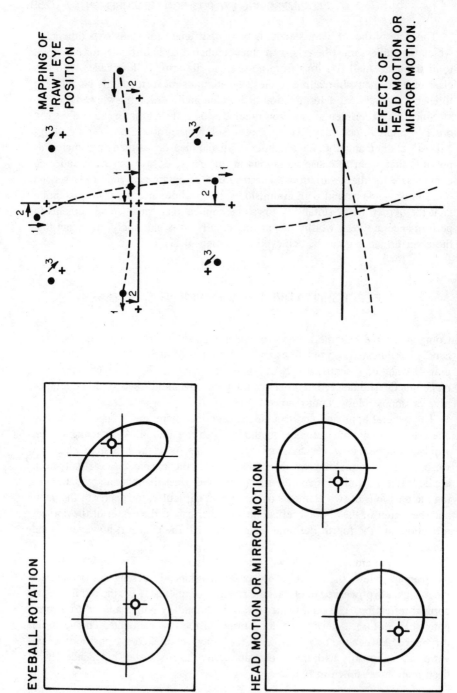

FIG. 2. Effects of eyeball rotation as opposed to head motion or mirror motion.

260

BASIC CALIBRATION

When the subject is instructed to view the 9 calibration target points indicated in Fig. 2, the raw eye position measurement obtained will fall on some distorted map of the calibration scene. This is shown in the figure. The first calibration step is to "stretch" this raw eye position "map" to fit the calibration point map. Considering only the horizontal axis, the "raw" eye position can be mapped into the scene by a simple quadratic relationship of the form:

$$EP_h = a + b\,X + c\,X^2 \tag{1}$$

where EP_h is the computed horizontal eye position and X is the "raw" horizontal eye position. This transformation produces the shift shown by the arrows labled "1" in Fig. 2.

The equation 1 transformation makes uniaxial corrections, and, as may be seen in the figure, some "crosstalk" remains in the mapping. This may have many sources such as the non-concurrence of the target vertical with the sensor vertical, slight asymmetries in the curvature of the cornea, etc. We must therefore add a crosstalk correction term as follows:

$$EP_h = \ldots\ldots + d\,Y + e\,Y^2 \tag{2}$$

where Y is "raw" vertical eye position. The effect is to "twist" the "raw" eye position axes so as to conform to those of the scene as indicated by the arrows labeled "2."

It should be pointed out that there is no intuitive reason for using quadratics in the equations 1 and 2 as opposed to cubics, quartics, etc. We have simply observed that the quadratics are sufficient.

Remaining, at this point, is a mismatch at the corners that can be corrected by the addition of a corner term:

$$EP_h = \ldots\ldots + f\,X\,Y \tag{3}$$

As might be expected, the necessary correction is usually different for each corner, and, in practice, a different "corner term" is needed for each quadrant. The result of "XY" term corner correction is shown, in Fig. 2, by the arrows labeled "3."

SECOND ORDER HEAD MOTION
AND MIRROR MOTION COMPENSATION

Head motion usually results in another overall shift between the mapped eye position space and the scene space as shown in Fig. 2. The approximation of head independent measurement is just that, an approximation that holds only if the scene being viewed is at infinity. When it is not, and the subject moves his head, there is a geometrical shift in the mapping. In addition to the geometrical effect, TV cameras or other sensors used to observe the eye are usually nonuniform, and change their response characteristics as the eye moves to different portions of the sensor "field." The total result is a mapping distortion due to head position change that can be corrected by the addition of axial and cross head motion compensation terms as follows:

$$EP_h = \ldots\ldots + g\,X_h + h\,X_h^2 + j\,Y_h + k\,Y_h^2 \tag{4}$$

where X_h and Y_h are the head position coordinates. The terms are, once again, quadratic.

In the particular "representative" system described in this chapter, a mirror is used to track the head. As the mirror moves, a translation and distortion similar to that caused by head motion is observed. This happens because the optical axis intersects the eye from different angles as the head moves about, and the features of the eye being observed, i.e., the pupil and the corneal reflection, are not in the same plane. An apparent change in separation results. To compensate for this effect, the following terms can be added:

$$EP_h = \ldots\ldots + m\,X_m + n\,X_m^2 + p\,Y_m + q\,Y_m^2 \tag{5}$$

where X_m and Y_m are mirror position coordinates.

DETERMINATION OF THE TRANSFORM COEFFICIENTS

The transform relation between "raw" eye position and the scene now has the form:

$$EP_h = a + b\,X + c\,X^2 + d\,Y + e\,Y^2 + f\,X\,Y + g\,X_h + h\,X_h^2 + j\,Y_h + k\,Y_h^2 + m\,X_m + n\,X_m^2 + p\,Y_m + q\,Y_m^2 \tag{6}$$

It should be emphasized that each of the correction terms that has been included represents a real effect and is not purely of mathematical interest.

In order to evaluate the 14 coefficients, it is necessary to generate 14 equations by appropriately exercising the subject. To insure a nonsingular solution, all parameters appearing in equation 6 must be varied. The first 6 coefficients operate on "raw" eye position measurements and sufficient data for these terms can be generated by requiring the subject to fixate the 5 axial target points (see Fig. 2), plus one corner point. If, as previously suggested, a different "f" (corner term coefficient) is to be used for each quadrant, the subject must fixate all 9 target points. To provide data for the head motion terms, the subject can be asked to fixate the center target point and move his head to different parts of the sensor (e.g., TV camera) field. Activating the mirror to follow the subject, as he moves his head in the allowable volume of space, provides data for the mirror motion terms.

The task of performing the computations to determine the various coefficients can be overwhelming, and this is where practical considerations become very important. An exact solution is virtually impossible within the limitations of practical computers, and a numerical solution, although quite satisfactory, can still require many minutes of processing—up to 15–20 minutes in some cases on a laboratory minicomputer.

This is prohibitive since good experimental practice requires that the calibration be as quick as possible in order to minimize subject fatigue and to reduce the time in which conditions can change. A more practical implementation becomes apparent with the realization that all terms other than the primary eye position quadratic (equation 1) are second order effects and can be varied independently of one another. They can, therefore, be very well approximated by additive corrections.

We begin with a simple linearization:

$$EP_{h0} = a' + b' X + c' X^2 \tag{7}$$

where X is "raw" horizontal eye position and EP_{h0} is an estimate of true eye position. Remember that true eye position is being determined only along the horizontal axis for simplicity of illustration. The subject fixates three known target points along the horizontal axis, and this provides the three values of X needed to solve for a', b', and c'.

Next, crosstalk (effect of vertical eye position on the horizontal measurement) is corrected with the following approximation:

$$EP_{h1} = EP_{h0} + c1 + d' Y + e' Y^2 \tag{8}$$

where Y is "raw" vertical eye position and EP_{h1} is a new estimate of true horizontal eye position. The subject fixates three target points along the vertical axis, providing three Y values and three corresponding values of EP_{h0} (calculated from eqn. 7), and allowing a simple quadratic solution for $c1$, d', and e'.

A corner correction (for one corner) is now added:

$$EP_{h2} = EP_{h1} + c2 + f' X Y \tag{9}$$

Subject fixation on one corner target point provides the additional data needed to calculate $c2$ and f'. Fixation data from the other three corner points can be used to calculate similar "corner terms" for the remaining quadrants.

Next, head motion and head motion crosstalk corrections are added:

$$EP_{h3} = EP_{h2} + c3 + g' X_h + h' X_h^2 \tag{10}$$

$$EP_{h4} = EP_{h3} + c4 + j' Y_h + k' Y_h^2 \tag{11}$$

where X_h and Y_h are horizontal and vertical head position coordinates. The three values of X_h and Y_h needed to solve for the coefficients in equations 10 and 11 can be generated by requiring the subject to move his head first laterally and then vertically as he fixates a single target point. The mirror must remain stationary during this procedure to allow the eye to translate with respect to the sensor (e.g., TV camera) field.

Finally, a mirror correction is added in a similar fashion:

$$EP_{h5} = EP_{h4} + c5 + m' X_m + n' X_m^2 \qquad (12)$$

$$EP_{h6} = EP_{h5} + c6 + p' Y_m + q' Y_m^2 \qquad (13)$$

Note that each new correction utilizes the results of the previous correction. coefficients for the additive correction process of equations 7 through 13, are evaluated by solving several small systems (maximum of three equations and three unknowns) instead of one 14 term system. An unwieldy procedure is thus reduced to a set of very manageable steps. In actual practice, a minicomputer can solve for these coefficients (i.e., perform a calibration) in less than one second.

The additive solution is mathematically precise only if the variables in equations 7 through 13 are completely independent of one another, but empirical results have shown this to be a very satisfactory approximation. For best performance, some care must be taken to maintain this independence during calibration (collection of data used to solve for the coefficients). For example, the vertical and horizontal axes of the calibration target must be aligned with the vertical and horizontal axes of the sensor, e.g., TV camera raster pattern; when varying head position during the calibration procedure, it is important that mirror position and eye fixation point remain fixed; etc.

REPRESENTATIVE RESULTS

Figure 3 is a representative example showing the effects of additive crosstalk and corner corrections. In this particular case, the nominal error is of the order of one degree of viewing angle, and these corrections reduce the error by a fraction of a degree. Although clearly a case of diminishing returns the improvement expands the usefulness of the instrument enough to make the effort quite worthwhile.

Figure 4 shows the improvement gained with the addition of head motion compensation. In this example, a subject was asked to fixate as he moved his head, and the figure shows variation in measured eye position with and without compensation. Clearly there is, once again, a gain on the order of a fraction of a degree. The mirror motion compensation produces very similar results.

The price for performing the type of additive calibration described, is a loss of flexibility during the calibration procedure since some care must be exercised to maintain the independence of the different variables. The advantage is a capability to implement very complicated calibrations in an extremely practical fashion, and, more importantly, the capability to include additional correction terms easily.

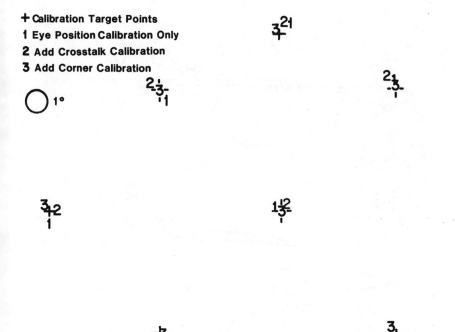

+ Calibration Target Points
1 Eye Position Calibration Only
2 Add Crosstalk Calibration
3 Add Corner Calibration

FIG. 3. Progression of calibration improvement as second order terms are added.

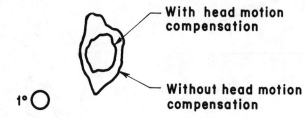

With head motion
compensation

Without head motion
compensation

FIG. 4. *X–Y* Recording of fixation points as subject moves his head.

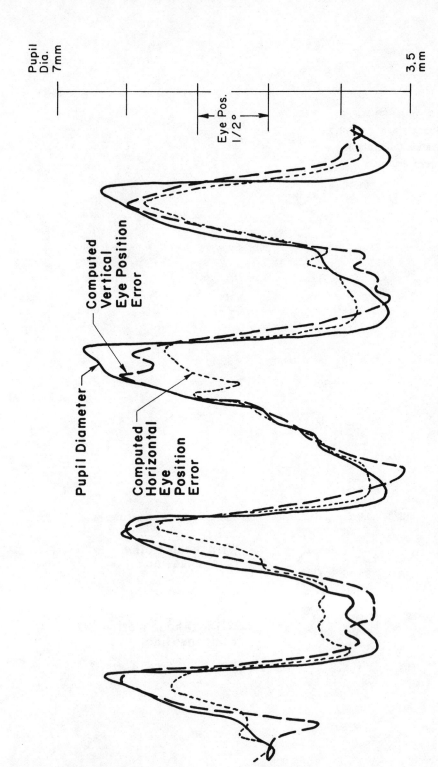

Pupil
Dia.
7mm

3.5
mm

Eye Pos.
1/2°

Computed
Vertical
Eye Position
Error

Pupil Diameter

Computed
Horizontal
Eye Position
Error

FIG. 5.   Effects of pupil diameter on eye position during fixation.

OTHER COMPENSATION CORRECTIONS

As anyone involved in eye movement measurement will attest, there is no dearth of remaining error, noise, and drift in the obtained measurement from any instrumentation used. This is the nature of physical measurement, and it becomes particularly pronounced as one tries to make "non-loading" measurements. We have, therefore, continued to seek out additional variables or parameters that have some relationship to the error in measured eye position.

In particular, a drift has been observed in the computed eye position that seems to correlate, in frequency, with pupil diameter variation, and some exploratory experiments have been conducted. Subjects were seated at a bite board and instructed to fixate while their pupils were stimulated by changes in the ambient light level. The measured eye position was plotted against the pupil diameter and the resulting variation is shown in Fig. 5. It shows a very dramatic correlation in the case of this extreme pupillary change. It is very important to note that this does not necessarily imply any physiological relationship between pupil diameter and pupil or foveal center, although some such relationship could exist. Most likely, the effect is purely a measurement artifact probably found in all eye position measurement instrumentation techniques and is a potential source of error in the computation that can now be removed.

The technique presented for additive corrective compensation offers a mechanism for doing this as follows:

$$EP_n = EP_{n-1} + cn + uPD + vPD^2 \tag{14}$$

where PD is the pupil diameter. The effect may actually involve more complex pupillary dynamics than the direct relationship to PD shown in equation 14, and this needs to be investigated further.

Other variables that have shown qualitative correlation to computed eye position include z-axis (distance between the sensor and the eye) variation, and corneal reflection shape changes caused by tear film changes.

CONCLUSION

As we try to increase subject freedom and reduce the obtrusiveness of eye movement measuring devices, additional variables are introduced to the measurement. It rapidly becomes impossible to achieve the kind of accuracy produced with very restrictive systems; however, by mathematically removing some of the variates, accuracy sufficient for many applications can be obtained. Although compensation for second order effects results in numerically small accuracy and precision gains, this is sometimes enough to cross the borderline of acceptability for certain uses and is therefore very worthwhile.

An additive method of calibration allows compensation for numerous second order errors in a very quick and practical fashion. While the additive procedure is mathematically imprecise, empirical results have shown the approximation to be quite satisfactory, yielding significant accuracy gains. It is likely that further improvements can be achieved by identifying and correcting for additional eye position measurement covariates.

ACKNOWLEDGMENT

This work is supported in part by contract DAAG29-79-C-0157 from the U.S. Army Research Office.

V SEARCH AND SCANNING

Are there developmental trends in visual search strategies? If so, are they dependent upon differential utilization of the periphery? During reading, is the text the only guide for information search? What within-word fixation dynamics occur as a function of word length? What is the nature of the scanning process? Is it flexible enough to allow for a variety of task demands?

In chapter V. 1, Cohen describes a match-to-standard feature search task in which children and adults attempt to match stimuli at various eccentricities to a central standard. Although children and adults are both selective in their use of detailed peripheral information on initial fixations off-standard during search, that selectivity is restricted to the 3° parafoveal region in children. Adults consistently prove far more efficient in overall task performance than children. In defining perceptual and decision phases of search Cohen describes a developmental model that includes—parsing, comparing, testing, and confirming processes.

In chapter V. 2, O'Regan describes information search from a "convenient viewing" position. Initial puzzlement evolved over the fact that fixations on short words are longer than fixations on long words. Although long words may be scanned differently than short words it seems as though the first fixation duration increases directly with the distance into the word that the eye lands. As O'Regan establishes a critical region for fixation the convenient viewing position hypothesis emerges. He describes the necessity for a subsequent fixation following an initial fixation at the beginning of a long word leading to two short fixations at either end of a long word, while only a single longer fixation is needed if the eye lands within the convenient viewing position where the entire word can be perceived. The probability of achieving the convenient viewing position is much more likely on short words hence the longer fixation. Although information about word identification comes from both the stimulus array and reader's knowledge of the rules of the language, the interaction of these two sources permits the appropriate compensatory eye movements to occur and facilitate identification.

In the final chapter of this section, Levy-Schoen examines the oculomotor control process during scanning. Her primary concern is in defining the response and seeking functions of exploration of the environment. She hypothesizes that prior to action a scanning ''routine'' is developed around which the subsequent oculomotor behavior will be organized. Evidence for the non-randomness of this routine is described as well as its operation on the local and global levels. More specifically, fixation duration during scanning seems directly related to availability of peripheral pre-processing. As task demands change so do the possible regulators of the scanning routine from a most general free-field pattern to global patterns with a few restrictions to those encountered in tasks like reading where moment-to-moment physical and cognitive factors intervene. Successful scanning depends upon good pre-established programs and the adapability of those programs when change occurs.

V.1 The Development of Strategies of Visual Search

Karen M. Cohen
Bell Laboratories

Perception is inherently selective. Selective processing of information from the visual environment reflects a constant interplay between perception and action. Global and detailed processing of visual arrays frequently guide subsequent information gathering activities that, in turn, provide new material for processing by the visual perceptual system. Selective sampling of available stimuli is an adaptive achievement enabling one to focus upon the most important aspects of the environment.

To be selective, one must process and integrate information from various parts of the visual environment. The small, 2°-region of the visual field projecting onto the fovea represents the area of greatest acuity and yields the most detailed processing. The peripheral retina, however, receives stimulation from a much larger region of the visual field (approximately 200° horizontally and 130° vertically) and is well-designed for selective sampling of a visual array because of its sensitivity to low levels of illumination and to movement.

Though information sampled from the visual periphery is relatively crude and indistinct, it presumably provides an important basis for the direction of focused attention. In fact, eye movements are frequently considered an attempt to orient objects detected in the periphery onto the fovea for closer examination. Despite its obvious importance, our current understanding of how peripheral information is actually selected and used in a planned sequence of activity, like directing fixations, is presently incomplete, while even less is known about how this ability develops.

The pattern of successive eye fixations is considered an observable indication of selective processing, especially in visual scanning tasks. Hence, examination of adults' and children's eye fixation records, when searching for a target in a visual display, should indicate ways in which selective processing abilities develop with age. Eye movement and fixation records, of course, provide voluminous data that can be subjected to many different types of analyses. In the research to be discussed, striking *similarities* in the way in which children and adults conduct their search will be reported based upon one type of analysis while systematic *differences* in search activity for various age groups will be described based upon another type of analysis. Finally, possible explanations for these observed developmental differences in search strategies will be provided by a third type of analysis. Examination of various analyses of eye movement and fixation records, then, will be a central theme in this chapter.

I will also discuss how information located in the visual periphery is used to guide overt search activity (eye movements) and a model of the processes involved in fixation-by-fixation decisions during search.

BACKGROUND

Despite the abundance and variety of literature on the role of eye movements in psychological processes, there is as yet an incomplete understanding of what operations or mechanisms control the actual redirection of gaze. Models have been postulated, ranging from local or global stimulus control to internal or cognitive control of eye fixation patterns (e.g., Rayner, 1978). A more plausible position is that a perceiver's intentions, expectations, and strategies of scanning are tempered by the particular task and stimulus materials with which one is confronted (Cohen, 1974).

This conclusion is intuitively obvious if one simply considers the difference in visual scanning between reading a newspaper or novel and reading a scientific article. The tempering force can best be described as a *plan* or *schema* of visual activity (Neisser, 1976); the plan reflects a cognitive strategy which is modifiable as a function of available stimulus information and task demands. Examples of modifiable scanning strategies abound and include adults who view a given painting differently in response to different probe questions (Yarbus, 1967), infants who scan a geometric figure in different ways with variation in its display size (Hainline, this volume), and adults who inspect various figures in an ambiguous picture in different ways (Stark, this volume).

The interaction of foveal and peripheral processing in conjunction with cognitive strategies has been frequently demonstrated in the literature on visual search. For example, Williams (1966) has shown that color cues can be used by adults to speed and by inference, direct visual search for a target. Such findings support the claim that scanning is not a random process and that the less detailed processing of peripherally-located information can be a major determinant of eye fixation patterns during visual search. The implication of this statement is that if searchers are given some prior knowledge regarding the relevance of particular stimulus information in a search task, they can selectively allocate attention and/or accompanying eye fixations to specific information which is most critical for task resolution.

The picture painted thus far of the searcher as a selective processor and integrator of multiple stimulus features is consonant with the characterization given by many visual perception theorists, whether their primary concern is information processing (Neisser, 1967), selective attention (Kahneman, 1973), visual scanning (Hochberg, 1970b), or perceptual development (Gibson, 1969). All these theoretical positions place a heavy burden on the perceiver both to appreciate figure-ground separations, invariant relations, or distinctive features in a stimulus array and to integrate these elements in the visual environment with strategies, expectations, or intentions. Such selective, integrative activity presumably underlies changes in the locus of gaze and results in efficient visual exploration with respect to stimulus properties and the task-at-hand. Such efficient visual exploration characterizes the mature perceiver; however, the same description does not accurately characterize the young perceiver.

DEVELOPMENTAL DIFFERENCES
IN VISUAL SCANNING

Differences between children and adults in the speed, efficiency, systematicity, and exhaustiveness of visual scanning have been previously summarized by Day (1975). Children do not fixate the most informative areas of a picture as frequently as adults (Mackworth & Bruner, 1970), and young children do not use the same criteria for judging similarity among visual stimuli as older children (Vurpillot, 1968). Based upon these generalizations, one might be tempted to conclude that children simply lack schemata for visual exploratory behavior or have a limited repertoire of visual scanning strategies.

This suggestion of restricted scanning strategies is somewhat naive given the last decade of research on infants' visual exploratory behavior (e.g., Haith, 1978). Moreover, an analytical review of the developmental literature indicates that young children do have a variety of scanning strategies, but they may apply these strategies inappropriately to the stimulus materials and/or the task-at-hand (Cohen, 1974). For example, Russian investigators (Zinchenko, Chzhi-Tsin, & Tarakanov, 1963) reported that in a visual inspection task young children focused only upon a limited area of an unfamiliar figure while older children carefully scanned the contours of the figure. However, in a subsequent recognition task, older children limited their visual scanning to a few features relevant to stimulus recognition while the younger children scanned the entire contour of the figure. This work demonstrated that children have various scanning strategies available to them, but they do not always use the most appropriate or efficient strategy for a particular task.

The research described demonstrates that exhaustive scanning is not always the strategy of choice for older subjects. Efficiency in visual scanning is a function of task demands, and for stimulus recognition or discrimination, *exhaustive* scanning may not be the most *efficient* scanning strategy. Venger (1971) has related these concepts of exhaustiveness and efficiency in his developmental model of visual scanning behavior. The developmental sequence proceeds from partial to exhaustive to efficient scanning. The major difference between the two types of incomplete scanning (partial and efficient) results from one's ability to limit scanning of a display to only the most task-relevant information. The empirical support for his model comes from research in which children were asked to match the length of a line with one embedded in a group of seriated lines. Prior knowledge of the concept of seriation enabled older children to ignore irrelevant aspects of the stimulus array and to make size comparisons only within a circumscribed area of the display. By contrast, younger children scanned a limited area of the display, but there was no systematic, logical basis for their limited scanning. Thus, the ability to determine relevance or informativeness of specific portions of a visual display for a given task may contribute to developmental differences in selective scanning.

Another hypothesized source of age differences in visual scanning is a size difference in the effective field of view (e.g., Fisher & Lefton, 1976; Mackworth & Bruner, 1970). Several recent tachistoscopic studies have reexamined this hypothesis (Cohen & Haith, 1977a; Holmes, Cohen, Haith, & Morrison, 1977). In such studies there was a consistent lack of differences from 5 years to adulthood in peripheral processing abilities over a 12°-square stimulus field. The experimental tasks ranged from judging similarity of peripherally-located figures to identifying such figures, with or without the presence of a foveally-located figure. This research does not, however, rule out the possibility that differential ability to process and integrate foveal and peripheral information simultaneously and to use such information to guide eye movements could account for reported age differences in visual scanning.

METHOD

The obvious next issue for empirical study, then, is to determine the way in which systematically varied information in the visual periphery is selected and used by children and adults to direct their overt search for a visual target. The research undertaken to address this issue (Cohen, 1978) was unique in 3 ways: (1) the use of a paradigm that required children and adults to select and use peripherally-located visual information for efficient task solution, (2) the employment of a novel, on-line technology for monitoring eye fixations, and (3) the systematic variation in the peripheral information available to the subject.

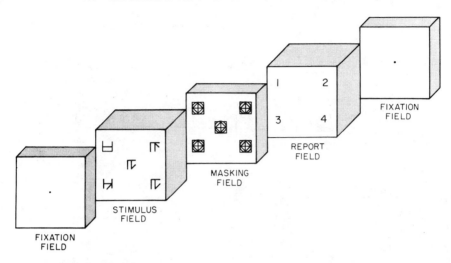

FIG. 1.   Diagram of experimental procedure.

Children, 5 and 8 years of age, and college adults participated in a visual search experiment (mean ages: 5.6, 8.7, and 19.7 years). The subjects' task was to identify as quickly as possible the location of a match between a centrally-located standard and one of four peripherally-located stimulus alternatives. Each trial was initiated by reminding subjects to look at a fixation dot located in the center of the display field, coincident with the upcoming location of the stimulus standard. Shortly thereafter, the stimulus array consisting of a centrally-located standard, a peripherally-located target, and 3 other peripherally-located alternatives was presented to the subject. When confident that target location had been found, the subject pressed a buzzer, which resulted in offset of the original array and the presentation of visual masks for 300 msec. Then, the numbers 1, 2, 3, and 4 replaced the masks in the periphery, and the subject simply reported the number that corresponded to target location (see Fig. 1).

The stimuli were unfamiliar, abstract figures that represented 2 levels of stimulus complexity, based upon the number of line segments, which were called features (see Fig. 2). The features were derived by dividing a square, a circle, and a diamond into 4 equivalent line segments each and by dividing a cross into 2 equivalent line segments. This process resulted in a set of 14 possible features. The visual mask was a composite of all possible features.

The peripheral alternatives differed systematically from the standard in terms of number of common features. While this similarity factor was operationally defined, the derived similarity relations among alternatives within a standard set were confirmed through ratings obtained from more than 100 subjects of various ages as well as from the subjects who participated in the experiment, following the completion of the search task. The alternatives were positioned equidistantly

FEATURAL TRANSFORMATIONS

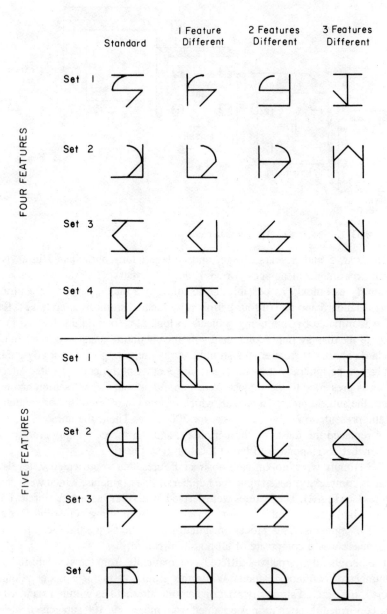

FIG. 2. Illustration of 4-feature and 5-feature standards and their respective set of alternatives.

276

from the standard (±36.87° radially from horizontal, the aspect ratio), with one figure in each quadrant. In blocked trials these peripheral alternatives were placed at 3°, 6°, or 9° from center of the display field.

Numerous dependent measures were computed based upon the location, frequency, and timing of observable eye fixations on various stimulus alternatives. Eye activity was monitored by an on-line, eye-tracking system, similar in external appearance to a tachistoscope (see Fig. 3). The subject looked through mirrors rotated 45° to his line of sight at a computer-generated display while a television camera and light source positioned perpendicular to his line of sight permitted simultaneous recording of his eye activity during search. Eye position was calculated every video field (16.6 msec). The on-line algorithm for selectively storing the eye position data was based upon comparison of successive eye position samples. When eye position on 2 successive samples differed by less than 0.5° of visual angle on both x- and y-axes, the eye was assumed to be fixated. When 2 successive samples differed by more than 1° of visual angle on either x- or y-axis, the eye was assumed to be moving to a new fixation region. Hence, the eye activity record consisted of the initial fixation on the standard, followed by the location and timing of subsequent eye movements and fixations.

EYE-TRACKING APPARATUS

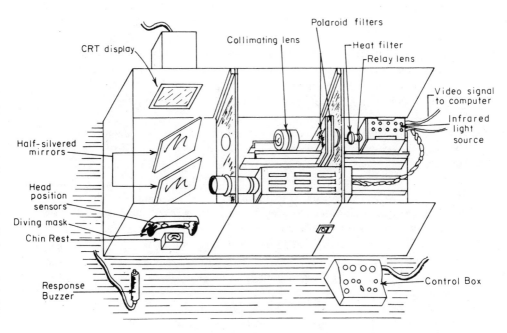

FIG. 3.   Illustration of eye-tracking apparatus.

RESULTS

Reported target location was, as expected, at ceiling for all subjects. All trials for which reported target location was in error or in which no eye movement off-standard was recorded were discarded from the analyses (2.1% and 1.0% of all trials, respectively).

The search data were examined in many different ways. At the most gross level of analysis, the results indicated that children made more fixations (mean total fixations: 3.2 vs. 1.7) and were generally slower (mean time: 4.2 vs. 2.7 sec.) to reach task solution, compared to adults. These findings refer to the overall distribution of eye fixations during search.

In order to analyze selectivity of fixations independent of the actual frequency of fixations, the percentage of each subject's fixations on various alternatives was computed. The results indicated that each age group looked most at the target, followed by the standard (see Fig. 4). These 2 stimulus items, the most relevant for task solution, attracted more than 60% of the total fixations. Thus, selective scanning by all age groups was demonstrated. In addition, comparable distributions of eye fixations on various alternatives were found for each age group at each distance.

Based upon the number of different stimulus alternatives looked at per trial, adults examined about 2.5 of the 5 possible stimuli per trial while children looked at about 3.4 items per trial. Hence, for each age group, scanning was not exhaustive. This task, then, is one which does not require exhaustive scanning for successful task completion. Based upon the age differences for this dependent measure and for the total number of fixations per trial, only the adult search patterns can be characterized as efficient. Thus far, then, the results indicate similarity between children and adults in their general *selectivity* of fixated items during visual search though adults differ from children in the *efficiency* of search.

The age differences in visual scanning reflect a difference in degree, not kind, because all age groups were somewhat selective and nonexhaustive. If the children had made fewer fixations and taken less time, they too could have been considered efficient searchers. In order to explore how the children's additional fixations were distributed, the search process was divided into 2 global phases. The time from stimulus onset to when the target was first fixated was called the Perceptual phase of search. The time from first fixating the target until deciding to report target location was called the Decision phase of search. The rationale behind this division was to explore whether children's additional fixations were made in order to locate the target initially or to decide that the target had indeed been found.

Analyses by phase indicated that all age groups had proportionally more fixations and time in the perceptual phase, rather than in the Decision phase of

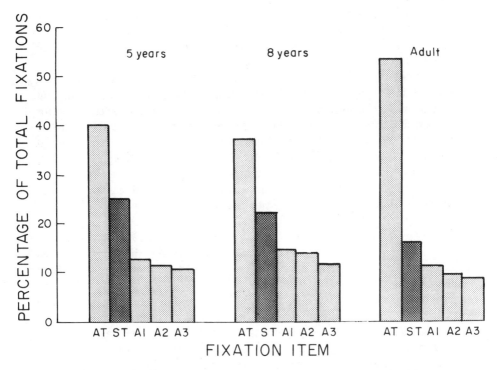

FIG. 4. Percentage of total fixations as a function of age and stimulus item. (ST = Standard, AT = 0 features different (target), A1=1 feature different, A2 = 2 features different, A3 = 3 features different).

search. For adults, 85% of their fixations occurred in the initial phase while children made 75% of their fixations in the Perceptual phase. These results may be viewed as confidence measures, especially for adults, in that once the target was first fixated, few confirmatory eye fixations were necessary to decide on reported target location. The allocation of time per phase paralleled these results (1.6 and 1.1 sec for the Perceptual and Decision phases, respectively). The difference in search time and percent of fixations between the two phases of search was most pronounced at the closest distance (3°). This finding most probably reflected simultaneous comparisons of foveal and peripheral information since stimuli were close together, and thus obviated the need for many confirmatory fixations or additional time during the Decision phase.

There were also important effects related to the complexity manipulation: Complex figures required more fixations and time to locate the target initially than did simpler figures. Recall that the complexity manipulation reflected the number of line segments or features in a stimulus set. The fact that more complex stimuli required more fixations to locate the target initially may be related to tunnel vision or foveal load. Prior research (Cohen & Haith, 1977a) has shown that as task complexity increases, the size of the effective visual field is reduced. Hence, if an increase in the number of features in a stimulus set represents an increment in task difficulty, then a task-induced shrinkage of the effective visual field should result. This tunnel vision effect (Mackworth, 1965) should lead to a lessened ability to process peripherally-located information and a consequent need to make eye movements in order to foveate peripheral alternatives for comparision with the standard. Of particular importance is the fact that this complexity effect for the Perceptual phase of search was reliable across the full age range tested. It should also be noted that the stimulus complexity effect occurred *only* in the Perceptual phase of search. Hence, once the standard has been examined and target location has been initially found, processing activities affected by the actual number of features in a stimulus array may become less critical in directing subsequent fixations. Other mental processes that are less affected by the stimulus complexity manipulation like memory for the location of the standard and target or cognitive criteria for judging similarity may then become more important in determining eye fixation patterns during the Decision phase of search.

Within each phase of search, there was some variation in the figures selected for fixation. In the Decision phase, all age groups refixated the standard more than any other figure, but especially 5-year-olds. These refixations of the standard and the target during the Decision phase became more numerous as distance of the peripheral alternatives extended beyond 3°.

In the Perceptual phase, children looked at more peripheral alternatives than adults did. In addition, the 5-year-old children reexamined the standard more frequently than other age groups. Since subjects in this phase were searching for the target, it is interesting to note what subjects did when their first off-standard fixation was not on the target. The location of the second eye fixation, when the first one was ''in error,'' provides evidence for developmental differences in search strategy. The 5-year-old children more frequently than older subjects or chance returned immediately to the standard whereas older subjects looked at another peripheral alternative. For these older subjects, there was a strong tendency relative to chance that the second eye fixation would be on the target ($p < .08$). This result suggests a bias for older subjects to continue their search by immediately fixating another peripheral alternative and selectively and accurately using peripheral information to direct the second fixation to the target.

Despite overall selectivity (percentage distribution of fixations) in visual search being comparable for children and adults, the age difference in the number of fixations required to find the target initially remains unexplained. To address this issue, a sensitive index of the integration and use of foveal and peripheral information was needed. Such a measure was computed by examining the choice of peripheral alternative first fixated on a trial. If one assumes that peripheral information is being used to guide fixations during search, then a subject's first

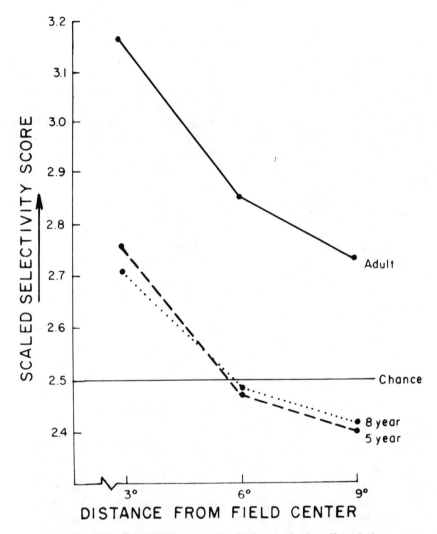

FIG. 5.   Mean scaled selectivity score for the first eye fixation off-standard as a function of age and stimulus distance.

off-standard fixation should be a highly probable choice—that is, on an alternative that is identical or very similar to the standard. Given this assumption, selectivity scores for initial eye movements for each subject were derived based upon the similarity of the peripheral alternative first fixated to the standard. Thus, if the first off-standard fixation was on the target, a score of 4 was assigned. If the subject had a position bias to look at a particular quadrant first, his average assigned score would be 2.5; this score was equivalent to chance, because the similarity of the alternatives to the standard was systematically varied with quadrant position. This measure, then, yielded a graded index of how featural information in the periphery was used to guide the initial off-standard eye fixation.

Analyses indicated that large differences in the mean scaled selectivity scores occurred as a function of both age and distance. Post hoc analyses of the age effects at each distance (see Fig. 5) indicated that children were indeed able to use peripheral information to guide their initial eye movement, but only when the information was close to the fovea (3°). Beyond this distance, their performance fell to chance. Adults, on the other hand, were far superior to children at 3° and did not decline to the children's 3° performance until stimulus alternatives were 3 times as eccentric.

The preceding finding was replicated when the dependent measure was the frequency with which various peripheral alternatives were fixated with the initial off-standard eye fixation (see Fig. 6). These data indicated that most of the age difference in initial selectivity of a peripheral alternative was attributable to adults' high frequency of fixating the target with the initial eye movement off-standard. Linear trend tests on this measure across peripheral distances provided supporting evidence for the better initial selectivity by adults compared to children. It is important to note, however, that the children's performance at 3° did reflect stable, linear trends different from zero ($-.5$), even though adult trend scores were far greater than that of the children at this distance (-1.3). In all of the analyses related to the initial eye movement, there was also a large effect of the distance factor, with usage of peripheral information declining most dramatically between 3° and farther distances.

The time between the onset of the stimulus array and the initiation of the first off-standard eye movement was longer at 3° than farther away (0.93 vs. 0.77 sec). This longer latency probably reflected the time required for simultaneous comparison of foveal and peripheral information. Presumably, it was possible to make more simultaneous comparisons when the standard and the alternatives were closer together than when they were more distant and sequential and/or memory comparisons were frequently required. Generally, within each distance, the latency to initiate the first eye movement was longer when the resultant first fixation was on a good choice or an alternative similar to the standard, compared to initial fixations on less similar alternatives. Longer latencies to initiate a saccade probably reflect more detailed processing of foveal and peripheral information while short latencies probably reflect more global information processing.

The examination of initial eye movement latencies as a function of age indicated that the 8-year-old children were comparable to adults on this measure at 3° while the 5-year-old children were slower (see Fig. 7). Since selectivity of the initial off-standard fixation was comparable for both groups of children and since several subsequent analyses of latency as a function of selectivity produced no reliable

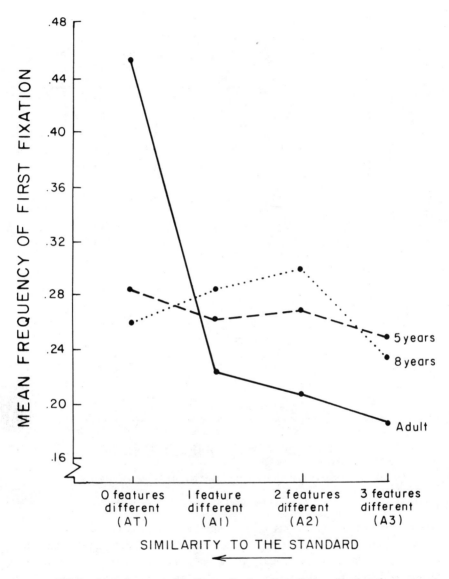

FIG. 6.   Mean frequency of the first eye fixation off-standard as a function of age and stimulus item. These data are collapsed over the 3 peripheral distances tested.

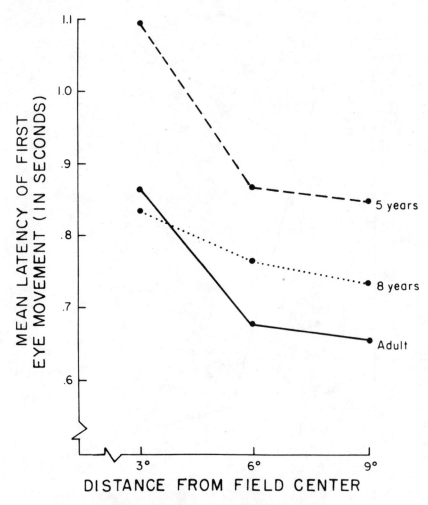

FIG. 7.   Mean latency of the first eye movement off-standard as a function of age and stimulus distance.

effects, these two components of the initial search process—selectivity and latency—were not related in a simple trade-off manner. It does appear that both components related to the initial off-standard fixation undergo considerable change with development.

In summary, the factors of age and peripheral distance produced the most dramatic effects in terms of the integration of foveal and peripheral information. The sharp differences in performance between 3° and greater distances parallel findings from recent reading research in which different types of peripheral input were useful to the reader at different distances from fixation (e.g., McConkie &

Rayner, 1975; Rayner, 1975). The age effects indicated selective, nonexhaustive scanning by all subjects, though only adults were efficient in their task performance. Adults were far superior to children in their ability to use detailed peripheral information to guide their initial eye movement off-standard at all eccentricities. However, children used detailed peripheral information to guide their initial eye movement off-standard when alternatives were restricted to the parafoveal region (3°).

MODEL OF VISUAL SEARCH PROCESSES

To better understand the nature of the age differences in this research, a model of visual search is needed that reflects the sequential activities the searcher engages in when looking for the target. The model is couched in terms of a perceptual activity cycle with component processes resembling those proposed by Neisser (1976) and Parker (1978). The processes in this model form a reiterative loop, and one process may directly influence another.

The first process is that of *Parsing* in which the subject must specify where visual information relevant to task solution is located in the display field. Since the display field is relatively uncrowded, the subject can easily make crude distinctions between figure and ground and thus can parse or isolate one figure from another.

The second process is that of *Comparing* in which the subject goes beyond mere isolation of stimuli and determines which stimuli are the most relevant for task solution. The ideal way to make this judgment is to compare simultaneously a foveated item with the information available in the visual periphery. This comparison process should result in hypotheses regarding which peripheral alternatives are most relevant to task solution, based upon the similarity of features in the standard and the alternatives.

The third process consists of *Testing* in which the subject goes beyond hypothesizing about the relevance of the stimulus and devises and implements a plan of action to verify prior hypotheses. In the visual search task, the testing process involves the direction of attention to the selected item, which may or may not be accompanied by an observable eye movement to the selected item. If an eye movement is made to the most relevant items in the display, then presumably the information derived from the first 2 processes is being used to guide the redirection of gaze. The plan and execution of fixations, then, is an observable verification or testing of the hypotheses generated by the comparison process.

The fourth and final process is that of *Confirming* in which the subject must decide whether he has sufficient information to confirm or disconfirm his hypothesis regarding the match of a peripheral alternative with the standard. This judgment will, to some extent, reflect criteria for certainty as well. When an alternative has been adequately processed and rejected as the match to the standard, the subject returns to the first process in which parsing of the array is undertaken and the entire cycle is repeated in searching for the target. On the other hand, if the subject is confident that target location has been found, search is terminated.

Hence, the model of fixations during visual search is composed of 4 processes: parsing, comparing, testing, and confirming. In some cases, the visual search process may be short-circuited; for example, testing may be unnecessary if the comparison process is sufficient for a confirmatory decision to be made. The integration of foveal and peripheral information clearly affects these processes.

With this model in mind, let us return to the data that reflected an age difference in the initial selection of a peripheral alternative. Prior research has shown that children can identify and judge similarity of geometric figures out to 6° as well as adults (Cohen & Haith, 1977a); hence, inadequate peripheral processing abilities per se are not considered to be the source of the children's poor initial selectivity. Prior research has also shown that children can generate hypotheses about bits of peripheral information as well as adults (Cohen & Haith, 1977b); hence, differences in inferential ability about the relevance of peripheral information are not considered to be the source of these age differences in initial selectivity. Also, children were able to appreciate the distinctive features of the unfamiliar stimuli as evidenced by the congruence of their similarity ratings with those of adults. The source is most likely, then, to be the generation of a plan of action whereby peripheral stimulation is used in conjunction with foveal stimulation to guide visual search.

Unfortunately, the data from the current study do not clearly isolate whether the age difference in initial eye movements is attributed to differences in simultaneous comparison of unfamiliar, peripheral and foveal stimulation or to differences in the generation and execution of a plan to assess the results of the comparison process. Here, both processes were indexed by what was first fixated. Subsequent research will be designed to tease apart these components by tachistoscopically presenting the arrays used here and asking subjects to identify the position of the target. Responses can then be scaled in terms of the similarity of the alternative selected to the standard. Should the performance of the children in this task surpass that of their scaled selectivity in the visual search task, then the argument will be strengthened that the source of age differences lies in the third process, that of generating and executing a plan of visual search based upon available peripheral input. If so, the reported age differences in the systematicity, efficiency, and speed of visual scanning (cf. Day, 1975) may be a result of children's less developed skill, compared to adults, in integrating and using foveal and peripheral information simultaneously to direct their sequences of eye movements.

A related conclusion was reached by Mackworth and Bruner (1970) based upon children having a larger number of short eye movements, compared to adults, when viewing a blurred photograph. These researchers suggested that children have more restricted peripheral vision and are unable to "examine details centrally and simultaneously monitor their peripheral fields for stimuli which might be candidates for closer inspection (p. 172)." Hence, they considered the source of developmental differences in visual scanning to be an inability to coordinate simultaneously the operations of foveal examination and peripheral monitoring. The research in this chapter provides more direct evidence related to this skill and further demonstrates that children can simultaneously coordinate such activities, albeit less well compared to adults and only when stimuli are located near the fovea. Moreover, coordination of information processing from different parts of the visual field is a necessary but not always sufficient skill to produce efficient visual search. It is also necessary to *use* the simultaneous processing of foveal and peripheral information to *plan* or *direct* subsequent information gathering activity. This plan or strategic activity in visual scanning, according to Brown and DeLoache (1978), represents the cognitive control over a naturally occurring response. "As the child matures, he develops the ability to control and coordinate scanning, to make scanning a strategic action tailored to changing task demands (p. 22)."

In conclusion, then, the research in this chapter provides a direct examination of how the availability and usage of particular peripheral information affects children's and adults' plans or anticipatory schemata for sampling the visual environment. Thus, this research enhances our understanding of the *relation* between available stimulus information and sequences of eye fixations—the link between perception and action. A promising avenue for future research is how plans or anticipatory schemata for visual exploration develop with age and how advanced training in other visuomotor domains affects this skill.

AFTERTHOUGHT

A question posed by Braddick (personal communication, 1980) was: Are there any data to refute the hypothesis that children were conducting a serial comparison of features, thereby necessitating more fixations and time during their search for the target? Though this study was not designed to test specifically feature-by-feature comparisons, there are some data available relevant to this issue. If one assumes that such a serial process is being conducted by subjects, then one would expect stimuli having more features to require more fixations and consequently, more time in order for subjects to determine which item is the perfect match with the standard. Recall that the complexity manipulation represented a difference in the number of features a standard and its associated alternatives contained. If serial feature-by-feature comparisons are being made, I would expect the more complex stimuli to require more fixations than simpler stimuli when searching for the target since there are more features in the stimulus set that must be compared. This is precisely the result obtained for the Perceptual phase of search. However, the effect occurred across the full age range tested; hence, the lack of significant interaction between the factors of age and stimulus complexity implies that there is no evidence in this research to support the developmental thrust of Braddick's suggestion.

ACKNOWLEDGMENTS

This research was based in part on a doctoral dissertation submitted to the Laboratory of Human Development, Harvard University, and was conducted in the Psychology Department, University of Denver. The research and author were supported in part by NIMH predoctoral fellowship MH 58205. The development and support of the eye monitoring laboratory was made possible by a Grant Foundation grant and NICHHD Research Grant HDO7232 to M. Haith. The author appreciates the cooperation of the children and college students who participated in this research as well as the helpful advice of Marshall Haith during the conduct of the research.

V.2 The "Convenient Viewing Position" Hypothesis

Kevin O'Regan
Laboratoire de Psychologie
Paris, FRANCE

My recent work on eye movement control in reading has been centered on the question: How quickly can information be extracted from the visual field and be put to use in controlling saccades and fixation durations. The conclusions that can be drawn at present are as follows.

1. Within three to four letters of the momentary fixation point, information about word type and identity is available sufficiently rapidly for it to modify the duration of the currently occurring fixation and the size of the next saccade. Thus for example, if the eye is fixating just left of the word THE, it will tend to make a shorter duration fixation and a larger saccade than if, everything else being the same, it is fixating just left of a three letter verb (c.f. O'Regan, 1979).

2. Beyond three to four letters from the momentary fixation point, the information extracted from the visual field is of poorer quality. Word length information is available sufficiently rapidly to influence the immediately following ocular behavior, the eye making larger saccades approaching and leaving long words than approaching or leaving short words. On the other hand, information about individual letters is nevertheless extracted and put to use, but it becomes available too slowly to influence the immediately following ocular behavior. It does, however, considerably speed up subsequent ocular behavior over a period of about one second, by variously increasing saccade sizes or diminishing fixation durations and regression probabilities (c.f. O'Regan, 1980).

DURATIONS ON LONG AND SHORT WORDS

While performing the experiments and analyzing the data leading to these conclusions, I was struck by a mysterious effect that, annoyingly, frequently proves stronger than the effects I am trying to demonstrate. The mean fixation duration

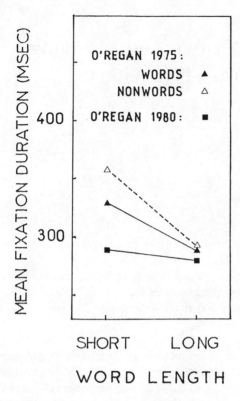

FIG. 1.   Mean fixation duration of fixations made on SHORT or LONG stimuli. O'Regan (1980): Fixation duration of the first fixation made, during reading, in the "critical region" of a sentence. This critical region was of 9–14 letters length, and was filled either with a 2-letter word followed by a medium length word (SHORT condition), or with a single 9–14 letter word (LONG condition). O'Regan (1975): Fixation duration of the first fixation made after the eye moved to an isolated stimulus presented 3 letter spaces right of the initial fixation point. Stimuli were of 8 letters (SHORT) or 10 letters (LONG) length. They were either words or nonwords. Nonwords were constructed by combining the first half of one of the words with the second half of a different word in the word set.

on short words tends to be 10–15 msec longer than those on long words. Though small, this difference has always been statistically significant. For example, in a recent experiment (O'Regan, 1980), a comparison was made of the way the eye fixated what was called a "critical region" of a given sentence as a function of whether this critical region consisted of a 9–14 letter word or of a 3-letter and a medium length word, everything else in the sentence being held constant. The square data points in Fig. 1 show that the first fixation made in the critical region is about 10 msec longer when it contains the 3-letter/medium combination than when it contains one long word. The differences are significant at $p < 0.05$. The other data points in Fig. 1 come from a completely different experiment (O'Regan, 1975). Here, the same effect is shown on the first fixation made on isolated short words being presented in a word-nonword decision task. The effect probably has nothing to do with word frequency differences, since it is found for both word (solid lines) and nonword (dotted lines) stimuli and the differences are significant at $p < 0.05$ or better.

A closer examination of the eye's behavior in these experiments reveals another interesting fact: The first fixation duration on a word increases directly with the distance into the word that the eye lands. For example, Fig. 2 shows this for the word-nonword decision experiment. As before, the effect exists for non-words as well as for words. The same dependence of fixation duration on position fixated was observed in the critical region experiment, where a more detailed analysis of eye movement behavior seems warranted.

Figure 3A shows the distribution of positions where the eye first landed in the critical region. Compared to the distribution for short words, the long word distribution is shifted to the right (and may even be bimodal). The most frequent landing positions are around the first letter of the short word when the critical region contained a short word followed by a medium length word, and around the second or third letter if it contained a long word. An analysis of variance showed that this 1-letter length effect was significant at $p < 0.05$. The existence of a length effect is expected from the earlier work showing longer saccades approaching and leaving long words as compared with short words (O'Regan, 1979). It is interesting to note that despite the significant length effect, the behaviors of the eye approaching long versus short words are not very different. The distribution for long words may in fact be bimodal, with one part being the same as for short words, and one part different. This suggests the existence of two distinct eye movement strategies for scanning long words.

Figure 3B shows the mean durations that the eye maintains during the first fixation in the critical region as a function of the position where it lands (fixations followed by regressions are excluded, since these probably play a special role). For long words, there is a trend for fixations to be longer when the landing

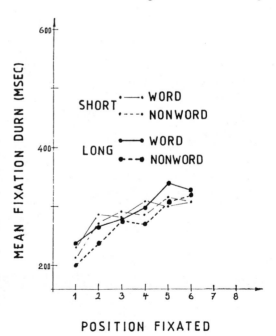

FIG. 2. Mean fixation durations of the first fixation made on the stimuli of the O'Regan (1975) experiment as a function of the position in the stimulus where this fixation occurred. Note that unequal numbers of records contribute to each data point. This explains how it is possible that, as shown in Fig. 1, mean durations are significantly longer for short words than for long words.

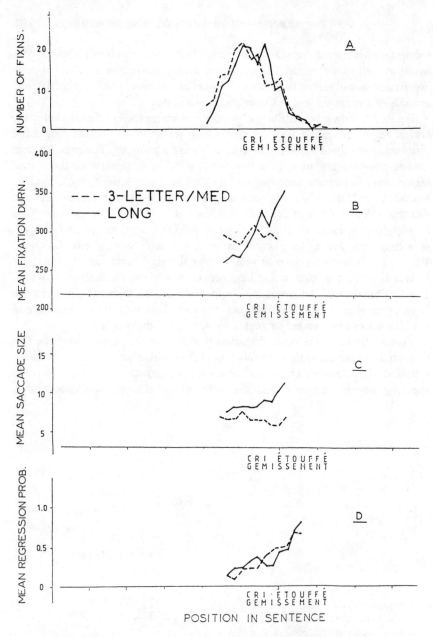

FIG. 3. Eye movement characteristics for the O'Regan (1980) experiment as a function of position where the eye first landed on first passing an imaginary boundary located 6 character spaces left of the critical region. Dotted curves are for the case where the critical region contained a 3-letter/medium length word combination, solid lines are for the case where it contained single long word. The abscissa shows the position in the sentence where fixations occurred or from which saccades started, relative to the critical region, indicated by a typical pair of alternative critical region contents (the experiment was performed in French).

position is further to the right. This is the same pattern found more clearly in the word-nonword decision task experiment (Fig. 2). Two mechanisms come to mind to explain the effect.

It could be that the farther into a word that the eye lands, the farther it has come, so the less information it had about the region it lands in; it would therefore tend to fixate longer. However this explanation would predict that the same effect should be found for short as for long words, but it is clear from Fig. 3B that the effect is strong only for long words. The explanation also predicts that a correlation between progression size and the following fixation duration should always be found in reading. Rayner and McConkie (1976) and Adriessen and de Voogd (1973) looked for but did not find strong correlations.

CONVENIENT VIEWING POSITION
AND DISTRIBUTED PROCESSING

An alternative explanation is to suppose that a fixation point too near the beginning of a long word does not allow the whole word to be identified: Only the first few letters are seen clearly; the eye foreshortens its fixation, and rapidly moves to the end of the word to complete identification. In this case, processing of the word is distributed over two short fixations located near each end of the word. If, on the other hand, the eye lands at a "convenient viewing position" near the middle or left of middle of a long word, the whole word can be perceived, and processing occurs in one longer fixation.

The convenient viewing position idea predicts that fixations too near the beginning of a long word should be followed by short progressions leading to near the end of the word. Confirmation is found in Fig. 3C, which shows the mean size of progressions made from each position in the critical region. It is seen that for long words, mean progressions are around seven to eight letters (i.e., lead to near the end of the word) unless the eye fixates beyond the fifth letter of the word, when mean progressions jump to 10 or 11 letters (leading out of the word). For short words however, fixations at the fifth and sixth letters of the critical region are not convenient viewing positions since they are at the beginning of the second word. Small progressions to another position in the second word are therefore made. Note that progressions leaving the beginning of long words lead the eye to near the end of the word and not to near the middle of the word. It therefore seems that when processing is distributed over two fixations, these are located near each end of the word.

What happens if the eye first lands near the end of the critical region? The convenient viewing position idea predicts that a short fixation should be made, and then the eye should regress to near the beginning of the region and make another short fixation. Figure 3D shows the probability of regressing from the first fixation point as a function of where it occurred. It is clear that, as predicted, the regression probability increases with the position where the eye landed.

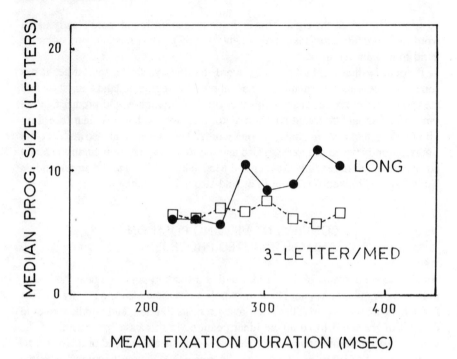

FIG. 4.   Median progression sizes made on leaving the first fixation in the critical region of the O'Regan (1980) experiment as a function of that fixation's mean duration.

Another prediction made by the convenient viewing position idea is that for long words, long fixation durations should be followed by large saccades leading out of the word. Figure 4 shows a graph of the median size of the progression that followed the first fixation in the critical region, plotted as a function of this fixation's duration. As predicted, for long words, progression size increases from about seven or eight letters to 10 or 11 letters when fixation duration goes beyond about 300 msec. Note that this result shows that locally a correlation between fixation duration and the following progression size can exist, even though, when averages over large bodies of text are taken, such correlations are not found (c.f. Andriessen & de Voogd, 1973; Rayner & McConkie, 1976).

Pending more direct experimental tests, the present data strongly suggest that processing takes place in one fixation if the eye lands at a convenient viewing position, but is distributed over two shorter fixations when the eye does not land at a convenient viewing position. It now becomes clear why fixations are generally longer for short words than for long words. Suppose, as was the case in this experiment (c.f. Fig. 3A), that fixations frequently fall near the first letters of a long word. Because this is probably not a convenient viewing position, fixations will usually be short (c.f. Fig. 3B). However, the first few letters of a short word constitute a good viewing position, and fixation durations tend to be long.

THE SENTENCE SHIFT EXPERIMENT

Further confirmation of the convenient viewing position idea occurs when a sentence is specially shifted during an eye movement. In this experiment, subjects read sentences of diverse structure. About one third of the sentences contained a long test word. Just as the eye was saccading to this test word, the computer did one of three things. It shifted the whole sentence either three letter spaces to the left (LEFT shift condition), three letter spaces to the right (RIGHT shift condition), or it did not shift the sentence at all (CENTER condition). Each subject saw a mixture of LEFT, RIGHT, and CENTER shifts. After the experiment, the subjects were asked if they had noticed anything odd about the way the sentences were displayed. They all answered ''No.''

An analysis of regression probability, fixation duration and saccade size for the two fixations preceding and the four fixations following the sentence shift showed that the eye is surprisingly unperturbed by the shifts. For LEFT shifts, 47% of the records showed no difference at all in ocular behavior as compared with the CENTER condition. The other 53% showed what appeared to be a corrective regression (mean size 4.4 letters, i.e., slightly larger than the 3–letter size expected of a movement to correct for the shift), but otherwise behaved in a way indistinguishable from those 20% of the CENTER shift records where a regression occurred after landing in the test word. For RIGHT shifts the only notable effects are shorter durations for the fixations following the shift, and a reduced progression size for the saccade following the shift (see Fig. 5).

The results are not compatible with a ''slow control'' model of eye movements in reading under which the eye globally compensates for changes in information intake rate by adjusting eye movement parameters over a fairly long time span. In particular, when a sentence shifts left, more information must be apprehended so fixation duration should increase or saccade size decrease. In fact saccade size does decrease, but fixation duration also decreases.

The results are, on the other hand, compatible with the convenient viewing position hypothesis. Table 1 gives the mean positions where the eye landed after the sentence shift. Assume, with Rayner (1979), that the convenient viewing position for a 10–letter word is near the fourth or fifth letter. In the CENTER condition the mean fixation made is quite near the convenient viewing position, and a fairly long (compared to global averages for reading) fixation is made (315 msec; c.f. Fig. 5B). In the RIGHT shift condition, the eye is too close to the beginning of the word, and a shorter fixation (compared to the CENTER condition) is made (275 msec), followed by a small progression (7 letters compared to 8.8 for the CENTER condition). In the LEFT shift condition, the eye is generally too close to the end of the word, and a regression is expected. As noted earlier, the regression probability after a LEFT shift is indeed significantly higher than in the CENTER condition (53% as compared to 20%). The duration (not indicated in Fig. 5) of the fixation preceding the regression is also shorter (275 msec) than for the records where no regression is made (300 msec, see Fig. 5). These latter

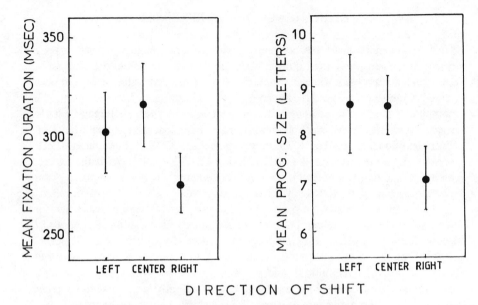

FIG. 5.   Mean fixation duration of the first fixation occurring after the sentence shift, and mean progression size of the progression following that fixation, as a function of the direction for the shift. All records where a regression occurs following the shift have been excluded from these graphs.

cases where no regression is made presumably correspond to the fraction of the fixations that, despite the leftward shift, fell near the convenient viewing position.

POSSIBLE MECHANISMS

Operationally, I have tried to show that when the eye first fixates near the middle of a long word, it makes a long fixation and jumps to the next word; but when it first fixates near an end of the word, it foreshortens its fixation and makes another fixation near the other end of the word before jumping to the next word. I have attributed this phenomenon to the existance of a convenient viewing position in words, which it is in some sense favorable to fixate.

Note that Rayner (1979) has suggested an idea similar to convenient viewing position. He found that medium length words tend to be fixated near their middles, and long words tend to be fixated just left of the middle. He called this the "preferred viewing position." The present convenient viewing position idea extends this notion by saying that when, for some reason, the favored viewing position is not fixated, processing will occur distributed over two shorter fixations. Now I would like to consider what might determine the convenient viewing position.

First, it is possible that the convenient viewing position behavior is *not* related directly to ongoing word identification, but is simply a consequence of a general oculomotor strategy driven by low level visual information like brightness, density of marks in the visual field, and position of blanks. Findlay (this volume) shows that in some circumstances saccade size and fixation duration depend on such purely physical aspects of the stimulus configuration.

However, the fact, shown by the THE-skipping experiment (O'Regan, 1979) described earlier, that saccade sizes and fixation durations can depend on the identity of words being fixated, suggests that the eye's behavior can, at least in certain cases, be driven by ongoing linguistic processing. What predictions can be made about fixation strategies if this is assumed to be generally true?

When the eye fixates in a word, information is available from two sources; the visual field, and the reader's knowledge of his language. These two sources of information interact to allow the fixated word to be identified. I suggest that it is the way this interaction proceeds in time that immediately determines the eye's behavior. Suppose, as is generally the case for long words, that from the position fixated, acuity and lateral masking effects act so that only some of the letters in the word are clearly visible. Then two options are open: Either the eye can move to the region where letter information is poor; or use can be made of the constraints in the lexicon to try to compensate for the lack of information in that region; the eye fixating longer while the process of narrowing down alternative in the lexicon occurs. Which option is chosen will depend on the interaction of lexical constraints and visibility conditions.

In general, around the fixation point, about five or six letters can be seen clearly. Those letters in near peripheral vision, which are flanked by spaces, can also be seen quite clearly. Constraints of the lexicon are variable, but in general it is true that the beginning of a word gives more clues to its identity than the end: Knowledge of the first five to seven letters can dramatically narrow down the number of alternatives in the lexicon. If knowledge of word length and end letter information as well as semantic context are added to this, the word will often be uniquely determined. Therefore a fixation near the fourth or fifth letter of the word can allow identification. On the other hand, a fixation too near the beginning or the end of the word would give too little letter information for the narrowing down of alternatives in the lexicon, and a second fixation in the word would be necessary.

While these considerations give general predictions about long-word scanning strategies, deviations from these predictions are expected in cases where lexical constraints of a word are abnormal. Consider for instance, what happens if the eye is fixating near the fourth or fifth letter of a word beginning with a frequently occurring prefix. Here, the word's beginning only weakly determines it's identity, and a second fixation will be required. On the other hand, a word whose beginning is very rare, like xylophone, would not require a second fixation. Experiments are underway to investigate such predictions. Preliminary favorable evidence comes from an experiment by Pavard (personal communication), who has subjects read texts containing words with spelling errors. The words could be either mono- or bimorphemic. For both word types, spelling errors were well detected during reading when they were located near the beginning of the words. But when spelling errors were near the ends of words, they were only detected well for bimorphemic words. This suggests that only for bimorphemic words are fixations made near word ends.

In summary, there appears to exist a convenient viewing position in long words such that when the eye fixates sufficiently near it, only one fairly long duration fixation need be made in the word. But when the eye does not fixate near it, two shorter duration fixations are made. The convenient viewing position is generally near the middle or left of the middle of a long word. Whereas this may be for reasons connected with some oculomotor strategy not related directly to ongoing cognitive processing, it is likely that the position of the convenient viewing position in a word depends on the extent to which information from the lexicon can be used to supplement poor quality visual clues gathered in non-central vision. This hypothesis needs more direct experimental testing.

V.3

Flexible and/or Rigid Control of Oculomotor Scanning Behavior

A. Levy-Schoen
Laboratoire de Psychologie Experimentale, Université René Descartes et EPHE 3ème Section associé au CNRS Paris, France

OUR EYES ARE NOT ONLY FOR RESPONDING TO RETINAL STIMULATION, OR ONLY FOR COLLECTING INFORMATION.

"Les yeux sont les fenêtres de l'âme," said the poet: "The eyes are the soul's windows." This could mean either that the captive soul can look out onto the world through the eyes, or that anyone can look into the soul's secrets through the eyes. Are not both of these statements more or less implicit assumptions made when one does scientific research on eye-movements?

Let me attempt to put my work into perspective so that our thinking about what individuals do with their eyes will not be limited purely to terms of information-collecting. Generally, an inventory of the functional roles of eye movements might at least include the three following categories.

1. *Exploration of the Environment.* This means *responding* to visual stimulation including what is new or changing, and initiating activity and moving toward things—*looking for* or searching in order to discover what is there. Eye movements may also create sensory renewal when there is no external change. It is known that vision quickly fades with stabilized retinal images. Those who participated in a laboratory experiment in which the gaze must be maintained on

299

a fixation point know that the surrounding objects, first visible in the periphery, rapidly fade away, and I assume that they experience, like me, an uncomfortable feeling and a strong tendency to want to move their eyes. It may be that, in daily life, a part of ocular activity corresponds neither to a response to visual stimulation nor to a search for visual information, but rather constitutes an ''activity of movement.'' Whereas normally one conceives of the active part of eye movements as being the process of moving from one fixation to the next, the present view suggests that an active part of the eye's business consists of suppressing the natural drive to move the eyes. Such a balance between active motion and active immobility is reminiscent of the agonist-antagonist mode of functioning of many biological systems.

2. *Participation in Body Movements and Postural Stabilization.* There are two basic ways eye movements contribute to the activity of an individual in his environment. The first is to guide gestures, like grasping an object, pointing to a target, directing locomotion (c.f. Paillard, 1974; Hay, 1979). Recent experimentation in cerebral pathology has brought strong support to the idea that part of this guiding function is accomplished not by ''normal'' viewing operations (i.e., visual information processing via visual cortex); but by a more basic non-cortical sensory-motor system (i.e., collicular neural paths mobilize the eyes, which in turn guide target-catching gestures). Secondly, eye movements participate in maintaining body balance and stabilizing the standing individual upon his precarious basis. Important roles are played by vestibulo-ocular interactions and oculomotor reflex activity as well as by visual perception of movement or ''ocular grasping'' of some spatial landmark (Lestienne, Berthoz, & Mascot, 1976).

3. *Action Upon People.* We cannot ignore the part played by gaze exchange in every-day life. It is probably the most fundamental role of eye movements at the beginning of life. Anyone who has watched a baby can notice that it not only responds to but also influences an adult's behavior towards itself by turning its eyes towards the adult. This remains true later in life: The role played by eye-contact in social relationships is well established. (Argyle, 1969).

No research can study reality on all fronts simultaneously, and mine concerns the first point afore mentioned. How do eye movements provide exploration of the visual environment? This activity is one of the principal interfaces between the individual and the environment that requires action and awareness. I consider visual exploratory behavior not as the passive response of the sensory-motor adaptive system, but as a self initiated prospective activity of an individual searching for new information relevant to short or long term intentions. Looking around consists not only of responding to the visual call of peripheral stimulation, but also in turning to the direction where significant information is expected, within a crowded visual field.

IN VISUAL EXPLORATION, GENERAL, EXPECTATION-CONTINGENT AND DISPLAY-CONTINGENT FACTORS CONTROL OCULOMOTOR BEHAVIOR.

It is my claim that, before beginning to scan a field, and as a function of the task and the expected properties of the material to be explored, a subject prepares a basic scanning "routine" around which oculomotor behavior will be organized.

For instance, while opening a book, a reader is setting up an "ocular reading routine," which involves scanning the successive lines of text from left to right, with certain basic organizational constraints related to text form, content, and to the aims of the particular reading task adopted. In another case, while searching for an object among many others, a "perceptual set" (i.e., some kind of mental image of the object) is established, together with an oculomotor routine. The latter includes rules like the following: "at each fixation, if there is some clue suggesting the presence of the searched-for object in periphery, jump to it, and verify its identify; if not, displace the fixation area to some other not yet visited place." Such routines imply certain functional constraints like: "choose the next fixation area at a distance that allows the new fixation to provide visual information *complementary* to previously acquired data, i.e., neither at too great a distance (which would mean fixating a non predictible target), nor to small (which would bring in material already processed in parifovea)." The routine does not determine absolute saccade length but rather criteria according to which saccade length will be programmed so that the eyes move in a way relevant to the task.

Once such a routine is determined as a function of the subject's intentions, many choices still remain open. These constitute the adjustments that adapt the general oculomotor routine to the particular situation. At each step, the ocular behavior arises from the conjunction of three factors: (1) the basic constraints of the oculomotor system, (2) the specific routine that has been set to work, and (3) the particular local (that entering in the instantaneous field of view, both foveal and peripheral, at this particular fixation) visual stimulation: physical characteristics and information content which has to be processed and coded in memory for further use.

What can be and what *actually are* these local adjustments are presently controversial topics. Which aspects of oculomotor behavior are rigidly fixed by the oculomotor system or by the prepared programs and which ones are flexible and adjustable while a scanning routine is at work? A second question is: What are the control agents that act upon these flexible characteristics to modify their values?

With these questions in mind, I will consider some experimental data that throw light on how the oculomotor system functions in various types of exploratory activity.

First I will discuss some experiments concerning the initial saccadic response to a patterned set of elements in a situation where there is a conflict between a prepared general program and the adjustment required by the instantaneous properties of the display. Secondly, the combined effects of a prepared program and of the current state of local information processing will be examined as manifested in the data of another experiment in which two objects have to be successively fixated. Finally, I will discuss the relative elasticity of the different components of eye movement behavior during reading.

EVIDENCE FOR THE EFFECT OF A GENERAL OCULOMOTOR ROUTINE ON THE FIRST OCULAR RESPONSE TO A DISPLAY.

At any moment of a scanning process, what is the flexibility in the choice of the next fixation or, stated differently, the next saccade to be executed?

Looking for trends in the spatial organization of oculomotor behavior, I ran a series of experiments (Levy-Schoen, 1974) in which physical as well as cognitive constraints were reduced to a minimum. I studied the order in which subjects spontaneously fixated two visual stimuli as a function of their relative positions in the visual field.

Each trial of an experimental session consisted of a pair of patches that appeared on a large blank field. The two patches (A and B), seen from the central fixation point (0), appeared as two equivalent luminous circles. Each one contained a randomly selected character, readable only in foveal vision. The task was to report the letters in the field, and required fixation of both elements (0–A–B or O–B–A). In a counter-balanced design, all paired combinations of several directions and several eccentricities were presented in unpredictible sequence.

The results gave clear evidence of non-random organization of oculomotor activity. First, a strong "centrifugal" order of fixation was found; for most of the trials, the element of the pair closest to the central departure point is fixated first. Combined with this trend, a stable "upwards first" tendency appears for all subjects. Regarding lateral tendencies however some subjects favor the left side and others the right. It is worth mentioning that both of these tendencies were found in 3- and 5-year-old children, which implies that they are not acquired through reading habits. This basic anisotropy of the organization of oculomotor activity may be related to sensory or motor properties of the ocular system, although neither visual sensitivity nor the ability to move the eyes seem to show

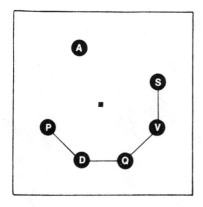 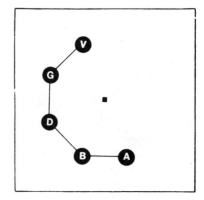

FIG. 1. An example of each of the displayed patterns of elements. Eight rotations of each of the two structures make sixteen different frames, with randomly selected letters appearing on the black patches. (The elements are not to scale: in reality, the eccentricity of each element from the central fixation point was 6°; a black patch was 1° diameter, and a white letter only 10′).

such dissymetries. The anisotropy also might be related to biological reinforcement of up versus down in daily life, as opposed to a left-right symmetric field of action. But what interests me is whether these asymmetries are compulsory or modifiable by the subject's intention or the immediate demands of the situation.

An experiment using a slightly more complex visual task provides some clues to this question. Each stimulus presented on a tachistoscope, consisted of a chain of black discs forming a half circle around the fixation point, each disc containing a white letter (as shown in Fig. 1). Different orientations of the half circles were used, and presented in unpredictible order. When reading the set of letters aloud, all subjects spontaneously began at one end of the chain. However, eye fixation records show that the gaze generally does not jump directly to the point read out first (see example shown in Fig. 2). Instead, the eye first jumps upward, and only then begins scanning in the natural reading order. Why is this so? Probably because, in this situation, the requirement to read the letters sequentially gives way to the general tendency to move upwards first. A pre-trial oculomotor program like the following is prepared: "Jump in the favored upwards direction if there is something there. If not, jump to the highest element of the chain." On appearance of the stimulus, the first saccade is triggered according to this rule, too fast for a more thorough analysis of the display to occur. It appears that the general eye movement tendency induced by the display configuration is not flexible enough to give way to a more adapted response.

It seems reasonable to suppose that in this very simple situation, the trends governing ocular behavior in an empty field are still acting, whereas if the visual display were meaningfully structured (filled with elements related in a significant

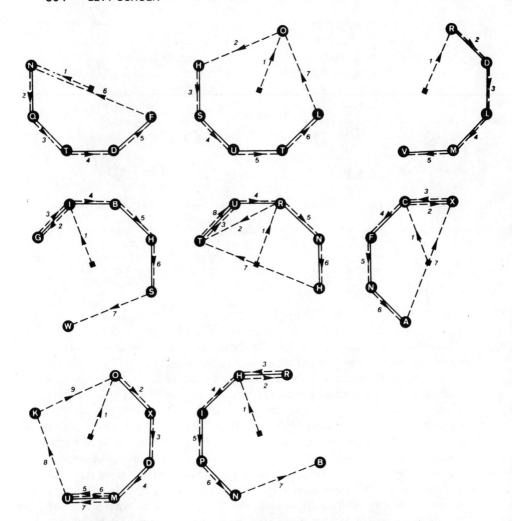

FIG. 2.   An example of the ocular scanning sequences of one of the subjects for 4
displays of each pattern. In four instances out of eight, the first saccade does not
aim to the first element of the subsequent reading sequence.

way for instance) these simple trends would be overridden. Thus here the repetition of trials in which the spatial configuration of elements is only slightly varied
gives rise to a powerful motor program and a high level of oculomotor preparation. Conceding to these two strong trends, the visual inspection needed to determine the optimal target is postponed until later, and the prepared movement is
executed first. General trends and expectation-contingent oculomotor routines
that are constant from trial to trial override trial-specific sensory data that take
longer to process. The incentive to move becomes stronger than the one to stay,

so that the saccade starts on the basis of spatial parameters only partially relevant to the given stimulus configuration. But by the time the first fixation is reached, the optimal choice is ready and can determine the second fixation.

Findlay's data (this volume) may be interpreted in an analogous way. When, because of a strong incentive to move, the ocular latency is brief, there is insufficient time to prepare a saccade to the single relevant target embedded in the double target configuration. This is the case in the "local examination" task, in which the most efficient behavior would be to aim with precision for the first target. Conversely, for the "global examination" task, less accurate fixation is required, leading to a weaker incentive to move, and consequently to longer oculomotor latency. This, paradoxically, gives time to compute the parameters of the saccade towards an isolated element of the target pair, thus explaining why contamination by the other target is less manifest in this second task than in the first one. Experimentation with variants of this situation is required before we can definitely support this hypothesis.

EVIDENCE FOR THE INFLUENCE OF LOCAL PROCESSING AND GLOBAL PROGRAMS UPON OCULOMOTOR SCANNING.

Thus far I have described how the choice of a first target in a simple scanning sequence depends on general eye movement trends. But now I would like to consider how the characteristics of one among a sequence of fixations may vary according to demands of local information processing. The question is to clarify whether or not fixation duration can be either prolonged or reduced when the processing of an object takes more or less time. This question is relevant to the current controversy about whether oculomotor behavior is controlled in a strict or lax fashion by cognitive processes during ocular scanning, and in particular during reading.

When the eyes foveally fixate an object that was seen in peripheral vision during the preceding fixation, the time necessary to complete its identification is reduced. This reduction of residual processing time is attributed to the fact that pre-processing of the object while it is located in peripheral vision contributes to its subsequent foveal processing. Experiments showing this effect, originally demonstrated by Dodge (1907), have been repeated under various conditions (generally verbal processing) by O'Regan (1975) and Rayner (1975). Using a nonverbal pattern identification situation, we have confirmed that this time-saving is indeed due to peripheral pre-processing of the object and cannot be attributed to a mere preparation effect. Evidence for this was provided by an experiment in which the object was presented under exactly the same conditions as normal, except that the distinctive feature necessary for its identification was absent until the moment when the eye was saccading towards it. In this condi-

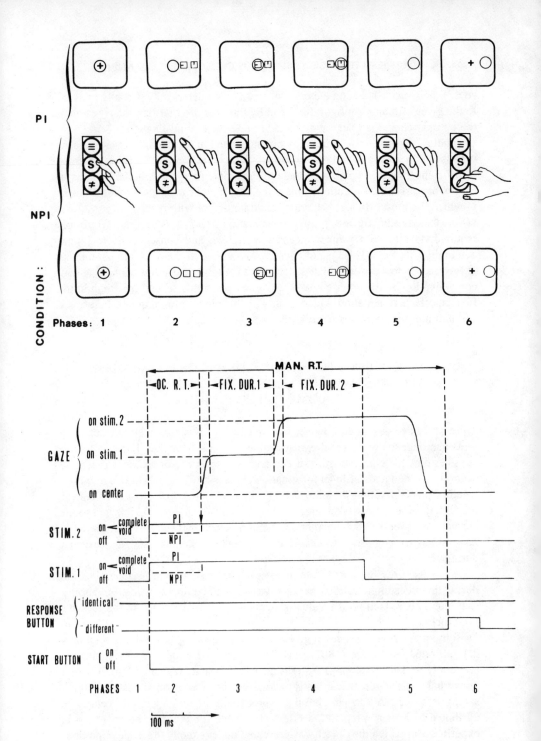

FIG. 3. The experimental situation for measuring the effect of peripheral pre-processing of an object on the duration of its fixation during scanning. (a) Hand and upper display phase sequence: PI condition. Hand and lower display sequence: NPI condition. The circle shows the eye-centering upon the display. (b) The corresponding trace of the recorded events along time abscissa.

tion, identification time, measured from the instant when the gaze landed on the object, was longer by 50 to 100 msec than the control. This extra time is a measure of the fixational processing time that is *saved* under conditions of normal peripheral vision (Levy-Schoen & Rigaut-Renard, 1979).

Now, in this type of situation, what happens to fixation duration on an object when scanning must immediately continue to another object? Will the saving in processing time also induce a reduction in duration of fixation on the first object? Or will this fixation duration be controlled primarily by the way basic oculomotor routines react to the physical organization of objects in the visual field?

An experiment was performed in which a comparison task required the successive fixation of two objects. As in the previous experiment, real time use of a laboratory computer allowed the visual stimuli to be changed as a function of the eye's behavior. In the "no-peripheral-identification" condition (NPI), both objects were displayed without their discriminative features until occurrence of the saccade which drove the eyes to the first object, whereas in the condition "with-peripheral-identification" (PI), both objects were complete from the beginning of the trial. The sequences are shown in Fig. 3.

The results show that as in the previous experiment, the total comparison time (manual response) is sensitive to whether peripheral pre-processing is possible during the oculomotor latency period preceding the first saccade: The total time spent fixating the stimuli before the manual response (around 800 msec duration) is about 60 msec shorter when peripheral pre-processing is possible than when it is not.

The more interesting part of the results concerns the fixation duration on the first stimulus fixated (i.e., the time measured from the end of the first saccade until the beginning of the second one). This duration also appears to be reduced when prior peripheral identification is possible, compared to its value when no prior peripheral identification is possible, as seen by the data in Fig. 4. Note that this reduction is slightly smaller than the time saved for the subsequent manual comparison response: an apparently paradoxical result, because after the moment the eyes get to the first object both conditions are exactly the same.

The objects in the experiment were displayed with different eccentricity and size characteristics so that their visibility when viewed from the initial fixation point would change. The plot shown in Fig. 5 of the saving in fixation times, is an increasing function of the first object's peripheral visibility: The more visible this object from the initial fixation point, the more the fixation duration is reduced in the peripheral-identification (PI) condition as compared with the no-peripheral-identification (NPI) condition. This relation supports our interpretation of the time saving effect in terms of peripheral pre-processing.

Another variable was considered in our experimental design to permit evaluation of the role of an overriding motor program. The experiment was always divided into blocks of 64 trials with identical stimulus size and eccentricity. Two sets of blocks were administered to the subjects: one set of "pure peripheral conditions," i.e., in which trials either all occurred in the NPI condition or all in the PI condition; and a second group of "mixed peripheral conditions," in which NPI and PI trials were randomly mixed. The results show that the effects are accentuated in pure conditions (c.f. again Fig. 5). This we interpret as the result of a general oculomotor routine active in a given block of trials. Under pure conditions a subject can optimize, from trial to trial, the processing time required at each step of the scan. During PI blocks he can minimize the duration of his first fixation, and maximize it during NPI blocks. In mixed conditions, since no prediction can be made, NPI and PI conditions contaminate each other, making differences less manifest. This is what appears in Fig. 5, in which the two curves for PI and NPI conditions are less separated for mixed blocks than for pure blocks.

What can be concluded from these data about our original question? During a scanning sequence, is the duration of a particular fixation sensitive to local information processing? First, evidence has clearly been provided that ocular pause duration can be modulated by the cognitive handling of the local visual input. The changes in duration are slight but stable: The eye stays longer when

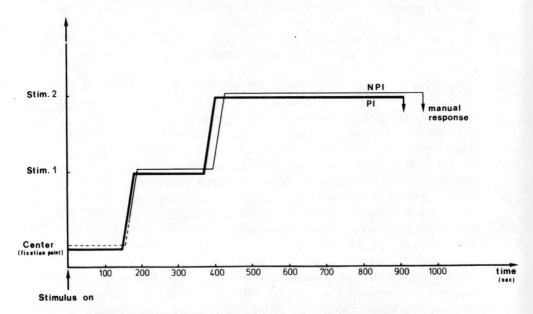

FIG. 4.   The averaged ocular behavior of 6 subjects, comparing the two conditions with or without peripheral pre-processing of the first object fixated. PI: with peripheral identification. NPI: no peripheral identification. Time in abscissa, and lateral eye displacement in ordinate (both sides pooled).

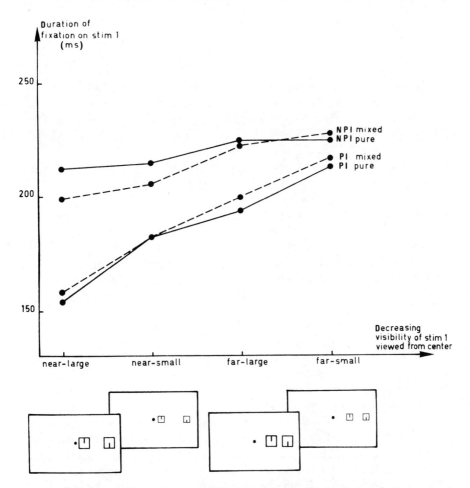

FIG. 5.   Detailed analysis of the difference between fixation duration on stimulus 1 in the two conditions with and without peripheral identification processing (resp. PI and NPI). Effects of visibility (size × distance of stimulus 1 to center) and of inter-trial homogeneity of conditions.

more processing must be done at a given position. Second: contamination appears between trials, enhancing or weakening the effects as a function of whether or not a prepared oculomotor program has been put to work ("pure vs. mixed blocks"). These observations support the idea that eye scanning is both partly pre-programmed as a function of task demands, and partly subsquently modulated according to the particularities of the visual field encountered at each step.

RELATIVE ELASTICITY OF VARIOUS ASPECTS OF OCULOMOTOR BEHAVIOR IN A COMPLEX ACTIVITY (READING).

The previous data provide support for the elasticity of oculomotor routines in simple repetitive tasks. Turning now to a more "natural" situation than repeated presentation of two similar objects, consider what happens in reading. Reading is not only an important part of daily life, it is also an activity of interest for the psychologist and the psycholinguist. Both are eager to use oculomotor behavior as a measurable clue to what happens inside the "black box" during reading. They hope that information processing, assumed to operate covertly while the subject is reading, is reflected overtly in the positions of fixations, in their durations, and in the backwards saccades occurring along the lines of text. Therefore, one of the most urgent problems is to formulate what those hypothesized cognitive operations are that might be detectable via their oculomotor effects. Another—although somewhat easier—problem is to discover which are those measurable oculomotor characteristics that are sufficiently flexible to be liable to change as a function of cognitive processing. The previous experiment showed that pause duration may be shortened or lengthened as a function of the current state of local information processing. But is it one of the most flexible characteristics or not?

Ever since classical studies performed in the 40's and 50's identified the main aspects of ocular behavior during reading, many detailed measurements of these basic characteristics have accumulated. In a recent review (O'Regan & Levy-Schoen, 1978), an attempt was made to extract from these data those characteristics that are most stable and those that are most variable for comparisons both within and between individuals. Figure 6 shows both within and between individual variabilities of the main oculomotor characteristics of four subjects reading many sentences (extracted from O'Regan's experimental data). The histograms show that within each individual fixation durations vary (standard deviation around 100 msec), but that the means and standard deviations of these distributions are much the same between individuals. On the other hand, saccade amplitudes, which vary greatly within each individual, also vary considerably from one reader to the other. Consequently, it may be inferred that saccade extents are more flexible characteristics than fixation duration. The latter seem to be a more invariant feature of oculomotor behavior.

Now, what can be said about the relative elasticity of these same aspects of oculomotor behavior within readers, when they are faced with different reading situations? The eye movements of eight subjects were recorded while they read passages of prose in three different conditions. In one condition they read silently at their own spontaneously chosen speed. In the other conditions, reading was paced in such a way as to obtain two reading rates, one twice as fast as the other

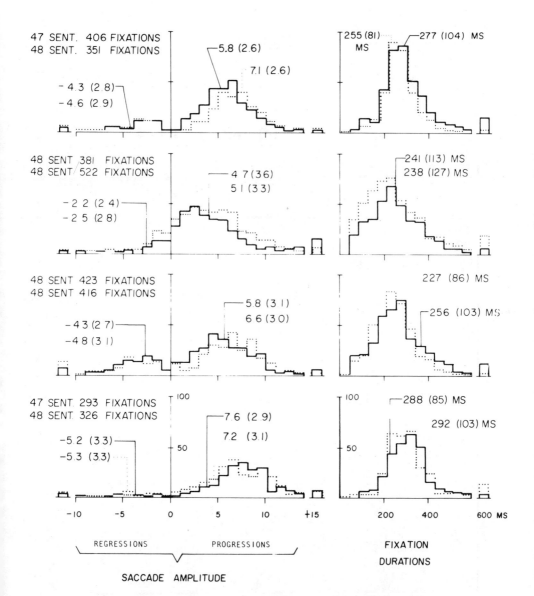

FIG. 6. Within and between subject variability of saccade amplitudes and of fixation durations during reading. The subjects read 48 one-line sentences, out of context, presented one by one in upper case on a computer screen. Solid lines show eye movement characteristics for the first reading, dotted lines for a second reading of the same sentences. Progression and regression sizes are defined as the distance, measured in number of characters, covered by the eye in moving from the end of a fixation to the end of the next fixation. Fixation duration is defined as the interval measured in milliseconds, between two successive saccades, and thus contains about 20 to 30 msec, corresponding to the duration of the saccade. The means and, in parentheses, the standard deviations, are shown for each histogram (From O'Regan & Levy-Schoen, 1978).

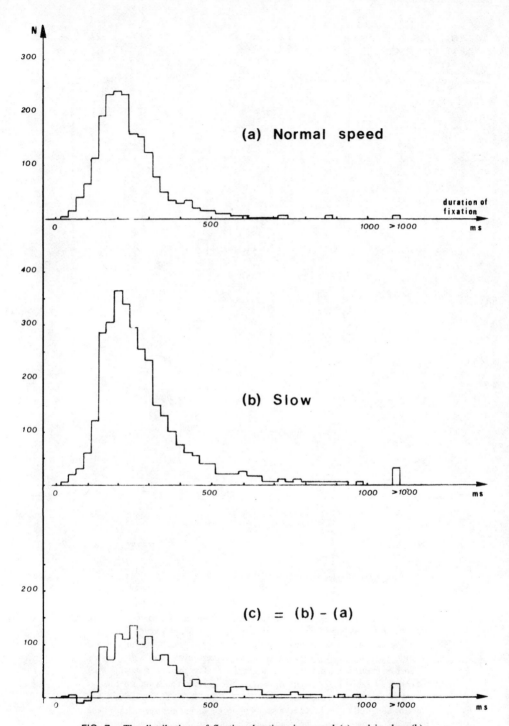

FIG. 7. The distributions of fixation durations in normal (a) and in slow (b) speed paced reading conditions, and the difference between these distributions (c) i.e., what is subtracted (below abscissa axis) or added (above abscissa axis) to normal reading distribution in order to change it into slow reading distribution.

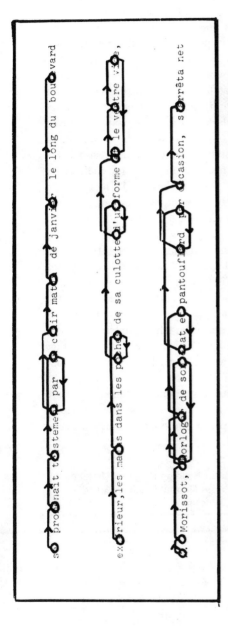

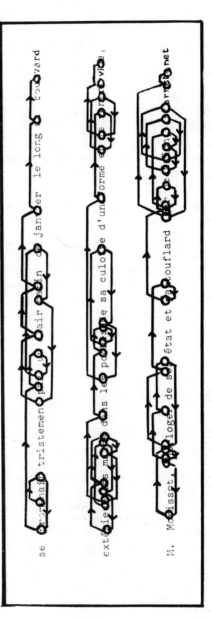

a

b

FIG. 8. An example of the ocular scanning pattern of a subject reading the same text in the two "paced reading" conditions, showing the succession of fixations along the lines. Progression saccades are arbitrarily symbolized as arrows above the line, regression saccades below it.

throughout the whole text. This was done by asking the subjects to read while they listened to a voice reading the same text, the task being to check that oral and written texts were identical. The number of progressive and regressive fixations, the amplitudes of saccades, and the durations of fixations were analyzed.

The speed of the "rapid paced reading" condition was about the same as spontaneous reading, and the data show that the oculomotor behavior is the same. For the "slow paced reading" condition, global reading speed was reduced by half. The question was: Which option would the subjects choose to double the time spent on the text? Would they keep constant the number of fixations along a line but double each pause duration? Or would they maintain the durations of the fixations and change their number? In this case they could either halve the size of each progression saccade size, or they could increase the number of regressions. The observed balance between these diverse options will give a measure of the relative elasticity or rigidity of each aspect of oculomotor behavior during reading.

The data (c.f. Table 1) clearly show that the parts taken by the different eye movement components in reducing the global speed are not equal. The average increase in mean fixation duration is 16%. The average increase in number of saccades is 64%, with progression and regression movements increasing by the same absolute number (an increase of approximately 3 per line); this implies that the relative increase is larger for the backward saccades, which are less numerous on the whole. Progression sizes are not reduced by half; the histograms (c.f. Fig. 7) show that small progressions are added to the normal speed distribution. Regressions, small and large, both increase in number.

Let me describe in more detail what happens to fixation durations. These are central to our preoccupations concerning general control processes in ocular scanning. By comparing the distribution of pause durations in the two paced

TABLE 1
Modifications in Characteristics of Oculomotor Reading Behavior Under
the Constraint of Reducing Global Speed from Normal Reading Speed
(3 sec/line) to Its Half (6 sec/line)

Condition of "Paced Reading"	Mean Duration of Fixations	Mean Number of Fixations Per Line	Progressions		Regressions	
			Number (per line)	Extent (characters)	Number (per line)	Extent (characters)
Normal speed	247ms	12.5	8.1	10.1	3.4	8.3
Slow speed	287ms	20.5	12.8	8.6	6.7	8.4
Percent average increase	+ 16%	+ 64%	+ 58%	− 15%	+ 97%	+ 0.1%

reading situations, it is seen that both have the same mode. This means that the first option mentioned is certainly not the right one: doubling the global reading time is not obtained by doubling each pause time. But, going from the normal speed to the slow speed, we observe that instead of replacing brief fixations by long ones, long fixations are simply added to the normal speed distribution. This means that slowing down does not work as brakes would in postponing the triggering of each saccade. Instead, slowing occurs by grossly maintaining saccade rate but increasing the number of saccades (see Fig. 7).

An illustration of the ocular behavior of the readers in the two conditions (Fig. 8) supports this interpretation. It can be seen that the scanning pattern along the lines becomes repetitive: Under the constraint to slow down, the typical reading pattern subsists, but with somewhat shorter saccades, and with an abundance of oscillatory backwards and forwards movements that resemble phases of waiting.

From these observations I conclude that in an activity as complex as reading a text, oculomotor behavior seems to be driven by a strongly organized routine that is adjusted both to the general physical properties of the text and to content processing requirements. When submitted to an external constraint to reduce global speed, pause duration tends to resist massive modification, and the saccades change in number but scarcely in amplitude. It seems that the basic reading routine is maintained, but that the speed constraint is obeyed by adding extra waiting phases to the main ocular pattern. Note that these extra phases adopt ocular patterns similar to the basic ones: They appear as repetitions of parts of the main routine.

CONCLUSION

I have considered three sources of regulation acting upon the scanning behavior of an individual engaged in ocular exploration: general free-field trends, global routines determined by the particular scanning task, and moment-to-moment physical and cognitive factors.

These three levels at which scanning is controlled may be regarded as mutually subordinated in such a way that when the most specifically adapted one is not at work it is the second more general level that becomes determinant. When this one also is not actively required, then free functioning is allowed, following the most general tendencies of the sensory-motor system. In this last case, the system functions without the intervention of cognitive control, which in the other cases modulates and adapts the rules, either to the requirements of the task as a whole, or to the way information is being locally collected and processed.

These three subordinated ways in which scanning is organized have been illustrated by the variety of situations that I have mentioned. The most general constraints of the saccadic system govern such a low level task as deciding where to look first when two objects appear somewhere in a blank field (c.f. the

"0-A-B or 0-B-A" experiment). As soon as spatial or temporal expectations can be formed (e.g., on the basis of similarities between successive trials), or as soon as the demands of the task are such that an anticipatory program is elaborated, then a more specific routine guides the ocular behavior (as appears in the scanning of partly repetitive displays, Fig. 2). Rules are set to work, preparing scanning of successive parts of the field, or at least preparing the first saccade and fixation. What remains open at this stage is the exact specification of the movements that have to be executed (direction, amplitude), and some modifications of their timing (shortening or lengthening of fixations). The duration of a fixation during scanning is sensitive to the local state of cognitive processing. This is demonstrated in the third experiment presented. The scanning routine at work is locally modulated in time: The modulation is slight but systematic (Figs. 4 and 5). During reading, the extent and direction of the saccades seem to be more "elastic" characteristics than their timing (c.f. last experiment).

More generally, that which determines the efficiency of exploratory oculomotor behavior may be the flexibility shown by these prepared routines: whether they can adjust to local requirements rapidly and in a manner appropriate to the particular demands of the task. Efficient scanning of the visual field as well as efficient reading imply a good pre-established program, but also its continuous adaptation to the visual material encountered as well as to the state of advancement of the processing of this material.

ACKNOWLEDGMENTS

I am thankful to Kevin O'Regan for his help in giving a proper form to this chapter, contributing to polishing up the ideas as well as the language.

VI CAN EYE MOVEMENTS SAVE THE EARTH?

This volume is the direct result of "The Last Whole Earth Eye Movement Conference" held in St. Petersburg, Florida in February, 1980. Many attendees queried the meaning of the title and whether or not it really signified the end of our series of conferences. Not necessarily. Our intention was merely to provide a light-hearted approach to the study of eye-movements, but "The Last" reflected our feeling that the three conferences taken together were successful in addressing most of the topics of interest to us up until the present time.

The study of eye movements tends to be intriguing and compelling. So much so that researchers exhibit myopia, or lose sight of the real world beyond the laboratory. For that reason we called upon E. Llewellyn-Thomas to utilize his unique sense of perspective and wit to tell us whether or not more eye movement research is worthwhile. The tone of his address has been carefully preserved, and, fortunately, he leaves us with the feeling that time spent in our eye movement laboratories, is indeed, worthwhile.

VI.1 "Can Eye Movements Save the Earth?"

E. Llewellyn-Thomas
Faculty of Medicine
University of Toronto

A keynote address coming at the end of conference can hardly strike a chord or set a theme. So at the end of this "Last Whole Earth Eye Movement Conference" I'll only try to sound a finale, and hope it'll serve as a rallying call for the next. I'll also try to answer the challenge the sponsors gave me as the title: "Can Eye Movements Save the Earth?"

I find these conferences unique because of the diverse backgrounds and the different talents of the people who come together to talk about something that fascinates us all—the movements of the eye and the movements within the eye. Something that fascinates each of us for different reasons, just as the eye itself has always fascinated poets, philosophers, artists, scientists, physicians, engineers, and warriors. Our conference includes samples of many such groups, plus some people who refuse to be classified.

Nature doesn't seem to recognize academic boundaries, but we humans must, because life's too short for any of us to learn all we'd like to learn, and for one person to understand the Eye Movement System he'd have to master many known disciplines and others still unknown. So the study of eye movements requires that people from different areas of knowledge try to understand and put up with each other. It is this interaction that gives these conferences their unique flavor and makes them important in their own right.

But because each of us is interested, and perhaps expert, in certain facets of the Eye Movement systems, and because the papers and discussions of the last three days have concentrated on particular aspects, we may forget the wonder of the whole in the same way that an expert analyzing the paint of one picture in the Louvre may forget the beauty all around him. So in this brief and final talk let me remind you of some of the almost incredible capabilities of the human visual system.

317

John Ruskin said "The greatest thing a human soul ever does in this world is to *see* something and tell what he *saw* in a plain way. Hundreds of people can talk for every one who can think. Thousands can think for every one who can *see*. To see clearly is poetry, prophecy, and religion—all in one!" Apart from the last overblown phrase I suggest John Ruskin had something. Again and again in the history of science only one person saw what was plain for all to see once shown. The hidden figure!

The Eye Movement System contains and exemplifies the major generalized unifying concepts of our age, the concepts whose application makes possible the computer, the modern aircraft, the ICBM, namely the concept of feedback and control, the concept of information and system. Explicitly or intuitively they are part of our thinking in almost every field as they are a physical part of almost all our hardware.

I'm from the Dark Ages when these were all unknown. It took some of the best brains in the world to see them but once seen they're rather obvious. Feedback reduces gain but it also offsets error so you can build high performance systems with low performance components: Systems that will correct for environmental changes and component deterioration: Systems that can accept some component failure, anticipate, and today select their own goals and choose how to reach them.

The concepts were developed to solve hardware problems in aiming guns, radar, and ships. Later we realized they were universal. Larry Stark and his colleagues showed how beautifully feedback and adaptive control are exemplified by the pupil of the eye. It took somebody like him to analyze the system, and his is a landmark paper. But anyone who has shown a narrow beam of light on the edge of the pupil and watched that pupil oscillate, looked at, but did not see, the essence of a servo system driven into oscillation. The ophthalmologists had a name for it: "Induced pupillary hippus." But they did not see the general concept hippus exemplified. What other generalized concepts are exemplified in the eye movement control systems? Concepts that we are looking at but not seeing? I find it amusing to think of Time as a one-way screen, with our invisible descendants studying us through the glass. What is exasperating them? Of what are they saying: "They've got an example right in front of them. Why can't the idiots see it?"

There are many wonders to wonder about in the eye movement system.

For example, Wayne Shebilsky showed that some of us can sometimes hit a baseball. It's astounding that any of us can hit one at all. A ball is travelling a hundred miles an hour. A visual sample is taken from a bad angle in a single fixation from which the batter has to compute and extrapolate the ball's trajectory while initiating the voluntary muscle movements to guide a round club along a convoluted curve so it impacts the ball hard at a unique point in time and space! Impossible—all those differential equations to solve, and curves to plot in milleseconds! The fact that a good batter can hit a third of the pitches demonstrates how fantastically efficient our visual and neuromuscular systems are. But then a monkey's eye movement control system solves almost instantly problems in higher mathematics when it leaps from bough to bough!

We have extraocular muscles which, like the wing muscles of insects, do not fatigue. Muscles that keep my eyes jumping constantly while I'm awake and much of the time I'm asleep, forever seeking information from the world around me, or following events in the world of my imagination. Muscles with an ample blood supply and the highest innervation of any muscles in the body. They can accelerate the eyeball up to 800° per second and they operate as an open loop bang-bang servo. There doesn't seem to be any checking action by the antagonists. There are stretch receptors—but what are they doing? And the system is probably computing the next saccade while the eye is still in flight. It computes, coordinates, and fires—but with anticipation! Anticipatory control? Feedforward? Bellman's dynamic programming in action? Markov chains?

We have a retina with about 150 million receptors and an optic nerve of about one million fibers. These facts alone suggest signal compression and that demands peripheral decision-making: a system of great overall accuracy built from fragile components exquisitely sensitive to pH, pO_2, pCO_2, Na^{++}, K^+, Ca^+, Glucose, Temp, et al.; an optical system with chromatic and other aberrations but that functions magnificently under gross insult.

We have an early warning system with an acoustic reflex and an ocular reflex to giving an instant response to a glimpsed threat. It is programmed to sense threatening information and to make fast decisions about pattern. Is it biased to use a "worse-case" strategy? To see not exactly the image that is there but the image of the most dangerous thing that could be there? As Shakespeare says:

> "Or in the night, imagining some fear.
> How easy is a bush supposed a bear?"

This system tries to extract information from a low-information scene. Staring into the darkness from a ship's bridge, or into the ganzfeld from an aircraft climbing through a cloud, the system turns its gain up for maximum sensitivity and may start to structure the increased noise into misinformation. Perhaps it hallucinates? For example, a radio operator listening for a faint signal through noise hears bursts of code. A paranoid patient hears threats in the murmur of an unintelligible conversation. Ecclesiastes sums it up ''The Eye is not satisfied with seeing.''

The opposite is perceptual defense. Our subconscious sometimes doesn't let us see things it thinks might damage our tender psyches. As Arien Levy-Schoen pointed out, eye movements represent more than a search for information. The eye is also a transmitter of information. In the words of the poet ''The eyes, the limpid mirrors of the soul.'' After proper lubrication at the bar even the less sentimental among us admit that there is something soulful about the Eye. ''Drink to me only with thine eyes, and I will pledge with mine!'', as Ben Jonson remarked to Celia and probably got a lot of mileage out of his line. The Poet knows that the Eye can express affect more effectively than any other mode of communication. It says things that, in Wittgenstein's words, "can't be said," and carries an immense load of emotional information. Brightness, blink-rate, pupil-size are signals of more than mere arousal.

When you record the eye movements of people looking at other people they look at the eyes most and then the mouth. This is particularly so when they are looking at living people—not pictures. As my boxing coach used to shout, "Watch his eyes—not his gloves!"

I have not yet answered the challenge given me with the title of this talk. "Can Eye Movements Save the Earth?" I have been reminding you about the wonders of the Eye Movement System, but save the Earth?

Our own futures will certainly be affected by whether both superpowers—and one in particular—have learned the prime survival lesson: NEVER TACKLE ANYONE YOUR OWN SIZE OR BIGGER! If they don't learn that, our futures become open-ended in every sense. If they do, the future of our race is going to be a function of our ability to live on easy terms with our own creations, and in particular the creations of engineers.

We—they—have put our lives on the line—twenty-four hours a day, three hundred and sixty-five days a year. We have created ballista that can drop a chunk of fusion into a trash-can on the other side of the world. At this moment a large number of ballista on both sides of the world are armed and aimed to do exactly that. We have been living for many years with the graticules of a telescopic sight aligned on our necks but it is only recently that the hair has again started to prickle.

It is not so much the knowledge that somebody is aiming at me all the time to which I object. After all, my ancestors lived out their lives in fear of battle, murder, and sudden death, to quote the Christian Litany. What makes me nervous is that the system being aimed is not up to specifications, that the rocketeers aiming it are insufficiently trained, that there's noise on their communication links, that their displays are designed after the manner of the average kitchen cooker, and that their target indentification is imperfect. In short they don't always see what they think they see.

The international treaty I want most is an agreement that no rocketeer of any nation be allowed to point an ICBM at anyone until he or she has been certified as having shown a high level of competence as judged by his or her peers drawn from among the nations at which he or she is most likely to point. A kind of "External Referee" system such as we have in Academe. And I further suggest that the Corps of Nuclear Engineers now being proposed as a result of the beer-bellies involved in the Three Mile Island fiasco, be expanded to an International Corps of Nuclear Engineers whose perceptual and multiple-choice decision making skills are at least up to the standard demanded by Admiral Rickover. Come to think of it, the Admiral would be the ideal man to lead such a Corps. And the spin-off would be an excuse to retire him from the Navy.

That is wishful thinking! But at least we could hope for a rule that anybody who wants to operate a nuclear reactor anywhere in the world must see well enough to read the dials—with glasses if worn. Because even in my gloomiest moments I doubt that anybody is going to start a nuclear melt-down or fire a nuclear broadside on purpose. But I'm getting increasingly suspicious that sooner or later somebody's going to misread a few inputs and do the wrong thing. You have only to apply Bayesian Statistics to the next hundred years to find that the probability somebody will fly the birds by accident approaches certainty.

I have, of course, used the dramatic to camouflage a chain of arguments so specious that it would make Markov himself shudder. But, valid or not, one has only to look to see the crunch that's tightening on us all. Ships are running into each other at a greater rate than ever in the past. Much bigger ships. There's a category called "Radar-assisted collisions!" Communication between men and machines, and communication between men through machines, is the weakest and yet most critical link in every high-technology system from airline booking to nuclear power. The air-traffic control system is operating at the limit of human perceptual ability. And the most important channel is still the visual. Man sees wonderfully well if he's given displays designed for men to read. In the new jargon we call it "optimization of information flow across the man-machine interface." And in order to optimize the flow from the display into the human mind the display must be designed to suit the physical, physiological, and psychological characteristics of the human being concerned. "Information impedance matching for optimum information transfer." In older terms "Make the alphanumerics big enough for the operator to read, illuminate them so he can, and put them where he looks." *Where he looks!*

The ability of machines to identify visual pattern is still primitive, though of course they've only been around less than thirty years while man's been using his eyes for at least a million. We have to learn everything we possibly can about how he uses them. High technology's still on an exponential rise and God knows what we'll have to look at before we can teach the machines to look for us. This justifies my answer to the question "Can Eye Movements Save the Earth?": Perhaps. Even if they don't actually save the Earth they can make its loss less traumatic. And without them Earth's a lost cause.

"Where there is no vision the people perish" was a metaphysical statement when made by the Old Testament prophet who wrote the Proverbs. Today it is an engineering forecast.

VII REFERENCES

Abrams, S. G., & Zuber, B. L. Some temporal characteristics of information processing during reading. *Reading Research Quarterly*, 1972, *8*, 40–51.

Adler, F. H., & Fliegelman, M. Influence of fixation on the visual acuity. *Archives of Ophthalmology*, 1934, *13*, 475–483.

Akin, O., & Reddy, R. Knowledge acquisition for image understanding research. *Computer Graphics and Image Processing*, 1977, *6*, 307–334.

Allum, J. H. J., Tole, J. R., & Weiss, A. D. MITNYS-II-A digital program for on-line analysis of nystagmus. *IEEE Transactions on Biomedical Engineering*, 1975, *22*, 196–202.

Alpern, M. The aftereffect of lateral duction testing on subsequent phoria measurements. *American Journal of Optometry*, 1946, *23*, 442–447.

Alpern, M. Types of movement. In H. Davson (Ed.), *The Eye* (2nd ed.), Vol. 3. New York: Academic Press, 1969.

Andriessen, J. J., & de Voogd, A. J. Analysis of eye movement patterns in silent reading. *I.P.O. Annual Progress Report*, 1973, *8*, 29–34.

Anstis, S. M., & Atkinson, J. Distortions in moving figures viewed through a stationary slit. *American Journal of Psychology*, 1967, *80*, 572–585.

Antes, J. R. The time course of picture viewing. *Journal of Experimental Psychology*, 1974, *103*, 62–70.

Antes, J. R. Recognizing and localizing features in brief picture presentations. *Memory and Cognition*, 1977, *5*, 155–161.

Antes, J. R., & Metzger, R. L. Influences of picture context on object recognition. *Acta Psychologica*, 1980, *44*, 21–30.

Antes, J. R., Penland, J. G., & Metzger, R. L. Context effects on the recognition of usual and unusual objects in pictures. Manuscript submitted for publication, 1980.

Appel, M. A., & Campos, J. J. Binocular disparity as a discriminable stimulus parameter for young infants. *Journal of Experimental Child Psychology*, 1977, *23*, 47–56.

Argyle, M. *Social interaction*. New York: Methuen, 1969.

Aslin, R. N. Development of binocular fixation in human infants. *Journal of Experimental Child Psychology*, 1977, *23*, 133–150.

Aslin, R. N., & Dumais, S. T. Binocular vision in infants: A review and a theoretical framework. In L. Lipsitt & H. Reese (Eds.), *Advances in Child Development and Behavior*. In Press.

Aslin, R. N., & Jackson, R. W. Accomodative-convergence in young infants: Development of a synergistic sensory-motor system. *Canadian Journal of Psychology*, 1979, *33*, 222–231.

Aslin, R. N., & Salapatek, P. Saccadic localization of visual targets by the very young human infant. *Perception and Psychophysics*, 1975, *17*, 293–302.

Atkinson, J. Development of optokinetic nystagmus in the human infant and monkey infant: An analogue to development in kittens. In R. D. Freeman (Ed.), *Developmental neurobiology of vision*, NATO Advanced Study Institutes Series. New York: Plenum Press, 1979.

Atkinson, J., & Braddick, O. Stereoscopic discrimination in infants. *Perception*, 1976, *5*, 29–38.

Attneave, F. Some informational aspects of visual perception. *Psychological Review*, 1954, *61*, 183–193.

Auerbach, F. Erklaerung der Brantano'schen optischen Tauschung. *Zeitschrift fur Psychologie*, 1894, *7*, 152–160.

Baddeley, A. D. The influence of semantic and acoustic similarity on long-term memory for word sequences. *Quarterly Journal of Experimental Psychology*, 1966, *8*, 302–304.

Bagust, J., Lewis, D. M., & Luck, J. D. Post-tetanic effects in motor units of fast and slow twitch muscle of the cat. *Journal of Physiology*, 1974, *237*, 115–121.

Bahill, T. A. Most naturally occurring human saccades have magnitudes of 15 degrees or less. *Investigative Ophthalmology*, 1975, *14*, 468–469.

Bahill, T. A., & Stark, L. Trajectories of saccadic eye movements. *Scientific American*, 1979, *240*, 84–93.

Bain, A. *The Senses and the Intellect*. London: Longmans, Green, 1855.

Bajcsy, R., & Rosenthal, D. Visual focusing and defocusing—an essential part of pattern recognition process. *Proceedings of the Computer Graphics, Pattern Recognition and Data Structure Conference*. Los Angeles, 1975.

Bajcsy, R., & Tavakoli, M. Image filtering—a content dependent process. *IEEE Transactions on Circuits and Systems*, 1975, *22*, 463–474.

Baker, R., & Berthoz, A. (Eds.) *Control of gaze by brain stem neurons*. Amsterdam: Elsevier/North Holland Press, 1977.

Ballard, D. H. *Strip trees: A hierarchial representation for map features. TR32*. University of Rochester: Computer Science Department, 1978.

Baloh, R. W., Kumley, W. E., & Honrubia, V. Algorithm for analysis of saccadic eye movements using a digital computer. *Aviation and Space Environmental Medicine*, 1976, *47*, 523–527.

Banks, M. S., & Salapatek, P. Infant pattern vision: A new approach based on the contrast sensitivity function. *Journal of Experimental Child Psychology*, in press.

Barlow, H. B. Eye-movements during fixation. *Journal of Physiology*, 1952, *116*, 290–306.

Barlow, H. B., Narasimhan, R., & Rosenfeld, A. Visual pattern analysis in machines and animals. *Science*, 1972, *177*, 567–575.

Barmack, N. H. Modification of eye movements by instantaneous changes in the velocity of visual targets. *Vision Research*, 1970, *10*, 1431–1441.

Barnes, J. A. *Analysis of pilot's eye movements during helicopter flight*. Technical Memorandum 11-72. Aberdeen Proving Ground, MD: U.S. Army Human Engineering Laboratory, 1972.

Barrett, R. F., & Magleby, K. L. Physiology of cholinergic transmission. In A. M. Goldberg & I. Hanin (Eds.), *Biology of cholinergic function*. New York: Raven, 1976.

Barrow, H. B., Ambles, A. P., & Bersh, R. M. Some techniques for recognizing structures in pictures. In S. Watanabe, *Frontiers of pattern recognition*, New York: Academic Press, 1972.

Barrow, H. B., and Tenenbaum, J. M. *Representation and uses of knowledge in vision*. Stanford Research Institute Technical Note 108, 1975.

Barten, S., Birns, B., & Ronch, J. Individual differences in the visual pursuit behavior of neonates. *Child Development*, 1971, *42*, 313–319.

Bartlett, J. R., & Doty, R. W. Response of units in striate cortex of squirrel monkeys to visual and electrical stimuli. *Journal of Neurophysiology*, 1974, *37*, 621–641.

Bartz, A. E. Eye-movement latency, duration, and response time as a function of angular displacement. *Journal of Experimental Psychology*, 1962, *64*, 318–324.

Beasley, W. C. Visual pursuit in 109 white and 142 Negro newborn infants. *Child Development*, 1933, *4*, 106–120.

Becker, W., & Jürgens, R. An analysis of the saccadic system by means of a double step stimuli. *Vision Research*, 1979, *19*, 976–983.

Bengi, H., & Thomas, J. G. Use of a piezo-accelerometer in studying eye-movements. *Journal of the Optical Society of America*, 1965, *55*, 534–537.

Bengi, H., & Thomas, J. G. Fixation tremor in relation to eyeball-muscle mechanics. *Nature*, 1968, *217*, 773–774.

Biederman, I. Perceiving real-word scenes. *Science*, 1972, *177*, 77–80.

Biederman, I. On the semantics of a glance at a scene. In M. Kubovy & J. R. Pomerantz (Eds.), *Perceptual organization*. Hillsdale, NJ: Lawrence Erlbaum Associates, 1980.

Biederman, I., Glass, A. L., & Stacy, E. W., Jr. Searching for objects in real-world scenes. *Journal of Experimental Psychology*, 1973, *97*, 22–27.

Biederman, I., Rabinowitz, J. C., Glass, A. L., & Stacy, E. W., Jr. On the information extracted from a glance at a scene. *Journal of Experimental Psychology*, 1974, *103*, 597–600.

Bielschowsky, A. Lectures on motor anomalies. I. The physiology of ocular movements. *American Journal of Ophthalmology*, 1938, *21*, 843–854.

Binet, A. La mesure des illusions visuelles chez les enfants. *Revue Philosophique*, 1895, *40*, 11–25.

Binford, T. O., & Tenenbaum, J. M. Computer vision. *IEEE Transactions on Computers*, 1973, *22*, 14–19.

Blum, H. Biological shape and visual science (Part I). *Theories of biology*, 1973, *38*, 205–287.

Bolles, R. C. *Verification vision within a programmable assembly suster: An introductory discussion.* Stanford Artificial Intelligence Laboratory, Memo AIM-275, 1975.

Bower, T. G. R. *Development in infancy.* San Francisco: Freeman, 1974.

Boyce, P. R. *An investigation of eye movements during fixation and tracking tasks.* Unpublished doctoral dissertation, University of Reading, U.K., 1965.

Boyce, P. R. Monocular fixation in eye-movements. *Proceedings of the Royal Society, Series B,* 1967, *167,* 293-315. (a)

Boyce, P. R. The effect of change of target luminance and colour on fixation eye-movements. *Optica Acta,* 1967, *14,* 119-126. (b)

Bozkov, V., Bohdanecky, Z., & Radil-Weiss, T. Eye movements and visual shape perception. *Activitas Nervosis Supplement,* 1973, *15,* 47-48.

Braddick, O. J., Atkinson, J., Julesz, B., Kropfl, W., Bodis-Wollner, I., & Raab, E. Cortical binocularity in infants: Evidence from evoked potentials with a cyclopean stimulus. In preparation.

Brandt, H. F. Ocular patterns and their psychological implications. *American Journal of Psychology,* 1940, *53,* 260-268.

Brandt, H. F. *The psychology of seeing.* New York: Philosophical Library 1945.

Braun, J. J., & Gault, F. P. Monocular and binocular control of horizontal optokinetic nystagmus in cats and rabbits. *Journal of Comparative and Physiological Psychology,* 1969, *69,* 12-16.

Brentano, F. Ueber ein optisches Paradoxen. *Journal of Psychology,* 1892, *3,* 349-358.

Breitmeyer, B. G., & Ganz, L. Implications of sustained and transient channels for theories of visual pattern masking, saccadic suppression, and information processing. *Psychological Review,* 1976, *83,* 1-36.

Bronson, G. The postnatal growth of visual capacity. *Child Development,* 1974, *45,* 873-890.

Brown, A. L., & DeLoache, J. S. Skills, plans, and self-regulation. In R. Siegler (Ed.), *Children's thinking: What develops?* Hillsdale, NJ: Lawrence Erlbaum Associates, 1978.

Brown, D. R., & Owen, D. H. The metrics of visual form: Methodological dyspepsia. *Psychological Bulletin,* 1967, *68,* 243-259.

Brown, G. L., & Von Euler, U. S. The aftereffects of a tetanus on mammalian muscle. *Journal of Physiology,* 1938, *93,* 39-60.

Bruce, D. J. Effects of context upon the intelligibility of heard speech. In C. Cherry (Ed.), *Information theory: Third London symposium.* London: Butterworth, 1956.

Bruell, J. H., & Albee, G. W. Notes toward a motor theory of visual egocentric localization. *Psychological Review,* 1955, *62,* 301-308.

Bullock, B. L., Dudani, S., Stafsudd, J., & Clark, C. Finding structure in outdoor scenes. Malibu: Hughes Research Laboratories, Report 498. Also in *Pattern recognition and artificial intelligence.* New York: Academic Press, 1976.

Burian, H. M. Fusional movements. *Archives of Ophthalmology,* 1939, *21,* 486-491.

Burnham, C. A. Decrement of the Mueller-Lyer illusion with saccadic and tracking eye movements. *Perception and Psychophysics,* 1968, *3,* 424-426.

Burr, D. C. Acuity for apparent vernier offset. *Vision Research,* 1979, *19,* 835-838.

Buswell, G. T. *How people look at pictures.* Chicago: University of Chicago Press, 1935.

Buttner, U., Hepp, K., & Henn, V. Neurons in the rostral mesencephalic and paramedian pontine reticular formation generating fast eye movements. In R. Baker & A. Berthoz (Eds.), *Control of gaze by brain stem neurons.* New York: Elsevier/North Holland Press, 1977, 309-318.

Campbell, F. W., & Robson, J. G. Application of Fourier analysis to the visibility of gratings. *Journal of Physiology,* 1968, *197,* 551-566.

Caron, A. J., Caron, R. F., Caldwell, R. C., & Weiss, S. J. Infant perception of the structural properties of the face. *Developmental Psychology,* 1973, *9,* 385-399.

Carpenter, P., & Just, M. Linguistic influences on picture scanning. In R. A. Monty and J. W. Senders (Eds.), *Eye movements and psychological processes.* Hillsdale, NJ: Lawrence Erlbaum Associates, 1976.

Carr, T. H., & Bacharach, V. R. Perceptual tuning and conscious attention: Systems of input regulation in visual information processing. *Cognition,* 1976, *4,* 281-302.

Carter, D. B. Fixation disparity and heterophoria following prolonged wearing of prisms. *American Journal of Optometry,* 1965, *42,* 141–151.

Cattell, J. McK. On the relations between time and space in vision. *Psychological Review,* 1900, *7,* 325–343.

Chomsky, N. *Syntactic structures.* The Hague: Mouton, 1957.

Clark, M. R., & Stark, L. Control of human eye movements III. Dynamic characteristics of the eye tracking mechanism. *Mathematical Biosciences,* 1974, *20,* 239–265.

Clark, M. R., & Stark, L. Time optimal behavior of human saccadic eye movement. *IEEE Transactions on Automatic Control,* 1975, *20,* 345–348.

Cohen, B., Goto, K., Shanzer, S., & Weis, A. H. Eye movements induced by electrical stimulation of the cerebellum in the alert cat. *Experimental Neurology,* 1965, *13,* 145–162.

Cohen, B., & Komatsuzaki, A. Eye movements induced by stimulation of the pontine reticular formation: Evidence for integration in oculomotor pathways. *Experimental Neurology,* 1972, *36,* 101–117.

Cohen, J., & Cohen, P. *Applied multiple regression/correlational analysis for the behavioral sciences.* Hillsdale, NJ: Lawrence Erlbaum Associates, 1975.

Cohen, K. M. *Eye movements and the development of psychological processes.* Unpublished paper commissioned in part by the National Institute of Education for their conference on Eye Movement Research and Technology, 1974.

Cohen, K. M. *The development of selective processing of information in the visual periphery.* Unpublished doctoral dissertation, Harvard University, 1978.

Cohen, K. M., & Haith, M. M. Peripheral vision: The effects of developmental, perceptual, and cognitive factors. *Journal of Experimental Child Psychology,* 1977, *24,* 373–394. (a)

Cohen, K. M., & Haith, M. M. *Processing wholes and parts in the visual periphery.* Paper presented at the Meetings of the American Psychological Association, San Francisco, 1977. (b)

Cohen, L. B. Attention-getting and attention-holding processes of infant visual preferences. *Child Development,* 1972, *43,* 869–879.

Collewijn, H. Optokinetic eye movements in the rabbit: Input-output relations. *Vision Research,* 1969, *9,* 117–132.

Collewijn, H. Direction-selective units in the rabbit's nucleus of the optic tract. *Brain Research,* 1975, *100,* 489–508.

Collier, R. M. An experimental study of form perception in indirect vision. *Journal of Comparative Psychology,* 1931, *11,* 281–290.

Conrad, R. Acoustic confusions in immediate memory. *British Journal of Psychology,* 1964, *55,* 75–83.

Cooper, R. The control of eye fixation by the meaning of spoken language. *Cognitive Psychology,* 1974, *6,* 84–107.

Corballis, M. C., & Beale, I. L. *The psychology of left and right.* Hillsdale, NJ: Lawrence Erlbaum Associates, 1976.

Corcoran, D. W. J. Serial and parallel classification. *British Journal of Psychology,* 1967, *58,* 197–203.

Coren, S. Lateral inhibition and geometric illusions. *Quarterly Journal of Experimental Psychology,* 1970, *22,* 274–278. (a)

Coren, S. Lateral inhibition and the Wundt-Hering illusion. *Psychonomic Science,* 1970, *18,* 341. (b)

Coren, S., Bradley, D. R., Hoenig, P., & Girgus, J. S. The effect of smooth tracking and saccadic eye movements on the perception of size: The shrinking circle illusion. *Vision Research,* 1975, *15,* 49–55.

Coren, S., & Festinger, L. An alternative view of the "Gibson normalization effect." *Perception and Psychophysics,* 1967, *2,* 621–626.

Coren, S., & Hoenig, P. Effect of non target stimuli upon length of voluntary saccades. *Perceptual and Motor Skills,* 1972, *34,* 499–508. (a)

Coren, S., & Hoenig, P. Eye movements and decrement in the Oppel-Kundt illusion. *Perception and Psychophysics*, 1972, *12*, 224–225. (b)

Craske, B., & Crawshaw, M. Spatial discordance is a sufficient condition for oculomotor adaptation to prisms: Eye muscle potentiation need not be a factor. *Perception and Psychophysics*, 1978, *23*, 75–79.

Craske, B., Crawshaw, M., & Heron, P. Disturbance of the oculomotor system due to lateral fixation. *Quarterly Journal of Experimental Psychology*, 1975, *27*, 459–465.

Craske, B., & Templeton, W. B. Prolonged oscillation of the eyes induced by conflicting position input. *Journal of Experimental Psychology*, 1968, *76*, 387–393.

Crone, R. A. Amblyopia: The pathology of motor disorders in amblyopic eyes. *Document of Ophthalmology Proceedings Series*. Experimental and Clinical Amblyopia XIIIth I.S.C.E.R.G. Symposium, 1977, *45*, 9–18.

Crovitz, H. F., & Davies, W. L. Tendencies to eye movement and perceptual accuracy. *Journal of Experimental Psychology*, 1962, *63*, 495–498.

Davies, W. L. *Electronic analysis and modeling of microtremor in normal and pathological cases*. Unpublished doctoral dissertation, University of Wales, University College, Cardiff, U.K., 1976.

Davies, W. L., & Plant, G. R. Recording and analysis of human ocular microtremor. *Journal of Physiology*, 1978, *276*, 21–22.

Davis, L. S. *Shape matching using relaxation techniques*. University of Maryland, College Park, Computer Science Center, TR–480, 1976.

Day, M.C. Developmental trends in visual scanning. In H. W. Reese (Ed.), *Advances in child developmental and behavior*. (Vol. 10) New York: Academic Press, 1975.

Dayton, G. O., & Jones, M. H. Analysis of characteristics of fixation reflexes in infants by use of direct current electrooculography. *Neurology*, 1964, *14*, 1152–1156.

Dayton, G. O., Jones, M. H., Aiu, P., Rawson, R. A., Steele, B., & Rose, M. Developmental study of coordinated eye movements in the human infant. I. Visual acuity in the newborn human: A study based on induced optokinetic nystagmus recorded by electrooculography. *Archives of Ophthalmology*, 1964, *71*, 865–870.

Dayton, G. O., Jones, M. H., Steele, B., & Rose, M. Developmental study of coordinated eye movements in the human infant. II. An electrooculographic study of the fixation reflex in the newborn. *Archives of Ophthalmology*, 1964, *71*, 871–875.

DeGroot, A. D. Perception and memory versus thought: Some old ideas and recent findings. In B. Kleinmunts (Ed.), *Problem solving: Research, method, and theory*. New York: Wiley, 1966.

DeLaBarre, E. B. A method of recording eye movements. *American Journal of Psychology*, 1897, *9*, 572–574.

DeSisto, M. J., & Moses, F. L. *Saccadic eye movement response to Mueller-Lyer stimuli*. Paper presented at the meeting of the Eastern Psychological Association, Washington, D.C., 1968.

Dewar, R. E. Stimulus determinants of the magnitude of the Mueller-Lyer illusion. *Perceptual and Motor Skills*, 1967, *24*, 708–710.

Dichgans, J., & Jung, R. Oculomotor abnormalities due to cerebellar lesions. In G. Lennerstrand & P. Bach-y-Rita (Eds.), *Basic mechanisms of ocular motility and their clinical implications*. Oxford: Pergamon Press, 1975.

Didday, R. L., & Arbib, M. A. *Eye movements and visual perception: A "two visual system" model*. COINS Technical Report 73C-9. University of Massachusetts, 1972.

Ditchburn, R. W. *Eye movements and visual perception*. Oxford: Clarendon Press, 1973.

Ditchburn, R. W. The function of small saccades. *Vision Research*, 1980, *20*, 271–272.

Ditchburn, R. W., & Drysdale, A. E. The effect of retinal image motion on vision. I. Step movements and pulse movements. *Proceedings of the Royal Society of Britain*, 1977, *197*, 131–144. (a)

Ditchburn, R. W., & Drysdale, A. E. The effect of retinal image motion on vision. II. Oscillatory movements. *Proceedings of the Royal Society of Britain*, 1977, *197*, 385–406. (b)

Ditchburn, R. W., Fender, D. H., & Mayne, S. Vision with controlled movements of the retinal image. *Journal of Physiology*, 1959, *145*, 98–107.

Ditchburn, R. W., & Foley-Fisher, J. A. *Effect of imposed eye movements on colour perception: Oscillatory movements*. In preparation.

Ditchburn, R. W., & Foley-Fisher, J. A. *Effect of imposed eye movements on colour perception: Step movements and pulse movements*. In preparation.

Ditchburn, R. W., & Ginsborg, B. L. Vision with a stabilized retinal image. *Nature*, 1952, *170*, 36–37.

Ditchburn, R. W., & Ginsborg, B. L. Involuntary eye movements during fixation. *Journal of Physiology (London)*, 1953, *119*, 1–17.

Dobson, V., & Teller, D. Y. Visual acuity in human infants: A review and comparison of behavioral and electrophysiological studies. *Vision Research*, 1978, *18*, 1469–1485.

Dodge, R. An experimental study of visual fixation. *Psychological Review Monograph Supplement*, 1907, *35*, 1–95.

Dodge, R., & Cline, T. S. The angle velocity of eye movements. *Psychological Review*, 1901, *8*, 145–157.

Donaldson, I. M. L., & Hawthorne, M. E. Coding of visual information by units in the cat cerebellar vermis. *Experimental Brain Research*, 1979, *34*, 27–48.

Doris, J., & Cooper, L. Brightness discrimination in infancy. *Journal of Experimental Child Psychology*, 1966, *3*, 31–39.

Dow, B. M. Functional classes of cells and their laminar distribution in monkey visual cortex. *Journal of Neurophysiology*, 1974, *37*, 927–946.

Down, R. M., & Stea, D. *Maps in minds*. New York: Harper & Row, 1977.

Duda, R., & Hart, P. *Pattern classification and scene analysis*. New York: Wiley, 1973.

Ebenholtz, S. M. The possible role of eye-muscle potentiation in several forms of prism adaptation. *Perception*, 1974, *3*, 477–485.

Ebenholtz, S. M. Additivity of aftereffects of maintained head and eye rotations: An alternative to recalibration. *Perception and Psychophysics*, 1976, *19*, 113–116.

Ebenholtz, S. M., & Shebilske, W. L. Instructions and the A and E effects in judgments of the vertical. *American Journal of Psychology*, 1973, *86*, 601–612.

Ebenholtz, S. M., & Shebilske, W. L. The doll reflex: Ocular counterrolling with head-body tilt in median plane. *Vision Research*, 1975, *15*, 713–717.

Ebenholtz, S. M., & Wolfson, P. M. Perceptual aftereffects of sustained convergence. *Perception and Psychophysics*, 1975, *17*, 485–491.

Egeth, H. E. Parallel versus serial processes in multidimensional stimulus discrimination. *Perceptive Psychophysiology*, 1966, *1*, 245–252.

Ellerbrock, V., & Fry, G. A. The aftereffect induced by vertical divergence. *American Journal of Optometry*, 1941, *18*, 450–454.

Ellis, S. R., & Stark, L. Eye movements while viewing Necker cubes. *Perception*, 1978, *7*, 575–581.

Ellis, S. R., & Stark, L. Reply to Piggins. *Perception*, 1979, *8*, 721–722.

Engel, F. L. *Visual conspicuity as an external determinant of eye movements and selective attention*. Eindhoven, Netherlands: Technische Hogeschool Eindhoven, 1976.

Engelken, E. J., & Wolfe, J. W. Analog processing of vestibular nystagmus for on-line cross-correlation data analysis. *Aviation and Space Environmental Medicine*, 1977, *48*, 210–214.

Epstein, W. Recalibration by pairing: A process of perceptual learning. *Perception*, 1975, *4*, 59–72.

Evans, C. R. Some studies of pattern perception using a stabilized retinal image. *British Journal of Psychology*, 1965, *56*, 121–133.

Evans, C. R., & Marsden, R. P. A study of the effect of perfect retinal stabilization on some well-known visual illusions, using the after-image as a method of compensating for eye movements. *British Journal of Physiological Optics*, 1966, *23*, 242–248.

Evans, J. E., & Gutmann, J. C. Minicomputer processing of dual Purkinje image eye-tracker data. *Behavior Research Methods and Instrumentation,* 1978, *10,* 701-704.

Evinger, C., Kaneko, C. M. S., Johanson, G. W., & Fuchs, A. F. Omnipauser cells in the cat. In R. Baker & A. Berthoz (Eds.), *Control of gaze by brain stem neurons.* New York: Elsevier/North Holland Press, 1977, 337-348.

Falk, G. Interpretation of imperfect line data as a three-dimensional scene. *Artificial Intelligence,* 1972, *3,* 77-100.

Fantz, R. L. A method for studying early visual development. *Perceptual and Motor Skills,* 1956, *3,* 13-15.

Fantz, R. L., Ordy, J. M., & Udelf, M. S. Maturation of pattern vision in infants during the first six months. *Journal of Comparative and Physiological Psychology,* 1962, *55,* 907-917.

Feigenbaum, E. A., & Feldman, J. *Computers and thought.* New York: McGraw-Hill, 1963.

Fender, D. H. *The function of eye movements in the visual process.* Unpublished doctoral dissertation. University of Reading, U.K., 1956.

Fender, D. H., & Nye, P. W. An investigation of the mechanism of eye-movement control. *Kybernetik,* 1961, *1,* 81-88.

Festinger, L., Burnham, C. A., Ono, H., & Bamber, D. Efference and the conscious experience of perception. *Journal of Experimental Psychology Monograph,* 1967, (Whole No. 637).

Festinger, L., Sedgwick, H. A., & Holtzman, J. D. Visual perception during smooth pursuit eye movements. *Vision Research,* 1976, *12,* 1377-1386.

Festinger, L., White, C. W., & Allyn, M. R. Eye movements and decrements in the Mueller-Lyer illusion. *Perception and Psychophysics,* 1968, *3,* 376-382.

Fick, E. Die Verlegung der Netzhautbidler mach aussen. *Zeitschrift fur Psychologie,* 1905, *XXXIX,* 102.

Findlay, J. M. Frequency analysis of human involuntary eye-movements. *Kybernetik,* 1971, *8,* 207-214.

Findlay, J. M. A simple apparatus for recording microsaccades during visual fixation. *Quarterly Journal of Experimental Psychology,* 1974, *26,* 167-170.

Findlay, J. M. The visual stimulus for saccadic eye movements in human observers. *Perception,* 1980, *9,* 7-21.

Firschein, O., & Fischer, M. A. A study in descriptive representation of pictorial data. *Pattern Recognition,* 1972, *4,* 361-377.

Fischler, H. A., & Elschlager, R. A. The representation and matching of pictorial structures. *IEE Transactions and Computations,* 1975, *22,* 67-92.

Fisher, D. F., & Lefton, L. A. Peripheral information extraction: A developmental examination of reading processes. *Journal of Experimental Child Psychology,* 1976, *21,* 77-93.

Fisher, D. F., Monty, R. A., & Perlmuter, L. C. Visual recognition memory for binary pictures: Another look. *Journal of Experimental Psychology: Human Learning and Memory,* 1978, *4,* 158-164.

Fisher, G. H. Perception and art: Why do we see the world as we do? *Aspects of Education,* 1971, *13,* 63-90.

Fitts, P. M., Jones, R. E., & Milton, J. L. Eye movements of aircraft pilots during instrument landing approaches. *Aeronautical Engineering Review,* 1950, *9,* 1-16.

Flagg, B. L. Children and television: Effect of stimulus repetition on eye activity. In J. Senders, D. F. Fisher, & R. A. Monty (Eds.), *Eye movements and the Higher psychological processes.* Hillsdale, NJ: Lawrence Erlbaum Associates, 1978.

Fodor, J. A., & Bever, T. The psychological reality of linguistic segments. *Journal of Verbal Learning and Verbal Behavior,* 1965, *4,* 414-420.

Fogelgren, L. A., & Shebilske, W. L. Central visual learning and illusory visual direction after backward head tilts. *Perception and Psychophysics,* 1979, *25,* 519-523.

Foley, J. M. Error in visually directed manual pointing. *Perception & Psychophysics,* 1975, *17,* 69-74.

Foley, J. M., & Held, R. Visually directed pointing as a function of target distance, direction, and available cues. *Perception & Psychophysics*, 1972, *12*, 263-268.

Fox, R., Aslin, R. N., Shea, S. L., & Dumais, S. T. Stereopsis in human infants. *Science*, 1980, *207*, 323-324.

Fraiberg, S. *Insights From the Blind: Comparative Studies of Blind and Sighted Infants*. New York: Basic Books, 1977.

Freedman, J., & Haber, R. One reason we rarely forget a face. *Bulletin of the Psychonomic Society*, 1974, *3*, 107-109.

Freeman, H. On the encoding of arbitrary geometric configurations. *IEEE Transactions on Electronic Computers*, 1961, *10*, 260-268.

Freksa, C., Ellis, S., & Stark, L. Simplified measurement of eye fixation. Submitted to *Computers in Biology and Medicine*, 1980.

Frender, E. C. *A computer system for visual recognition using active knowledge*. Doctoral dissertation AI-TR-345. MIT, Cambridge, MA, 1976.

Friedman, A. Framing pictures: The role of knowledge in automatized encoding and memory for gist. *Journal of Experimental Psychology: General*, 1979, *108*, 316-355.

Fu, K. S. *Syntactic methods in pattern recognition*. New York: Academic Press, 1974.

Fu, K. S., & Pavlides, T. *Biomedical pattern recognition and image processing*. Weinhem: Verlag Chemie, 1979.

Fuchs, A. F. Periodic eye tracking in the monkey. *Journal of Physiology (London)*, 1967, *193*, 161-171. (a)

Fuchs, A. F. Saccadic and smooth pursuit eye movements in the monkey. *Journal of Physiology*, 1967, *191*, 609-631. (b)

Fukuda, T. The unidirectionality of the labyrinthine reflex in relation to the unidirectionality of the optokinetic reflex. *Acta Oto-laryngology (Stockholm)*, 1959, *50*, 507-516.

Fukushima, K. Visual feature extraction by a multilayered network of analog threshold elements. *IEEE Transactions of Systems Science and Cybernetics*, 1969, *5*, 322-333.

Fukushima, K. A feature extractor for curvilinear patterns: A design suggested by the mammalian visual system. *Cybernetic*, 1970, *7*, 153-160.

Garvey, T. D. Artificial intelligence strategies for purposive vision. *SRI International*, Note 117, 1976.

Gentles, W. *Application of automated techniques to the study of vestibular function in man*. Unpublished doctoral dissertation, Department of Electrical Engineering, University of Toronto, June, 1974.

Gerrits, H. J. M., & Vendrik, A. J. H. Artificial movements of a retinal image. *Vision Research*, 1970, *10*, 1443-1456.

Gerrits, H. J. M., & Vendrik, A. J. H. The influence of stimulus movement on perception in parafoveal stabilized vision. *Vision Research*, 1974, *14*, 175-180.

Gibson, E. J. *Principle learning and development*. New York: Appleton, 1969.

Gibson, J. J. *The perception of The visual world*. Boston: Houghton-Mifflin, 1950.

Gibson, J. J. *The senses considered as perceptual systems*. Boston: Houghton-Mifflin, 1966.

Gibson, J. J. *The ecological approach to visual perception*. Boston: Houghton-Mifflin, 1979.

Glezer, V. D. *Pattern recognition mechanisms*. Leningrad: Nauka Academy, 1970. (in Russian).

Gliem, H. Beitrag zur Kenntnis der unwillkurlichen Fixationsbewegungen. *Graefes Archives fur Ophthalomologie*, 1964, *167*, 307-316.

Gliem, Das Verhalten der Fixationsbewegungen bei herabgesetzter Helligkeit der Fixationsobjektes. *Klinische Monatsblatter fur Augenheilkunde*, 1967, *150*, 334-341.

Gliem, H., & Gunther, G. Das Verhalten der Fixationsbewegungen des Auges bei zentrallen Ausfallen. *Graefes Archiv fur Klinische und Experimentelle Ophthalomologie*, 1965, *168*, 322-329.

Gogel, W. C., & Sturm, R. D. A comparison of accommodative and fusional convergence as cues to distance. *Perception & Psychophysics*, 1972, *11*, 166-168.

Goldberg, M. E., & Robinson, D. L. Visual mechanisms underlying gaze: Function of the cerebral cortex. In R. Baker & A. Berthoz (Eds.), *Control of gaze by brain stem neurons*. New York: Elsevier/North Holland Press, 1977, 469–476.

Gopher, D. Eye movement patterns in selective listening tasks of focal attention. *Perception and Psychophysics*, 1973, *14*, 259–263.

Gorman, J. J., Cogan, D. G., & Gellis, S. S. An apparatus for grading the visual acuity of infants on the basis of optokinetic nystagmus. *Pediatrics*, 1957, *19*, 1088–1092.

Gough, P. B. The verification of sentences: The effects of delay of evidence and sentence length. *Journal of Verbal Learning and Verbal Behavior*, 1966, *5*, 492–496.

Gould, J. D. Pattern recognition and eye-movement parameters. *Perception and Psychophysics*, 1967, *2*, 399–407.

Gould, J. D., & Dill, A. B. Eye movement patterns and pattern discrimination. *Perception and Psychophysics*, 1969, *6*, 311–320.

Gregory, R. Cognitive contours. *Nature*, 1972, *238*, 51–52.

Grindley, G. C. Psychological factors in peripheral vision. *Medical Research Council, Special Reports Series, No. 163*. London: His Majesty's Stationery Office, 1931.

Grobstein, P., & Chow, K. L. Receptive field organization in the mammalian visual cortex: The role of individual experience in development. In G. Gottlieb (Ed.), *Neural and behavioral specificity*. New York: Academic Press, 1976.

Guernsey, M. A. A quantitative study of the eye reflexes in infants. *Psychological Bulletin*, 1929, *26*, 160–161.

Guitton, D., & Mandl, G. The effect of frontal eye field stimulation on unit responses in the superior colliculus of the cat. *Brain Research*, 1974, *68*, 330–334.

Guitton, D., & Mandl, G. The frontal eye field in cat. In R. Baker & A. Berthoz (Eds.), *Control of gaze by brain stem neurons*. New York: Elsevier/North Holland Press, 1977, 463–467.

Guzman, A. *Computer recognition of three dimensional objects in a visual scene*. Doctoral dissertation MAC-TR-59. MIT, Cambridge, MA, 1968.

Haber, R. N. Eidetic images. *Scientific American*, April, 1969, *220*, 36–44.

Haith, M. M. Visual competence in early infancy. In R. Held, H. Liebowitz, & H. L. Teuber (Eds.), *Handbook of sensory physiology: Perception, Vol. VIII*. New York: Springer-Verlag, 1978.

Haith, M. M., & Campos, J. J. Human infancy. In M. R. Rosenzweig & L. W. Porter (Eds.), *Annual review of psychology, Vol. 28*. Palo Alto: Annual Reviews, Inc., 1977.

Haith, M. M., Morrison, F. J., & Sheingold, K. Tachistoscope recognition of geometric forms by children and adults. *Psychonomic Science*, 1970, *19*, 345–347.

Hanson, A. R., & Riseman, E. M. *Processing cones: A parallel computational structure for scene analysis*. COINS Technical Report 74-C7. University of Massachusetts, 1974.

Harris, P., & MacFarlane, A. The growth of the effective visual field from birth to seven weeks. *Journal of Experimental Child Psychology*, 1974, *18*, 340–348.

Hay, L. Le mouvement dirige vers un objectif visuel, chez l'adulte et chez l'enfant. *L'Annee Psychologique*, 1979, *79*, 559–588.

Hayes, K. C. Effects of fatiguing isometric exercise upon achilles tendon reflex and plantar flexion reaction time components in man. *European Journal of Applied Psychology*, 1975, *34*, 69–79.

Head, H. *Studies in neurology*. London: Hodder and Stoughton, 1920.

Hebb, D. O. *The organization of behavior*. New York: Wiley, 1949.

Hebb, D. O. Concerning imagery. *Psychological Review*, 1968, *75*, 466–477.

Hein, A., Vital-Durand, F., Salinger, W., & Diamond, R. Eye movements initiate visual-motor development in the cat. *Science*, 1979, *204*, 1321–1322.

Helmholtz, H. von Handbuch der physiologischen optik (3rd ed.). In J. P. C. Southall (Ed. & trans.), *A Treatise on physiological optics (Vol. III)*. New York: Dover, 1962. (Originally published, 1909).

Hering, E. Theory of binocular vision. In B. Bridgeman & L. Stark (Eds.), *Theory of binocular vision*. New York: Plenum Press, 1977, 1–210. (English Edition, 1868).

Heymans, G. Quantitative Untersuchungen ueber das optische Paradoxen. *Zeitschrift fur Psychologie*, 1896, *9*, 221–255.

Hicks, G. D., & Rivers, W. H. R. The illusion of compared horizontal and vertical lines. *British Journal of Psychology*, 1908, *2*, 243–260.

Hochberg, J. In the mind's eye. In R. N. Haber (Ed.), *Contemporary theory and research in visual perception*. New York: Holt, Rinehart, & Winston, 1968.

Hochberg, J. Attention, organization, and consciousness. In D. I. Mostofsky (Ed.), *Attention: Contemporary theory and analysis*. New York: Appleton-Century-Crofts, 1970. (a)

Hochberg, J. Components of literacy: Speculation and exploratory research. In H. Levin & J. P. Williams (Eds.), *Basic studies on reading*. New York: Basic Books, 1970. (b)

Hochberg, J. Perception. I. Color and shape. In J. W. Kling & L. A. Riggs (Eds.), *Woodworth & Schlosberg's experimental psychology*. New York: Holt, Rinehart and Winston, 1971.

Hochberg, J. *Perception*. Englewood, NJ: Prentice-Hall, 1978 (Second ed.).

Hochberg, J., & Brooks, V. Film cutting and visual momentum. In J. W. Senders, D. F. Fisher, & R. A. Monty (Eds.), *Eye movements and the higher psychological functions*. Hillsdale, NJ: Lawrence Erlbaum Associates, 1978.

Hoffmann, K. P. Visual response of neurons in the nucleus of the optic tract of visually deprived cats. *7th Annual Meeting of the Society for Neuroscience, Abstracts (Vol. III)*, 1977.

Hoffmann, K. P. Optokinetic mystagmus and single-cell responses in the nucleus tractus opticus after early monocular deprivation in the cat. In R. D. Freeman (Ed.), *Developmental neurobiology of vision*, NATO Advanced Study Institute Series. New York: Plenum Press, 1979.

Hoffmann, K. P., & Schoppmann, A. Retinal input to the direction-selective cells of the nucleus tractus opticus of the cat. *Brain Research*, 1975, *99*, 359–366.

Hofsten, C. von. Recalibration of the convergence system. *Perception*, 1979, *8*, 37–42.

Hollerbach, J. M. *Hierarchical shape description of objects by selection and modification on prototypes*. M.S. thesis A1-TR-346. MIT, Cambridge, MA, 1975.

Holmes, D. L., Cohen, K. M., Haith, M. M., & Morrison, F. J. Peripheral visual processing. *Perception and Psychophysics*, 1977, *22*, 571–577.

Holst, E. von, & Mittelstaedt, H. Das Reafferenzprinzip (Wechselwirkugen zwischen Zentralnerven-system und Peripheric). *Naturwissen*, 1950, *37*, 464–476. Cited by Evarts, EV., Feedback and corollary discharge: A merging of the concepts. *Neurosciences Research Progression Bulletin*, 1971, *9*, 86–112.

Horowitz, S. L. A general peak detection algorithm with applications in the computer analysis of electrocardiograms. *Communications of the Association for Computing Machinery*, 1975, *18*, 281–285.

Horowitz, S. L., & Pavlides, T. A graph-theoretic approach to picture processing. *Computer Graphics and Image Processing*, 1978, *7*, 282–291.

Howard, I. P. Displacing the optical array. In S. J. Freedman (Ed.), *The neurophysiology of spatially oriented behavior*. Chicago: Dorsey Press, 1968.

Hubel, D. H., & Weisel, T. N. Receptive fields, binocular interaction and functional architecture in the cat's visual cortex. *Journal of Physiology (London)*, 1962, *160*, 106–154.

Hubel, D. H., Wiesel, T. N., & LeVay, S. Plasticity of ocular dominance columns in monkey striate cortex. *Philosophical Transactions of the Royal Society of London, Series B*, 1977, *278*, 377–410.

Hughes, J. R. Post-tetanic potentiation. *Psychological Review*, 1958, *38*, 91–113.

Hughes, J. R., & Morrell, R. M. Post-tetanic changes in the human neuromuscular system. *Journal of Applied Physiology*, 1957, *11*, 51–57.

Hutton, R. S., Smith, J. L., & Eldred, E. Postcontraction sensory discharge from muscle and its source. *Journal of Neurophysiology*, 1973, *36*, 1090–1103.

Hyde, J. E. Some characteristics of voluntary human ocular movements in the horizontal plane. *American Journal of Ophthalmology*, 1959, *48*, 85–94.

REFERENCES

D. *Infants' perception of incomplete faces.* (in preparation)

D., & Lewis, T. L. Peripheral discrimination by three-month-old infants. *Child Develop-* , 1979, *50,* 276–279.

key, M., & Watkins, M. J. The seeing-more-than-is-there phenomenon: Implications for the s of iconic storage. *Journal of Experimental Psychology, Human Perception and Perfor-* ce, 1978, *4,* 553–564.

kie, G. K., & Rayner, K. The span of the effective stimulus during a fixation in reading. ception and Psychophysics, 1975, *17,* 578–586.

och, W., & Pitts, W. A logical calculus imminent in nerve nets. *Bulletin of Mathematical* hysics, 1943, *5,* 115–133.

and, J. H. "Parts" of perceived visual forms: New evidence. *Perception and Psychophysics,* 8, *3,* 118–120.

nis, J. M. Eye movements and optic nystagmus in early infancy. *Genetic Psychology Mono-* phs, 1930, *8,* 321–430.

vie, S. The meaningfulness and meaning of schematic faces. *Perception and Psychophysics,* 73, *14,* 343–348.

l, J. A., & Jones, G. M. Dependence of visual tracking capability upon stimulus predictabil- . *Vision Research,* 1966, *6,* 707–716.

els, D. L., & Tole, J. R. A microprocessor based instrument for nystagmus analysis. *Proceed-* s of the IEEE, 1977, *65,* 730–735.

ls, K. M., & Zusne, L. The metrics of visual form. *Psychology Bulletin,* 1965, *63,* 74–86.

n, H. T. *The application of control theory to physiological systems.* Philadelphia: Saunders, 66.

, G. A., Galanter, E., & Pribram, K. *Plan and the structure of behavior.* New York: Holt, nehart & Winston, 1960.

, L. Developmental differences in the field of view during tachistoscopic presentation. *Child* evelopment, 1971, *42,* 1543–1551.

y, M. L. Steps toward artificial intelligence. *Proceedings of the Institute of Radio Engineers,* 61, *49,* 8–30.

y, M. L. A framework for representing knowledge. In P. H. Winston (Ed.), *Psychology of* omputer Vision. New York: McGraw-Hill, 1975.

y, M. L., & Pappart, S. *Perceptrons.* Cambridge, MA: MIT Press, 1969.

ni, L., & Dimitrov, G. Pursuit movements of a disappearing moving target. *Vision Research,* 978, 537–538.

er, C. W., Goldberg, M. E., & Wurtz, R. H. Visual receptive fields of frontal eye field eurons. *Brain Research,* 1973, *61,* 385–389.

y, R. A., & Senders, J. W. (Eds.) *Eye movements and psychological processes.* Hillsdale, NJ: awrence Erlbaum Associates, 1976.

ney, C. M. Closure with negative afterimages under flickering light. *Canadian Journal of* sychology, 1956, *10,* 191–199.

ney, C. M. Recognition of novel visual configurations with and without eye movements. ournal of Experimental Psychology, 1958, *56,* 113–138.

rs, J., & Vendrick, A. J. H. Responses of single units in the monkey superior colliculus to stationary flashing stimuli. *Experimental Brain Research,* 1979, *35,* 333–347. (a)

rs, J., & Vendrick, A. J. H. Responses of single units in the monkey superior colliculus to moving stimuli. *Experimental Brain Research,* 1979, *35,* 349–369. (b)

gan, M. J. Pulfrich effect and the filling in of apparent motion. *Perception,* 1976, *5,* 187–195.

gan, M. J. Spatio-temporal filtering and the interpolation effect in apparent motion. *Perception,* 1980, (in press).

gan, M. J., & Turnbull, D. F. Smooth eye tracking and the perception of movement in the absence of real movement. *Vision Research,* 1978, *18,* 1053–1059.

Intraub, H. *Rapid semantic identification of pictures.* Presented at the 50th Annual Meeting of the Eastern Psychological Association, Philadelphia, PA, 1979. (a)

Intraub, H. *Selective attention for a subset of sequentially presented scenes.* Presented at the 87th Annual Meeting of the American Psychological Association, New York, 1979 (b).

Intraub, H. The role of implicit naming in pictorial encoding. *Journal of Experimental Psychology: Human Learning and Memory,* 1979, *5,* 78–87. (c)

Intraub, H. Presentation rate and the representation of briefly glimpsed pictures in memory. *Journal of Experimental Psychology: Human Learning and Memory,* 1980, *6,* 1–12.

Jain, R., & Nagel, H. H. Analyzing a real world scene sequence using fuzziness. *Proceedings of the 1977 IEEE Conference on Decision and Control.* New Orleans, 1977.

Jeannerod, M., Gerin, P., & Pernier, J. Deplacements et fixation du regard dans l'exploration libre d'une scene visuelle. *Vision Research,* 1968, *8,* 81–97.

Jernigan, M. E. Visual field plotting using eye movement response. *IEEE Transactions on Biomedical Engineering,* 1979, *26,* 11.

Johnson, C. A., Keltner, J. L., & Balestrery, F. Effects of target size and eccentricity on visual detection and resolution. *Vision Research,* 1978, *18,* 1217–1222.

Judd, C. H. The Mueller-Lyer illusion. *Psychological Review Monograph Supplement,* 1905, *29,* 55–82.

Just, M. A., & Carpenter, P. A. Eye fixations and cognitive processes. *Cognitive Psychology,* 1976, *8,* 441–480.

Kahneman, D. *Attention and effort.* Englewood Cliffs, NJ: Prentice-Hall, 1973.

Kaplan, I. T., & Schoenfeld, W. N. Ocularmotor patterns during viewing of visually displayed anagrams. *Journal of Experimental Psychology,* 1966, *72,* 447–451.

Karp, R. M. Probabilistic analysis of partitioning algorithms for the traveling-salesman problem in the plane. *Mathematics of Operations Research,* 1977, *2,* 209–224.

Kaufman, L., & Richards, W. Spontaneous fixation tendencies for visual forms. *Perception and Psychophysics,* 1969, *5,* 85–88.

Keller, E. L. Participation of medial pontine reticular formation in eye movement generation in monkeys. *Journal of Neurophysiology,* 1974, *37,* 316–332.

Keller, E. L. Control of saccadic eye movements by midline brain stem neurons. In R. Baker & A. Berthoz (Eds.), *Control of gaze by brain stem neurons.* New York: Elsevier/North Holland Press, 1977, 327–336.

King-Smith, P. E., & Riggs, L. A. Visual sensitivity to controlled movements of a line or edge. *Vision Research,* 1978, *18,* 1509–1520.

Kleitman, N., & Blier, Z. A. Color and form discrimination in the periphery of the retina. *American Journal of Physiology,* 1928, *85,* 178–190.

Klinger, A., & Dyer, C. R. Experiences in picture representation using regular decomposition. *Computer Graphics and Image Processing,* 1976, *5,* 68–105.

Kohler, W. *Gestalt psychology.* New York: Liveright, 1929.

Kornhuber, H. H., & Deecke, L. Hirnpotentialanderungen bei Willkurbewegungen und passiven Bewegungen des Menschen: Bereitschaftspotential und reafferente Potentiale. *Pfulgers Archives,* 1965, *284,* 1–17.

Kosslyn, S. M., Ball, T. M., & Reiser, B. J. Visual images preserves metric spatial information: Evidence from studies of imagery scanning. *Journal of Experimental Psychology: Human Perception and Performance,* 1978, *4,* 47–60.

Kowler, E., & Steinman, R. M. The role of small saccades in counting. *Vision Research,* 1977, *17,* 141–146.

Kowler, E., & Steinman, R. M. The effect of expectations on slow occulomotor control. II. Single target displacements. *Vision Research,* 1979, *19,* 633–646.

Kraft, C. L., & Elworth, C. L. Flight deck work load and night visual approach performance. In *Measurement of Aircrew Performance: The Flight Deck Workload and Its Relation to Pilot Performance.* (NTIS 70-19779/AD 699934-DTIC), 1969.

Kremenitzer, J. P., Vaughan, H. G., Kurtzberg, D., & Dowling, K. Smooth-pursuit eye movements in the newborn infant. *Child Development*, 1979, *50*, 442–448.

Krishan, V. V., & Stark, L. A heuristic model for the human vergence eye movement system. *IEEE Transactions on Biomedical Engineering*, 1977, *24*, 44–49.

Kuipers, B. J. *Representing knowledge of large-scale space*. Unpublished doctoral dissertation A1-TR-418. MIT, Cambridge, MA, 1977.

Lai, D. C. *Biocybernetic factors in human perception and memory*. Stanford University Center for Systems Research, Technical Report, 1975, 6741–6745.

Larrabee, M. G., & Bronk, D. W. Long-lasting effects of activity on ganglionic transmission. *American Journal of Physiology*, 1938, *123*, 126.

Larrabee, M. G., & Bronk, D. W. Prolonged facilitation of synaptic excitation in sympathetic ganglia. *Journal of Neurophysiology*, 1947, *10*, 139–154.

Lashley, K. S. The problem of the serial order of behavior. In L. A. Jefferess (Ed.), *Cerebral mechanism in behavior*. New York: Wiley, 1951.

Leask, J., & Haber, R. N. Eidetic images in children II: Longitudinal and experimental results. *Psychonomic Monograph Supplement*, 1969, *3*, 25–48.

Lestienne, F., Berthoz, A., & Mascot, J. C. Etude Biomecanique de la contribution de la vision a la stabilisation posturale chez l'homme. *Le Travail Humain*, 1976, *39*, 180–183.

Lettvin, J. Y., Maturana, H. R., McCulloch, W. S., & Pitts, W. H. What the frog's eye tells the frog's brain. *Proceedings of the Institute of Radio Engineers*, 1966, *47*, 1940–1951.

Levin, J. A., & Hutchins, E. L. *The structure and process of talking about doing*. Proceedings of the 17th Annual Meeting of the Association for Computation of Linguistics, 1979, 79–81.

Levy, J. Autokinesis direction during and after eye turn. *Perception and Psychophysics*, 1973, *13*, 337–343.

Lévy-Schoen, A. Le champ d'activite du regard; donnees experimentales. *L'annee Psychologique*, 1974, *74*, 43–66.

Lévy-Schoen, A., & Rigaut-Renard, C. Pre-perception on activation motrice au cours du T. R. oculomoteur? In J. Requin (Ed.), *Anticipation et Comportement*. Paris: Editions du CNRS, 1979.

Lewis, E. O. The effect of practice on the perception of the Mueller-Lyer illusion. *British Journal of Psychology*, 1908, *2*, 294–306.

Lewis, E. O. Confluxion and contrast effects in the Mueller-Lyer illusion. *British Journal of Psychology*, 1909, *3*, 21–41.

Lindsay, R. K., & Lindsay, J. M. Reaction time and serial versus parallel information processing. *Journal of Experimental Psychology*, 1966, *71*, 294–303.

Ling, B. C. A genetic study of sustained fixation and associated behavior in the human infant from birth to six months. *Journal of Genetic Psychology*, 1942, *61*, 227–277.

Linksz, A. Physiology of the eye. *Vision*, 1952, *2*, 380.

Lipps, T. *Raumausthetik und Geometrisch-optische Taeuschungen*. Leipzig: Barth, 1897.

Llewellyn-Thomas, E. Eye movements and fixations during initial viewing of Rorschach cards. *Journal of Projective Techniques and Personality Assessment*, 1963, *27*, 345–349.

Llewellyn-Thomas, E. Movements of the eye. *Scientific American*, 1968, *219*, 88–95.

Llinas, R. Motor aspects of cerebellar control. *The Physiologist*, 1974, *17*, 19–46.

Lloyd, D. P. C. Post-tetanic potentiation of response in monosynaptic reflex pathways of the spinal cord. *Journal of General Physiology*, 1949, *33*, 147–170.

Locher, P., & Nodine, C. The influence of visual symmetry on visual scanning patterns. *Perception and Psychophysics*, 1973, *13*, 408–412.

Loftus, G. R. Eye fixations and recognition memory for pictures. *Cognitive Psychology*, 1972, *3*, 525–551.

Loftus, G. R. A framework for a theory of picture recognition. In R. A. Monty & J. W. Senders (Eds.), *Eye movements and psychological processes*. Hillsdale, NJ: Lawrence Erlbaum Associates, 1976.

Loftus, G. R. Cognitive factors controlling visual search in pictu... *Symposium of the Center for Visual Science*. Rochester, NY, 1...

Loftus, G. R., & Kallman, H. J. Encoding and use of detail info... *Journal of Experimental Psychology: Human Learning and Mer*...

Loftus, G. R., & Mackworth, N. H. Cognitive determinants of f... viewing. *Journal of Experimental Psychology: Human Percepti*... 565–572.

Luria, S. M., & Strauss, M. S. Comparison of eye movements over... and negatives. *Perception*, 1978, *7*, 349–358.

Luschei, E. S., & Fuchs, A. F. Activity of brain stem neurons d... monkeys. *Journal of Neurophysiology*, 1972, *35*, 445–461.

Lynch, J. C., Mountcastle, V. B., Talbot, W. H., & Yin, T. C. T... directed visual attention. *Journal of Neurophysiology*, 1977, *40*,...

MacFarlane, A., Harris, P., & Barnes, I. Central and peripheral visi... *Experimental Child Psychology*, 1976, *21*, 532–538.

Mach, E. Uber Analogy der personlichen Differenz Awischen beiden A... desselben Auges. *Sitzungsberichte der konliche Bohmischen Ge*... (Prag), 1872, 65–75.

Mach, E. *The analysis of sensations*. New York: Dover, 1959. (Orig...

MacKay, D. M. Visual stability and voluntary eye movements. In R. Ju... of visual information. New York: Springer-Verlag, 1973.

Mackworth, A. K. On reading sketch maps. *Proceedings of the 5th I*...

Mackworth, A. K. How to see a simple world: An exegesis of some... analysis. *Machine Intelligence*, 1978, *8*, 510–537.

Mackworth, J. F., & Mackworth, N. H. Eye fixations recorded on c... television eye marker. *Journal of the Optometric Society of Ameri*...

Mackworth, N. H. Visual noise causes tunnel vision. *Psychonomic Sc*...

Mackworth, N. H. Stimulus density limits the useful field of view. In R... (Eds.), *Eye movements and psychological processes*. Hillsdale, N... sociates, 1976.

Mackworth, N. H., & Bruner, J. S. How adults and children search and... *Development*, 1970, *13*, 149–177.

Mackworth, N. H., & Morandi, A. J. The gaze selects informative details... and *Psychophysics*, 1967, *2*, 547–552.

Mandelbrot, B. B. *Fractals*. San Francisco: W. H. Freeman, 1977.

Mann, I. *The Development of the Human Eye*. London: British Medical...

Marks, D. F. Visual image-y differences and eye movements in recall o... *Psychophysics*, 1973, *14*, 407–412.

Marr, D., & Poggio, T. A computational theory of human stereo vision.... *Society*, London, 1979, *204B*, 301–328.

Martin, M. Local and global processing: The role of sparsity. *Memory*... 476–484.

Martin, L. A. A possible hybrid mechanism for modification of visual dir... movements: The paralyzed-eye experiments reconsidered. *Perception*,...

Matin, L. A., & MacKinnon, G. E. Autokinetic movement: Selective m... components by image stabilization. *Science*, 1964, *143*, 147–148.

Matin, L. A., Matin, E., & Pearce, D. G. Visual perception of direction... occur: I. Relation of visual direction of a fixation target extinguished... presented during the saccade. *Perception and Psychophysics*, 1969, *5*,...

Maurer, D. Infant's visual perception. In L. Cohen & P. Salapatek (Eds.),... *sensation to cognition*. New York: Academic Press, 1975.

Mountcastle, V. B., Lynch, J. C., Georgopoulos, A., Sakata, H., & Acuna, D. Posterior parietal association cortex of monkey: Command functions for operations withing extrapersonal space. *Journal of Neurophysiology*, 1975, *38*, 871–908.

Mowrer, O. H. A comparison of the reaction mechanisms mediating optokinetic nystagmus in human beings and in pigeons. *Psychological Monographs*, 1936, *47*, 294–305.

Muchnik, I. B. Local characteristic formation algorithms for visual patterns. *Automated Remote Control*, 1966, *27*, 1737–1747.

Muensterberg, H. The physiological basis of mental life. *Science*, 1899, *9*, 442–447.

Munn, N. L., & Geil, G. A. A note on peripheral form discrimination. *Journal of General Psychology*, 1931, *5*, 78–88.

Nachmias, J. Two dimensional motions of the retinal image during monocular fixation. *Journal of the Optical Society of America*, 1959, *49*, 901–908.

Nagel, H. H. *Formation of an object concept by analysis of systematic time variations in the optically perceptible environment*. Berich I and I-HH-27-26. Institue fur Informatik, Universitat Hamburg, 1976.

Nakagawa, D. Mueller-Lyer illusion and retinal induction. *Psychologia*, 1958, *1*, 167–174.

Navon, D. Forest before trees: The precedence of global features in visual perception. *Cognitive Psychology*, 1977, *9*, 353–383.

Navon, D., & Gopher, D. On the economy of the human-processing system. *Psychological Review*, 1979, *86*, 214–255.

Neisser, U. *Cognitive psychology*. New York: Appleton, 1967.

Neisser, U. *Cognition and reality*. San Francisco: W. H. Freeman, 1976.

Nevabia, R., & Binford, T. O. Description and recognition of curved objects. *Artificial Intelligence*, 1977, *8*, 77–98.

Newell, A., & Simon, H. A. *Human problem solving*. Englewood Cliffs, NJ: Prentice-Hall, 1972.

Nickerson, R. S. Short-term memory for complex meaningful visual configurations: A demonstration of capacity. *Canadian Journal of Psychology*, 1965, *19*, 155–160.

Nickerson, R. S., & Adams, M. J. Long-term memory for a common object. *Cognitive Psychology*, 1979, *11*, 287–307.

Nicolai, H. Differenzen zwischen optokinetischem Rechts- und Linksynstagmus bei einseitiger (Schiel-) Amblyopie. *Klinische Monatsblatter fur Augenheilkunde*, 1959, *134*, 245–250.

Nilsson, N. J. *Learning machines*. New York: McGraw-Hill, 1965.

Noda, H., Asoh, R., & Shibaki, M. Floccular unit activity associated with eye movements and fixation. In R. Baker & A. Berthoz (Eds.), *Control of gaze by brain stem neurons*. New York: Elsevier/North Holland Press, 1977, 371–380.

Noorden, G. K. von., Burian-von Noorden's *Binocular vision and ocular motility: Theory and management of strabismus*. St. Louis: C. V. Mosby, 1980.

Norman, D. A., & Rumelhart, D. E. (Eds.), *Explorations in cognition*. San Francisco: W. H. Freeman, 1975.

Noton, D., & Stark, L. Eye movements and visual perception. *Scientific American*, 1971, *224*, 34–43. (a)

Noton, D., & Stark, L. Scanpaths in eye movements during pattern perception. *Science*, 1971, *171*, 308–311. (b)

Noton, D., & Stark, L. Scanpaths in saccadic eye movements while viewing and recognizing patterns. *Vision Research*, 1971, *11*, 929–942. (c)

O'Regan, J. K. *Structural and contextual constraints on eye movements in reading*. Unpublished doctoral thesis, University of Cambridge, Cambridge, England, 1975.

O'Regan, J. K. Saccade size control in reading: Evidence for the linguistic control hypothesis. *Perception and Psychophysics*, 1979, *25*, 501–509.

O'Regan, J. K. The control of saccade size and fixation duration in reading: The limits of linguistic control. *Perception and Psychophysics*, 1980, *28*, 112–117.

O'Regan, J. K., & Levy-Schoen, A. Les mouvements des yeux dans la lecture. *L'Annee Psychologique*, 1978, *78*, 459–492.

Ogle, K. N., Martens, T. G., & Dyer, J. A. *Oculomotor imbalance in binocular vision and fixation disparity*. Philadelphia: Lea & Febiger, 1967.

Ogle, K. N., & Prangen, A. Observations on vertical divergences and hyperphorias. *American Journal of Ophthalmology*, 1953, *49*, 313–334.

Ohlander, R. B. *Analysis of natural scenes*. Unpublished doctoral dissertation, Carnegie-Mellon University, 1975.

Okajima, M., Stark, L., Whipple, G. H., & Yasui, S. Computer pattern recognition techniques: Some results with real electrocardiographic data. *IEEE Transactions on Biomedical Electronics*, 1963, *10* 106–114.

Paap, K. R. *Perceptual consequences of post-tetanic-potentiation: An alternative explanation for adaptation to wedge prisms*. Unpublished doctoral dissertation, University of Wisconsin, 1975.

Paap, K. R., & Ebenholtz, S. M. Perceptual consequences of potentiation in the extraocular muscles: An alternative explanation for adaptation to wedge prisms. *Journal of Experimental Psychology: Human Perception and Performance*, 1976, *2*, 457–468.

Paap, K. R., & Ebenholtz, S. M. Concomitant direction and distance aftereffects of sustained convergence. A muscle potentiation explanation for eye-specific adaptation. *Perception and Psychophysics*, 1977, *21*, 307–314.

Paillard, J. Le traitement des informations spatiales. In F. Bresson, et al. (Eds.), *De l'espace corporel a l'espace ecologique*. Paris: Presses Universitaires de France, 1974.

Palmer, S. E. The effects of contextual scenes on the identification of objects. *Memory and Cognition*, 1975, *3*, 519–526. (a)

Palmer, S. E. The nature of perceptual representation: An examination of the analog/propositional controversy. In R. C. Schank & B. Nash-Webber (Eds.), *Theoretical issues in natural language processing*. Arlington, VA: Tinlap Press, 1975. (b)

Palmer, S. E. Visual perception and world knowledge: Notes on a model of sensory-cognitive interaction. In: D. A. Norman & K. E. Rumelhart (Eds.), *Explorations in cognition*. San Francisco: W. H. Freeman, 1975. (c)

Palmer, S. E., Baty, D., & O'Conner, S. Perception of aircraft separation with various symbols on CDTI. *Proceedings of the 15th Annual Conference on Manual Control*, 1978, AFFDL-TR-79-3134, 650–655.

Park, J. N. Displacement of appacent straight ahead as an aftereffect of deviation of the eyes from normal position. *Perceptual and Motor Skill*, 1969, *28*, 591–597.

Parker, R. E. Picture processing during recognition. *Journal of Experimental Psychology: Human Perception and Performance*, 1978, *4*, 284–293.

Pavlides, T. Hierarchies in structural pattern recognition. *Structural pattern recognition*. New York: Springer, 1977.

Pavlides, T., & Ali, F. A hierarchical syntactic shape analyzer. *IEEE Transactions on Pattern Analysis and Machine Intelligence*, 1979, 2–8.

Pavlides, T., & Horowitz, S. L. Segmentation of plane curves. *IEEE Transactions and Computations*, 1974, *23*, 860–870.

Pettigrew, J. D. The paradox of the critical period for striate cortex. In C. Cotman (Ed.), *Neural plasticity*. New York: Raven Press, 1978.

Plateau, J. A. F. Quatrième note sur de nouvelles applications curieuses de la persistance des impressions de la rétine. *Bulletin of the Academy of Science Belgium*, 1850, *16*, 254–60.

Porter, P. B. Another picture puzzle. *American Journal of Psychology*, 1954, *67*, 550–551.

Potter, M. C. Meaning in visual search. *Science*, 1975, *187*, 965–966.

Potter, M. C. Short-term conceptual memory for pictures. *Journal of Experimental Psychology: Human Learning and Memory*, 1976, *2*, 509–522.

Potter, M. C., & Levy, E. I. Recognition memory for a rapid sequence of pictures. *Journal of Experimental Psychology*, 1969, *81*, 10–15.

Pritchard, R. M. Visual illusions viewed as stabilized retinal images. *Quarterly Journal of Experimental Psychology*, 1958, *10*, 77–81.

Prokoski, F. J. *A model for human eye movements during viewing of a general, two-dimensional, dynamic display*. Unpublished doctoral dissertation, University of Connecticut, 1971.

Pylyshyn, Z. W. What the mind's eye tells the mind's brain: A critique of mental imagery. *Psychological Bulletin*, 1973, *80*, 1–24.

Rashbass, C. The relationship between saccadic and smooth tracking eye movements. *Journal of Physiology (London)*, 1961, *159*, 326–338.

Rashbass, C. Second thoughts on smooth pursuit. In P. Bach-y-Rita and C. C. Collins (Eds.), *The control of eye movements*. New York: Academic Press, 1971.

Rashbass, C., & Westheimer, G. Disjunctive eye movements. *Journal of Physiology*, 1961, *159*, 339–360.

Ratliff, F., & Riggs, L. A. Involuntary motions of the eye during monocular fixation. *Journal of Experimental Psychology*, 1950, *40*, 687–701.

Rattle, J. D. Effect of target size on monocular fixation. *Optica Acta*, 1969, *16*, 183–192.

Rayner, K. Parafoveal identification during a fixation in reading. *Acta Psychologica*, 1975, *39*, 271–282. (a)

Rayner, K. The perceptual span and peripheral cues in reading. *Cognitive Psychology*, 1975, *7*, 65–81. (b)

Rayner, K. Eye movements in reading and information processing. *Psychological Bulletin*, 1978, *85*, 616–660.

Rayner, K. Eye guidance in reading: Fixation locations within words. *Perception*, 1979, *8*, 21–30.

Rayner, K., & McConkie, G. W. What guides a reader's eye movements? *Vision Research*, 1976, *16*, 829–837.

Regal, D. M. Critical flicker frequency (CFF) in human infants. Paper presented at the Society for Research in Child Development. San Francisco, March, 1979.

Remond, A., Lesevre, N., & Gaversek, V. Approche d'une semeiologie electrographique du regard. *Revue Neurologique*, 1957, *96*, 536–546.

Restle, F., & Decker, J. Size of the Mueller-Lyer illusion as a function of its dimensions: Theory and data. *Perception and Psychophysics*, 1977, *21*, 489–503.

Richards, W., & Kaufman, L. "Center-of-gravity" tendencies for fixations and flow patterns. *Perception and Psychophysics*, 1969, *5*, 81–84.

Riggs, L. A., Armington, J. C., & Ratliff, F. Motions of the retinal image during fixation. *Journal of the Optical Society of America*, 1954, *44*, 315–321.

Riseman, E. *Computer vision*. New York: Academic Press, 1978.

Roberts, L. G. Machine perception of three-dimensional solids. In J. T. Tippett, et al. (Eds.), *Optical and electro-optical information processing*, Cambridge, MA: MIT Press, 1965.

Robinson, D. A. The mechanics of human saccadic eye movement. *Journal of Physiology*, 1964, *171*, 245–264.

Robinson, D. A. The mechanics of human smooth pursuit eye movement. *Journal of Physiology (London)*, 1965, *180*, 569–591.

Robinson, D. A. Oculomotor unit behaviour in the monkey. *Journal of Neurophysiology*, 1970, *33*, 393–404.

Robinson, D. A. Models of oculomotor neural organization. In P. Bach-y-rita & C. C. Collins (Eds.), *The control of eye movements*. New York: Academic Press, 1971.

Robinson, D. A. Eye movements evoked by collicular stimulation in the alert monkey. *Vision Research*, 1972, *12*, 1795–1808.

Robinson, D. A. Models of the saccadic eye movement control system. *Kybernetik*, 1973, *14*, 71–83.

Robinson, D. A. The physiology of pursuit eye movements. In R. A. Monty & J. W. Senders (Eds.), *Eye movements and psychological processes*. Hillsdale, NJ: Lawrence Erlbaum Associates, 1976.

Robinson, D. A., & Fuchs, A. F. Eye movements evoked by stimulation of frontal eye fields. *Journal of Neurophysiology,* 1969, *32,* 637–648.

Robinson, D. L., & Goldberg, M. E. Visual mechanisms underlying gaze: Function of the superior colliculus. In R. Baker & A. Berthoz (Eds.), *Control of gaze by brain stem neurons.* New York: Elsevier/North Holland Press, 1977, 445–451.

Rock, I. *The nature of perceptual adaptation.* New York: Basic Books, 1966.

Rock, I., & Gilchrist, A. Induced form. *American Journal of Psychology,* 1975, *88,* 475–482.

Rock, I., & Sigman, E. Intelligence factors in the perception of form through a moving slit. *Perception,* 1973, *2,* 357–369.

Ron, S., & Robinson, D. A. Eye movements evoked by cerebellar stimulation in the alert monkey. *Journal of Neurophysiology,* 1973, *36,* 1004–1022.

Rosenblatt, F. The perceptron. *Psychological Review,* 1958, *5,* 386–407.

Rosenblood, L. K., & Pulton, T. W. Recognition after tachistoscopic presentations of complex pictorial stimuli. *Canadian Journal of Psychology,* 1975, *29,* 195–200.

Ross, J. A new type of display relying on vision's sensitivity to motion. *Proceedings of the Physiological Society,* 1977, 2P–3P.

Russo, J. E. Adaptation of cognitive processes to the eye movement system. In J. W. Senders, D. F. Fisher, & R. A. Monty (Eds.), *Eye movements and the higher psychological functions.* Hillsdale, NJ: Lawrence Erlbaum Associates, 1978.

Salaman, M. Reports of the committee upon the physiology of vision. VI. Some experiments on peripheral vision. *Medical Research Council, Special Report Series No. 136.* London: His Majesty's Stationery Office, 1929.

Salapatek, P. Visual scanning of geometric figures by the human newborn. *Journal of Comparative and Physiological Psychology,* 1968, *66,* 247–258.

Salapatek, P. *The visual investigation of geometric patterns by the one-month and two-month old infant.* Paper presented at Meetings of AAAS, Boston, 1969.

Salapatek, P. Pattern perception in early infancy. In L. B. Cohen & P. Salapatek (Eds.), *Infant perception: From sensation to cognition, Vol. 1.* New York: Academic Press, 1975.

Salapatek, P., Aslin, R. N., Simonson, J., & Pulos, E. Infant saccadic eye movements to visible and previously visible targets. *Child Development,* in press.

Salapatek, P., & Banks, M. S. Infant sensory assessment: Vision. In F. D. Minifie & L. L. Lloyd (Eds.), *Communicative and cognitive abilities—Early behavioral assessment.* Baltimore, MD: University Press, 1977.

Salapatek, P., & Kessen, W. Visual scanning of triangles by the human newborn. *Journal of Experimental Child Psychology,* 1966, *3,* 155–167.

Schank, R. C., & Abelson, R. Scripts, plans, and knowledge. *Proceedings of the Fourth International Joint Conference on Artificial Intelligence.* Tbilisi, USSR, 1975.

Schifferli, P. Etude par enregistrement photographique de le motricite oculaire dans l'exploration, dans la reconnaissance et dans la representation visuelles. *Monatschrift fur Psychiatrie und Neurologie,* 1953, *126,* 65–118.

Schiller, P. H., & Koerner, F. Discharge characteristics of single units in the superior colliculus of the alert rhesus monkey. *Journal of Neurophysiology,* 1972, *34,* 920–926.

Schiller, P. H., & Stryker, M. Single-unit recording and stimulation in superior colliculus of the alert rhesus monkey. *Journal of Neurophysiology,* 1972, *35,* 915–924.

Schlag, J., Lehtinen, I., & Schlag-Rey, M. Neuronal activity before and during eye movements in thalamic internal medullary lamina of cat. *Journal of Neurophysiology,* 1974, *37,* 982–995.

Schlag, J., & Schlag-Rey, M. Visuomotor properties of cells in cat thalamic internal medullary lamina. In R. Baker & A. Berthoz (Eds.), *Control of gaze by brain stem neurons.* New York: Elsevier/North Holland Press, 1977, 453–462.

Schneider, G. E. Two visual systems. *Science,* 1969, *163,* 895–902.

Schor, C. M. The influence of rapid prism adaptation upon fixation disparity. *Vision Research,* 1979, *19,* 757–765. (a)

Schor, C. M. The relationship between fusional vergency eye movements and fixation disparity. *Vision Research*, 1979, *9*, 1359–1367. (b)

Schwede, G. W., & Kandel, A. Fuzzy maps. *IEEE Transactions for Systems, Man, & Cybernetics*, 1977, *7*, 669–674.

Sekuler, R. W. Spatial vision. *Annual of Review of Psychology*, 1974, *25*, 195–233.

Selfridge, O. G., & Neisser, U. Pattern recognition by matrice. *Scientific American*, 1960, *203*, 60–68.

Senders, J. W. The human operator as a monitor and controller of multidegree of freedom systems. *IEEE Transactions on Human Factors in Electronics*, 1964, *5*, 2–5.

Senders, J. W., Fisher, D. F., & Monty, R. A. (Eds.), *Eye movements and the higher psychological processes*. Hillsdale, NJ: Lawrence Erlbaum Associates, 1978.

Senders, J. W., Elkind, J. I., Grignetti, M. C., & Smallwood, R. *An Investigation of the Visual Sampling Behavior of Human Observers*, NASA CR 434, 1966.

Shaknovich, A. R. *The brain and regulation of eye movement*. New York: Plenum Press, 1977.

Shantz, M. J., & McCann, G. D. Computational morphology: Three-dimensional computer graphics for electron microscopy. *IEEE Transactions of Biomedical Engineering*, 1976, *25*, 99–103.

Shebilske, W. L. Directional scanning biases and shifts of apparent visual direction. *Vision Research*, 1977, *17*, 495–497. (a)

Shebilske, W. L. Visuomotor coordination in visual direction and position constancies. In W. Epstein (Ed.), *Perceptual stability and constancy: Mechanisms and processes*. New York: Wiley, 1977. (b).

Shebilske, W. L. Sensory feedback during eye movements reconsidered. *The Behavioral and Brain Sciences*, 1978, *1*, 160–161.

Shebilske, W. L., & Fogelgren, L. A. Eye-position aftereffects of backwards head tilt manifested by illusory visual direction. *Perception and Psychophysics*, 1977, *21*, 77–82.

Shebilske, W. L., & Karmiohl, C. M. Illusory visual direction during and after backward head tilts. *Perception and Psychophysics*, 1978, *24*, 543–545.

Shebilske, W. L., & Nice, R. S. Optical insignificance of the nose and the Pinnochio effect in free scan visual straight ahead judgments. *Perception and Psychophysics*, 1976, *20*, 17–20.

Sheena, D. Pattern-recognition techniques for extraction of features of the eye from a conventional television scan. In R. A. Monty & J. W. Senders (Eds.), *Eye movements and psychological processes*. Hillsdale, N.J.: Lawrence Erlbaum Associates, 1976.

Shephard, R. N. Recognition memory for words, sentences, and pictures. *Journal of Verbal Learning and Verbal Behavior*, 1967, *6*, 156–163.

Shepard, R. N., & Judd, S. A. Perceptual illusion of rotation of three dimensional objects. *Science*, 1976, *191*, 952–954.

Shepard, R. N., & Metzler, J. Mental rotation of three dimensional objects. *Science*, 1971, *186*, 701–703.

Shirai, Y. A heterarchical program for recognition of polyhedra. *Bulletin of the Electrotechnical Laboratory*, 1972, *36*, 655–672.

Shulman, G. L., Remington, R. W., & McLean, J. P. Moving attention through visual space. *Journal of Experimental Psychology; Human Perception and Performance*, 1979, *5*, 522–526.

Sills, A. W., Honrubia, V., & Kumley, W. E. Algorithm for the multi-parameter analysis of nystagmus using a digital computer. *Aviation and Space Environmental Medicine*, 1975, *46*, 934–942.

Singer, J., Greenberg, S., & Antrobus, J. Looking at the mind eye: Experimental studies of ocular motility during day dreaming. *Transactions of the New York Academy of Science*, 1971, *33*, 694–709.

Skavinski, A. A. The nature and role of extra-retinal eye position information in visual localization. In R. A. Monty & J. W. Senders (Eds.), *Eye movements and psychological processes*. Hillsdale, NJ: Lawrence Erlbaum Associates, 1976.

Skavinski, A. A., & Steinman, R. M. Control of eye position in the dark. *Vision Research*, 1970, *10*, 193–203.

Slater, A. M., & Findlay, J. M. The measurement of fixation position in the newborn baby. *Journal of Experimental Child Psychology*, 1972, *14*, 349–364.

Slater, A. M., & Findlay, J. M. Binocular fixation in the newborn baby. *Journal of Experimental Child Psychology*, 1975, *20*, 248–273. (a)

Slater, A. M., & Findlay, J. M. The corneal-reflection technique and the visual preference method: Sources of error. *Journal of Experimental Child Psychology*, 1975, *20*, 240–247. (b)

Slobin, D. I. Grammatical transformations in childhood and adulthood. *Journal of Verbal Learning and Verbal Behavior*, 1966, *5*, 219–227.

Smith, K. U., & Bridgman, M. The neural mechanisms of movement vision and optic nystagmus. *Journal of Experimental Psychology*, 1943, *33*, 165–187.

Snow, C. P. *A postscript to science and government*, Oxford: Oxford University Press, 1962.

Sobel, I. On calibrating computer controlled cameras for perceiving 3-D scenes. *Artificial Intelligence*, 1974, *5*, 185–198.

Spady, Jr., A. A. *Airline pilots' scan behavior during simulated ILS approaches*. Paper presented at the 2nd U.S. Army Human Engineering Laboratory Conference: Eye Movements and the Higher Psychological Processes. Monterey, CA, 1977.

Spady, Jr., A. A. *Airline pilot scan patterns during simulated ILS approaches*. NASA Technical Paper 1250, 1978, 1–69.

Sparks, D., Holland, R., & Guthrie, B. L. Size and distribution of movement fields in the monkey superior colliculus. *Brain Research*, 1976, *113*, 21–34.

Sperling, G. The information available in brief visual presentation. *Psychological Monographs*, 1960, *74*, (whole #498).

Sperry, R. Neurology and the mind-brain problem. *American Scientist*, 1952, *40*, 291–312.

Standing, L., Conezio, J., & Haber, R. N. Perception and memory for pictures: Single-trial learning of 2560 visual stimuli. *Psychonomic Science*, 1970, *19*, 73–74.

Stark, L., & Dickson, J. F. Mathematical concepts of central nervous system function. *Neurosciences Research Program Bulletin*, 1965, *3*, 1–72. (also *Neurosciences Research Symposium Summaries*, 1966, *1*, 109–178.)

Stark, L., Ellis, S. R., Inoue, H., Freksa, C. R., & Zeevi, J. Cognitive models direct scanpath eye movements. XII International Conference on Medical and Biological Engineering, Jerusalem, Israel, 1979.

Stark, L., Hoyt, W., Cuiffreda, K., Kenyon, R., & Hsu, F. Time optimal saccadic trajectory model and voluntary nystagmus. In B. L. Luber (Ed.), *Models of oculomotor behavior and control*. West Palm Beach, FL: CRC Press, 1980.

Stark, L., Okajima, M., & Whipple, G. H. Computer pattern recognition techniques: Electrocardiograph diagnosis. *Communications of the Association for Computing Machinery*, 1962, *5*, 527–532.

Stark, L., Vossius, G., & Young, L. R. Predictive control of eye tracking movements. *IRE Transactions of Human Factors in Electronics*, 1962, *3*, 52–57.

Steinman, R. M. Effect of target size, luminance and colour on monocular fixation. *Journal of the Optical Society of America*, 1965, *55*, 1158–1165.

Steinman, R. M., & Cunitz, R. J. Fixation of targets near the absolute threshold. *Vision Research*, 1968, *8*, 277–286.

Steinman, R. M., Haddad, G. M., Skavinski, A. A., & Wyman, D. Miniature eye movement. *Science*, 1973, *181*, 810–819.

Steinman, R. M., & Kowler, E. Miniature saccades: Eye movements that do not count. *Vision Research*, 1979, *19*, 105–108.

Stevens, J. K., Emerson, R. C., Gerstein, T. K., Neufeld, G. R., Nichols, C. W., & Rosenquist, A. C. Paralysis of the awake human: Visual perceptions. *Vision Research*, 1976, *16*, 93–98.

Straschill, M., & Schick, F. Neuronal activity during eye movements in a visual association area of cat cerebral cortex. *Experimental Brain Research*, 1974, *19*, 467–477.

Stratton, G. M. Symmetry, linear illusions, and the movements of the eye. *Psychological Review*, 1906, *13*, 81-96.

St. Cyr, G. J., & Fender, D. H. Nonlinearities of the human oculomotor system: Gain. *Vision Research*, 1969, *9*, 1235-1246. (a)

St. Cyr, G. J., & Fender, D. H. Nonlinearities of the human oculomotor system: Time delays. *Vision Research*, 1969, *9*, 1491-1503. (b)

St. Cyr, G. J., & Fender, D. H. The interplay of drifts and flicks in binocular fixation. *Vision Research*, 1969, *9*, 245-265. (c)

Sutro, L. L., & Lerman, J. B. Robot vision. In E. Heer (Ed.), *1st National Conference on Remote Manned Systems*. Pasadena, CA: California Institute of Technology, 1973, 251-282.

Tanimoto, S., & Pavilides, T. Hierarchical data structure for picture processing. *Complete Graphics and Image Processing*, 1975, *4*, 104-119.

Tauber, E. S., & Koffler, S. Optomotor response in human infants to apparent motion: Evidence of innateness. *Science*, 1966, *152*, 382-383.

Teller, D. Y. A forced-choice preferential looking procedure: A psychophysical technique for use with human infants. *Infant Behavior and Development*, 1979, *2*, 135-153.

Tenenbaum, J. M. On locating objects by their distinguishing features in multisensory images. Technical Note 84, SRI AI-Center, 1973.

Tenenbaum, J. M., & Barrow, H. G. MSYS: A system for reasoning about scenes. SRI Report, 1975.

Thomas, J. G. An electrical method for recording eye movements. *Journal of Physiology*, 1958, *141*, 7.

Thomas, J. G. The torque-angle transfer function of the eye. *Kybernetik*, 1967, *3*, 254-263.

Thomas, J. G. The dynamics of small saccadic eye-movements. *Journal of Physiology*, 1969, *200*, 109-127.

Toates, F. M. Vergence eye movements. *Documenta Ophthalmologica*, 1974, *37*, 153-241.

Tolman, E. C. Cognitive maps in rats and men. *Psychological Review*, 1948, *53*, 189-208.

Turner, K. J. *Computer perception of curved objects using a television camera*. Unpublished doctoral dissertation. School of Artificial Intelligence, University of Edinburgh, 1975.

Turvey, M. T. Contrasting orientations to the theory of visual information processing. *Psychological Review*, 1977, *84*, 67-78.

Turvey, M. T. The thesis of the efference-mediation of vision cannot be rationalized. *The Behavioral and Brain Sciences*, 1979, *2*, 59-94.

Van Biervliet, J. J. Nouvelles measures des illusions visuelles chez les adultes et chez les enfants. *Revue Philosophique*, 1896, *41*, 169-181.

Van Hof-van Duin, J. Development of visuomotor behavior in normal and dark reared cats. *Brain Research*, 1976, *104*, 233-241. (a)

Van Hof-van Duin, J. Early and permanent effects of monocular deprivation on pattern discrimination and visuomotor behavior in cats. *Brain Research*, 1976, *111*, 261-276. (b)

Van Hof-van Duin, J. Direction preference of optokinetic responses in monocularly tested and normal kittens and light-deprived cats. *Archives of Italian Biology*, 1978, *116*, 471-477.

Venger, L. A. Selections from perception and learning. *Soviet Psychology*, 1971, *10*, 5-108.

Virsu, V. Tendencies to eye movement and misperception of curvature, direction and length. *Perception and Psychophysics*, 1971, *9*, 65-72.

von Holst, E., & Mittelstaedt, H. Das Reafferenzprinzip (Wechselwirkugen swischen Zentralnerven-system und Peripheric). *Naturwissen*, 1950, *37*, 464-476. Cited by Evarts, E. V., Feedback and corollary discharge: A merging of the concepts. *Neurosciences Research Progression Bulletin*, 1971, *9*, 86-112.

von Kries, J. Notes on perception of depth, 1925. In H. von Helmholtz, *Treatise on physiological optics*, J. P. C. Southall (Ed.), Vol. 3. New York: Dover, 1962.

Voots, R. J. Computerless automatic data reduction for electronystagmography. *Aerospace Medicine*, 1969, *40*, 1080-1086.

Vurpillot, E. The development of scanning strategies and their relation to visual differentiation. *Journal of Experimental Child Psychology*, 1968, *6*, 632–656.

Walker-Smith, G. J., Gale, A. G., & Findlay, J. M. Eye movement strategies involved in face perceptions. *Perception*, 1977, *6*, 313–326.

Wallach, H., & Frey, K. J. Adaptation in distance perception based on oculomotor cues. *Perception & Psychophysics*, 1972, *11*, 77–83.

Wallach, H., Frey, K. J., & Bode, K. A. The nature of adaptation in distance perception based on oculomotor cues. *Perception & Psychophysics*, 1972, *11*, 110–116.

Wallach, H., & Halperin, P. Eye muscle potentiation does not account for adaptation in distance perception based on oculomotor cues. *Perception & Psychophysics*, 1977, *22*, 427–430.

Washburn, M. F. *Movement and mental imagery*. Boston: Houghton Mifflin, 1916.

Watson, J. B. *Behaviorism*. Chicago: University of Chicago Press, 1930.

Webber, R., & Stark, L. Fitting an image to the eye: A conceptual basis for processing radiographs. *Oral Surgery, Oral Medicine, Oral Pathology*, 1971, *31*, 831–837.

Webber, R., & Stark, L. Influence of fogging radiation and mode of display of the interpretation of dental caries from conventional radiographs. *Investigative Radiology*, 1972, *7*, 506–560.

Weber, R. B., & Daroff, R. B. The metrics of normal human saccadic eye movements. *Vision Research*, 1971, *11*, 921–928.

Weber, R. J., & Malstrom, F. V. Measuring the size of mental images. *Journal of Experimental Psychology: Human Perception and Performance*, 1979, *5*, 1–12.

Webster, R. G., & Haslerud, M. Influence on extreme peripheral vision of attention to a visual or auditory task. *Journal of Experimental Psychology*, 1964, *68*, 269–272.

Weiner, S., & Ehrlichman, H. Ocular motility and cognitive process. *Cognition*, 1976, *4*, 31–43.

Weir, J., & Klein, R. H. The measurement and analysis of pilot scanning and control behavior during simulated instrument approaches. NASA CR-1535, 1970.

Weisman, S., & Neisser, U. Perceptual organization as a determinant of visual recognition memory. *American Journal of Psychology*, 1974, 675–681.

Weisstein, N., & Harris, C. S. Visual detection of line segments: An object-superiority effect. *Science*, 1974, *186*, 752–755.

Westheimer, G. Eye movement response to a horizontally moving visual stimulus. *AMA Archives of Ophthalmology*, 1954, *52*, 932–941.

Westheimer, G., & McKee, S. P. Visual acuity in the presence of retinal image motion. *Journal of the Optometric Society of America*, 1975, *65*, 847–850.

Wheeler, D. D. Processes in word recognition. *Cognitive Psychology*, 1970, *1*, 59–85.

Wheeless, L. L., Cohen, G. H., & Boynton, R. M. Luminance as a parameter of the eye-movement control system. *Journal of the Optical Society of America*, 1967, *57*, 394–400.

White, C. T., Eason, R. G., & Bartlett, N. R. Latency and duration of eye movements in the horizontal plane. *Journal of the Optical Society of America*, 1962, *52*, 210–213.

White, K. G. Implicit contours in the Zoellner illusion. *American Journal of Psychology*, 1972, *85*, 421–424.

Whitmer, C. A. Peripheral form discrimination under dark-adaptation. *Journal of General Psychology*, 1933, *9*, 405–419.

Wickelgren, W. A. Acoustic similarity and intrusion errors in short term memory for English vowels. *Journal of the Acoustical Society of America*, 1966, *70*, 102–108.

Willey, R., Gyr, J. W., & Henry, A. Changes in the perception of spatial location: A test of potentiation vs. recalibration theory. *Perception and Psychophysics*, 1978, *24*, 356–360.

Williams, L. G. The effect of target specification on objects fixated during visual search. *Perception and Psychophysics*, 1966, *1*, 315–318.

Winston, P. H. *Leaving structural description from examples*. Doctoral dissertation report AI TR-231. MIT, Cambridge, MA, 1970.

Winston, P. H. *The psychology of computer vision*. New York: McGraw-Hill, 1975.

Winterson, B. J., & Steinman, R. M. The effect of luminance on human smooth pursuit of perifoveal and foveal targets. *Vision Research,* 1978, *18,* 1165–1172.

Wolfe, J. Relationship of cerebellar potentials to saccadic eye movements. *Brain Research,* 1971, *30,* 204–207.

Wood, C. C., Spear, P. D., & Braun, J. J. Direction-specific deficits in horizontal optokinetic nystagmus following removal of visual cortex in the cat. *Brain Research,* 1973, *60,* 231–237.

Wundt, W. Die goemetrisch-optischen Taeuschungen. *Akademie der Saechs, Wissenschaften.* Leipzig: Abnandlungem, 1898, *24,* 53–178.

Wurtz, R. H., & Goldberg, M. E. Activity of superior colliculus in behaving monkey. III. Cells discharging before eye movements. *Journal of Neurophysiology,* 1972, *35,* 575–586.

Wurtz, R. H., & Mohler, C. W. Selection of visual targets for the initiation of saccadic eye movements. *Brain Research,* 1974, *71,* 209–214.

Wurtz, R. H., & Mohler, C. W. Organization of monkey superior colliculus: Enhanced visual response of superficial layer cells. *Journal of Neurophysiology,* 1976, *39,* 745–765. (a)

Wurtz, R. H., & Mohler, C. W. Enhancement of visual responses in monkey striate cortex and frontal eye fields. *Journal of Neurophysiology,* 1976, *39,* 766–772. (b)

Yarbus, A. L. *Eye movements and vision.* New York: Plenum Press, 1967.

Young, L. R. Pursuit eye tracking movements. In P. Bach-y-Rita & C. C. Collins (Eds.), *The Control of Eye Movements.* New York: Academic Press, 1971.

Young, L. R. Pursuit eye movement—What is being pursued? In R. Baker & A. Berthoz (Eds.), *Control of gaze by brain stem neurons.* Amsterdam: Elsevier/North Holland Press, 1977.

Young, L. R., & Sheena, D. Survey of eye movement recording methods. *Behavioral Research Methods and Instrumentation,* 1975, *7,* 397–429.

Young, L. R., & Stark, L. Variable feedback experiments testing a sampled data model for eye tracking movements. *IEEE Transactions of Human Factors in Electronics,* 1963, *4,* 38–51.

Zavalishin, N. V. Hypothesis concerning the distribution of eye fixation points during the examination of pictures. *Automatic Remote Control,* 1968, *29,* 1944–1951.

Zinchenko, V. P., Chzhi-Tsin, V., & Tarakanov, V. V. The formation and development of perceptual activity. *Soviet Psychology and Psychiatry,* 1963, *2,* 3–12.

Zigler, M. J., Cook, B., Miller, D., & Wemple, L. The perception of form in peripheral vision. *American Journal of Psychology,* 1930, 42, 246–259.

Zollner, F. Uber eine neue Art anortoskopischer Zerrbilder. *Annalen der Physic,* 1862, *117,* 477–484.

Zuber, B. L., Stark, L., & Cook, G. Microsaccades and the velocity amplitude relationship for saccadic eye movement. *Science,* 1965, *15,* 1459–1460.

Zusne, L., & Michels, K. M. Nonrepresentational shapes and eye movements. *Perceptual and Motor Skill,* 1964, *18,* 11–20.

Author Index

Italics denote pages with complete bibliographic information.

Subject Index